MODERN WOMAN'S MEDICAL ENCYCLOPEDIA

Modern Woman's
MEDICAL
ENCYCLOPEDIA

Edited by Anna Mantel Fishbein

Illustrated by Lou Barlow

DOUBLEDAY & COMPANY, INC.
GARDEN CITY, NEW YORK

To Laura Orford Runyon

whose way of life with family,
friends and the welfare of others
has made her dear to me.

PREFACE

Several years have passed since Dr. Morris Fishbein and Peter Briggs in a conference with Milton Runyon and Ken McCormick of the Doubleday organization developed the idea of a Medical Encyclopedia written by women physicians for women. With my husband, Dr. Fishbein, I participated in the development of the book and was assigned the exceedingly pleasant task of editing the chapters written by distinguished women physicians and teachers so as to give the book uniformity in expression and to clarify difficult technical terms.

After having read and carefully edited these chapters, I wished that such a book had been available long years ago.

Many of the chapters will be late for some but timely for others. All, however, I am sure, will bring not only understanding and hope in problems which seemed unsurmountable but also inspiration, contentment, happiness and longer lives—not especially to aging women but to women growing older.

This volume also provides an encyclopedia; as such, I believe it will be consulted periodically. The information is interesting, instructive and dependable.

I am sincerely grateful for having had the privilege and opportunity to participate in editing this book.

Anna Mantel Fishbein

Chicago
1966

AUTHORS

MARJORIE JANE MCKUSICK, M.D., Wilmington, Delaware: graduate of Harvard Medical School. Pediatrician in St. Francis Hospital, General Hospital and Delaware Hospital in Wilmington, Delaware.

IDA NAKASHIMA SCHNECK, M.D., Denver, Colorado: graduate of Woman's Medical College, Philadelphia, Pennsylvania. Pediatrician to Colorado General Hospital.

ESTHER M. GREISHEIMER, M.D., Philadelphia, Pennsylvania: professor, Woman's Medical College, Philadelphia, Pennsylvania.

CATHERINE L. DOBSON, M.D., Chicago, Illinois: graduate of Rush Medical College, Chicago. On the staff of the Chicago Lying-In Hospital, Chicago, University of Illinois College of Medicine and Chicago Maternity Center.

CHARLOTTE H. KERR, M.D., Michigan City, Indiana: graduate of University of Illinois College of Medicine. Master of Science in Nutrition. Member of the staff of Passavant Hospital, Chicago; instructor in obstetrics and gynecology, Northwestern University Medical College.

RUTH R. RAUSCHKOLB, M.D., Cleveland, Ohio: graduate of Western Reserve University College of Medicine. Associate clinical professor of dermatology in Western Reserve University Medical School.

KLARA G. TULSKY, M.D., Chicago, Illinois: graduate of Universite de Antioquia, Medellin, Colombia, South America. Presently doing research in gynecology and endocrinology at Michael Reese Hospital, Chicago, Illinois.

ELOISE PARSONS, M.D., Chicago, Illinois: graduate of Rush Medical College. On the staff of Chicago Lying-In Hospital; attending gynecologist, Mary Thompson Hospital, Chicago.

BEATRICE E. TUCKER, M.D., Chicago, Illinois: graduate of Rush Medical College. Attending obstetrician, Chicago Lying-In Hospital, Wesley Memorial Hospital; associate professor of obstetrics and gynecology, Northwestern University Medical School; director Chicago Maternity Center.

JANET R. KINNEY, M.D., Chicago, Illinois: graduate of Northwestern University Medical School. Attending staff Cook County Hospital and Presbyterian-St. Luke's Hospital, Chicago. Associate professor of medicine, University of Illinois College of Medicine.

CONTENTS

LIST OF ILLUSTRATIONS

PART ONE

A Medical Adviser for Women

Chapter I

HEALTH DURING CHILDHOOD AND INTO ADOLESCENCE

Marjorie Jane McKusick, M.D.

INTRODUCTION

Never has the American child had a greater opportunity for good health and a long life. The tremendous advances in preventive medicine with the development of immunization procedures, the discovery of antibiotics and the recognition of abnormalities arising from genetic mutation (inherited structural differences) are some of the reasons for this great opportunity. However, infants and children must have routine physical checkups with their private physicians or at well-baby centers to take full advantage of this unique state of events. Only by regular visits can the child be fully immunized, and abnormalities and diseases be detected early in their course so that proper treatment can be instituted before complications develop and possibly irreversible damage or even death result.

What are some of the factors that determine the continuing good health of our children from birth into adolescence?

THE NEWBORN INFANT

The health of the newborn infant depends greatly on factors present long before birth. Even at the moment of conception, his genetic (ancestral) inheritance is determined. In addition to the brown eyes of his mother and the curly hair of his father, the fertilized egg may carry genes (biologic units of heredity) of familial disease such as Cooley's anemia (blood disorder), phenylketonuria (PKU—an acid which appears in the urine—is associated with mental retardation), or fibrocystic disease of the pancreas, often called cystic fibrosis. Increasing knowledge of these abnormalities and how they arise in the fetus has made "genetic counseling" an important new field in preventive medicine.

The health and nutrition of the mother during pregnancy may influence the condition of the infant at birth. If she had German measles (rubella) during the first three months of her pregnancy, her infant

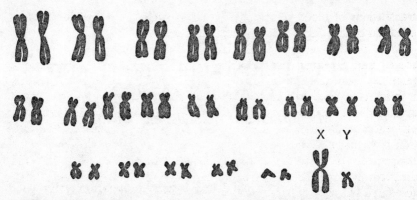

Fig. 1. Chromosomes—the material of inheritance. Each cell has 46, or 23 pairs, of X and Y chromosomes. Derived from both the male and female sex cells, they make the child resemble its parents.

runs the risk of being born with cataracts, deafness, or abnormalities of the heart. Babies born of mothers with diabetes are much more likely to suffer from respiratory distress after birth than if the mother did not have this disease. Insufficient iodine in the mother's diet may result in cretinism in the newborn infant. Also, drugs may influence the baby in utero, the most striking example in recent years being thalidomide, which can cause severe deformities of the baby's limbs if taken by the mother in the early weeks of pregnancy. Thus, prenatal care of the mother is just as important for her unborn baby as it is for her own health.

The infant may be born with a great variety of congenital anomalies for which predisposing factors are unknown. Abnormalities of almost every organ can occur. A continuing search is being made for an explanation of these anomalies, in an effort to reduce their occurrence. Two diseases seen in the newborn period which have been virtually conquered by just such studies are retrolental fibroplasia (scarring of the retina) and erythroblastosis fetalis, a serious blood disorder. The first of these results in blindness, notably in premature infants. This disease is now rarely seen, since we know that it is caused by excessive oxygen administered early in life. This form of treatment is carefully monitored when it has to be used, so that the baby is not exposed to excessive amounts of oxygen which may damage his eyes. The second, erythroblastosis fetalis, or Rh disease, is caused by an incompatibility between the mother's blood and her baby's. We can often anticipate the serious developments and give the baby one or more exchange transfusions of blood shortly after birth to avoid the most serious complication of this disease, namely, mental deficiency.

Most babies are now born in hospitals where the well-trained personnel and excellent facilities make the care of the newborn infant a relatively easy task for mother and doctor. If the baby is premature, it is taken at once to a nursery which is fully equipped to attend to all special needs. Incubators are here, in which the heat, moisture, and oxygen concentration are carefully controlled, and bacterial contamination is virtually absent. Special equipment is available to regulate body temperature in the very small premature infant so that it does not fall dangerously low. The heart and respiratory rates can also be monitored in a seriously ill baby.

In the hospital nursery, daily examinations by the physician and constant nursing care of babies result in prevention of infection, a decrease in the number of feeding problems and early detection of illness or anomalies which may be correctable. Usually the mother receives instruction in the care of her new baby and gets a much-needed rest before she returns home and assumes complete responsibility of her infant.

NUTRITION

The feeding of infants has become greatly simplified during recent years. The oldest method, breast feeding, still remains the simplest, the safest, and the best method for most infants. In cases in which the mother is unwilling or unable to nurse her baby, formulas, simulating breast milk, can be purchased already prepared, sterilized, and in a disposable bottle ready to warm and serve. There is some debate whether or not the milk even needs to be heated, since babies apparently thrive on cold milk. Most nurseries now serve formulas at room temperature, and mothers may do the same. Formulas are also easily prepared from evaporated milk, water, and added carbohydrate such as sugar or corn syrup. These formulas are safer and easier to prepare by the terminal method of sterilization than by the older "aseptic technique."

During the first month, most infants require only formula, water, and a supplement of vitamins A, C, and D in a liquid form. Fluoride may be incorporated in this preparation if it is not already added to the local water supply in order to retard tooth decay in later years.

After the first month, solid foods are gradually added, so that by six months of age the infant is given many varieties of strained food such as meats, vegetables, fruits, cereal, egg yolk, and fruit juices. By this age he should have three or four bottles of milk daily and three meals a day. Pasteurized whole cow's milk is usually well tolerated at this age and many doctors believe that rigid sterilization procedures are no longer necessary.

Before the age of six months, propping a baby's bottle and leaving him unattended while feeding should not be condoned, regardless of how busy the mother may be. The danger is great that the milk will come too fast, choke the baby, and make him aspirate the fluid into his lungs. This may cause sudden death by suffocation or severe pneumonia. Moreover, it is highly desirable that the mother sit down and hold her baby for its feedings three or four times a day. This not only gives the mother a few moments of rest and relaxation but, according to psychologists, a warm, close relationship is likely to develop which benefits both mother and child.

The use of pacifiers during infancy is controversial. Probably these devices do no harm other than cause excess air to be swallowed which may cause pain and give vent to screaming. As long as pacifiers are not continued too long, they may serve a useful purpose during the early weeks of life in making a more peaceful environment for both mother and baby.

During the second half of the first year, the baby is gradually introduced to coarser diets. Chopped canned foods, the "Junior Foods," are an easy way to start the transition from strained baby edibles to foods from the table. Babies differ in ability to handle these foods so that the transition from strained baby foods to table meals may occur anywhere from six to eighteen months of age. The age at which teeth appear seems to have little to do with this change. An important factor, however, may be the ease with which the infant's schedule can be adapted to the family mealtimes. As far as the infant's nutrition is concerned, little difference occurs between strained and table food as long as the child can handle the coarser meats, which become its chief source of iron. During infancy, the well-fortified infant cereals provide adequate iron for the average baby, and meats do not assume importance until the child stops taking such cereal in favor of the adult-type ones which often do not have added iron.

During the second year, babies are no longer growing as rapidly as they did during the first year. They may gain only five or six pounds, increasing their weight by one quarter to one third, compared to the former rapid rate of growth during the first year, when they increased their weight threefold. Consequently, appetites diminish and a mother often feels that her child is sick or malnourished as a result of this normal physiological change in appetite of the one- to two-year-old child. It is helpful to remember that never has a case been recorded of a healthy child starving to death if an adequate diet was offered to him.

What constitutes an adequate diet during the toddler years? Milk is still the backbone of the diet, but should not exceed three or four cups a day for fear of suppressing appetite for other foods which are important in providing iron, roughage, and certain vitamins not occurring naturally in milk. A well-balanced diet should also include at least one serving of each of the other three basic food groups—protein, carbohydrates, and fat.

THE FOUR NECESSARY FOOD GROUPS

The Milk Group	*milk, cheese, and ice cream*
The Meat Group	*beef, veal, lamb, pork, poultry, eggs, and fish*
The Vegetable-Fruit Group	*fruits and vegetables rich in vitamins A & C*
The Bread-Cereal Group	*whole grain, enriched or restored*

If these recommendations are followed, the caloric requirements of the child will be met and their approximate distribution will be: protein 15 per cent, carbohydrate 50 per cent, and fat 35 per cent.

Considerable discussion continues concerning the addition of more vitamins to a well-balanced diet. At the present time so many foods such as bread and cereals are fortified with B complex vitamins, and milk with vitamin D, that a child usually does not require supplementary vitamin drops or tablets. However, most physicians recommend extra vitamins as a safety factor. Sickness or hot weather may cause poor appetite and keep a child from getting a full complement of vitamins in his diet. Personal taste or allergy may induce elimination of citrus fruit from his diet, causing deficiency of vitamin C (ascorbic acid). Salt is also an essential food, but need not be added to the ordinary diet since it occurs abundantly in natural and processed foods. The use of iodized salt in regions which lack iodine in local foodstuffs has so substantially reduced the growth of goiters in these areas as to banish it as a problem.

During the school years and adolescence, the same dietary requirements should be met as during the toddler years. If good eating habits are established early, feeding problems are rarely encountered at this time. Usually, too, during these years a great spurt of appetite seems to develop which carries over into teen-age. Moreover, many children seem to be influenced then by other children rather than by their parents and may thus suffer nutritionally from food fads. These fads include the popular frequent between-meal snacks of soft drinks, potato chips, candy, and other foods that are high in calories but low in nutritional value. Sometimes the children may even wish to lose weight and adapt nutritionally poor weight-losing diets. Important habits that should be formed early in childhood are: little or no eating between meals; a minimum of sweet foods such as cake, cookies, candy and chewing gum; and regular mealtime hours. If these rules are followed, children will have better teeth, healthier bodies, and fewer skin problems during the adolescent years.

Special Problems of Nutrition: One of the most common problems that arises during the baby's first few months is infant colic. The usual history is that the baby nurses and falls asleep but soon awakens screaming. He draws up his knees and seems to have a lot of "gas." He is rarely consoled by being held or by simply passing gas. Such an attack may last an hour or two between feedings, and may recur several times a day. Parents become distraught and doctors anxious in their desire to seek a cause and a cure. As yet a single cause or a single cure has not been found. What may help one infant often does not help another. A change of formula or hormones, sedatives, muscle relaxants, heat to the abdomen, psychotherapy for the mother, and a host of other "cures" may be tried. The condition is usually self-limited and may stop as suddenly as it began, which has led to the term "three-month colic." This is a most reassuring fact to remember when a baby with colic is given the best of care by parents and doctor and does not seem to respond.

Another problem encountered frequently during infancy is commonly called cow's milk "allergy." A better term might be cow's milk "intolerance" since considerable debate continues as to whether or not this syndrome represents a true allergy. These babies have symptoms of colic, may vomit persistently or may have intractable diarrhea. Sometimes a rash will appear on the face and spread over the neck and shoulders. Often the infant will show dramatic improvement when given a formula based on goat's milk, meat, or soy beans. This sensitization is usually self-limited and after six months or a year, cow's milk can be given again without any recurrence of distressing symptoms.

Much has been written about infant diarrhea. Epidemics of this disease have occurred in nurseries and at times have resulted in many deaths. Fortunately this is no longer a problem, but isolated cases of vomiting and diarrhea still occur and babies may become rapidly dehydrated and require hospitalization for intravenous replacement of fluids and salts.

Constipation in infants and children is not unusual. This condition seldom causes any distressing symptoms, and harsh laxatives and huge enemas are to be deplored. If, after two or three days, the child has not had a bowel movement, a simple glycerine suppository is recommended. If this fails, a warm salt-water enema, using ½ teaspoon of salt to a pint of water, may be given. The diet should be checked and adequate amounts of fruits and roughage should be included. Prunes, raisins, and other laxative foods may be given, and one of the stool softeners can be used on advice of the physician.

Anemia is often encountered in the nine- to eighteen-month age group. This may be due to inadequate iron storage during fetal life, such as is seen in prematurely born infants, but more often it is due to faulty diet. The usual history is that the baby has been fed large amounts of milk, which has little iron, and he has had insufficient quantities of other foods containing iron and other minerals important in blood formation. These babies may appear fat, since their caloric intake has been adequate, but usually they are pale and may have only half the amount of hemoglobin they should have at this age. They are often listless and fussy and, due to their inability to fight off infection, may become quite sick with only a minor illness such as a common cold. Indeed, this cold may be the reason that the physician is consulted and nutritional anemia is discovered. If the infection is severe, the infant may need an immediate blood transfusion to save his life. More often, judicious use of antibiotics and supportive care are all that are required to overcome the infection and the baby can then be treated with oral iron preparations. The milk intake should be reduced and iron-rich foods added to the diet. After a month or two, a dramatic rise of hemoglobin level is observed as iron stores are increased and, with them, good health and vitality return.

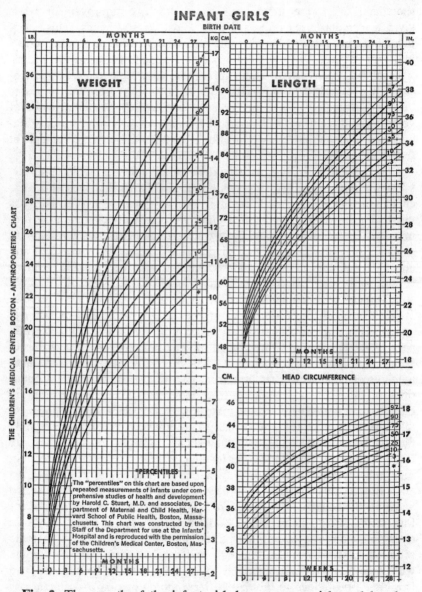

Fig. 2. The growth of the infant girl, her average weight and length from birth through thirty months, plus head circumference.

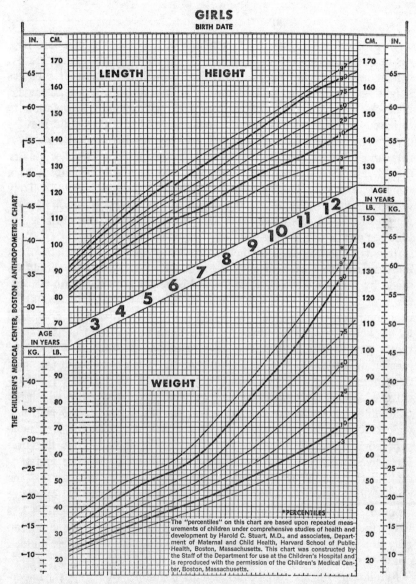

Fig. 3. The growth of the girl, her average length, height, and weight from three years of age through twelve.

GROWTH AND DEVELOPMENT

In evaluating the growth of a child it is important to compare him, not to his peers or his siblings, but to himself. Growth charts are excellent help in visualizing the individual growth of a child. If a child's height and weight are plotted on an anthropometric chart at regular intervals, one can see how he compares with himself in relation to hundreds of other children of the same age and sex. One child may be continually above average and fall consistently between the seventy-fifth and ninetieth percentile, whereas another child of smaller stature may fall constantly between the tenth and twenty-fifth percentile in height and weight. During periods of illness a drop in weight is likely to occur but usually is rapidly regained on return of good health. Rarely, however, does gain in height drop except in the most severe illnesses or in cases of long-standing chronic disorders.

If a wide discrepancy in the percentiles of height and weight of an individual child occurs, a careful examination of this child should be made by a physician. For example, if his height is in the tenth percentile and his weight is in the ninetieth percentile, the child should be evaluated for obesity. Has he recently become overweight compared to his height or has he always shown these body proportions? Is the recent gain in weight secondary to a metabolic disorder or is it due to overeating? If the gain is due to overeating, what has caused this sudden change in appetite? Is it an exaggeration of his normal physiological needs, or is there an underlying psychological problem in which the child finds an outlet by overeating? If the child has always shown a wide discrepancy between his height and weight percentiles, one must proceed more cautiously. Are the parents overweight? If so, this presents two theories. First, heredity may be influencing his size and general stature, and second, the table from which he derives his nourishment may well be loaded with inappropriate or excessive amounts of food. The child who is constitutionally overweight is less likely to respond to treatment of any kind and, indeed, the condition may not be as urgent as in the case of the child with the more sudden onset of obesity.

Similar arguments can be applied to the child who appears underweight in relation to his height. If it seems to be a constitutional condition, one is less likely to be concerned than if the child suddenly begins to lose weight or gain less rapidly, and thus begins to drop from a higher to a lower percentile. Does this child have an underlying, perhaps unsuspected, illness? Is it physiological, psychological, or organic? These are the questions that arise when the individual child's growth is followed and charted and plotted at periodic intervals on his own growth chart. These charts do much to correlate the findings with the growth of the child as a whole.

The routine measuring and charting of the head circumference of the child is helpful in the early detection of abnormally small heads (microcephaly) or abnormally large heads (hydrocephaly). As the child grows, an unexpected jump in the percentile of his head size may indicate an abnormal increase in fluid or a mass within the cranium.

Developmental charts such as the Wetzel Grid have also been devised on which can be plotted various milestones of the child's development, such as when and how he sits alone and when and how he walks without support. These can then be compared with the development of other children of the same sex and age. Since the individual variation in children is so great, with rapid strides in motor and mental development alternating with periods when they do not seem to progress, this type of charting has only limited usefulness. Therefore, in this area, clinical judgment coupled with careful physical examination and environmental evaluation is important in deciding whether or not the child is advancing at a normal rate. The following chart illustrates a wide range of normal for various milestones in neuromuscular development during the first year. Apparently, these milestones are also achieved in regular progression in any individual child. Thus, an infant will gain head control before hand control; he will roll over before he

MILESTONES DURING FIRST YEAR*

	Range of Normal	Average Age
1. Smiles purposefully	3 weeks– 2 months	1 month
2. Vocalizes	1–2 mo.	1.5 mo.
3. Lifts head from supine position	2–4 mo.	3 mo.
4. Reaches for and grasps toy	3–5 mo.	4 mo.
5. Rolls from back to stomach	4–7 mo.	5 mo.
6. Sits briefly without support	5–8 mo.	6 mo.
7. Crawls on hands and knees	6–9 mo.	7 mo.
8. Grasps objects with thumb and forefinger	6–10 mo.	8 mo.
9. Pulls to a standing position	7–11 mo.	9 mo.
10. Walks with support	8–12 mo.	10 mo.
11. Stands briefly alone	9–13 mo.	11 mo.
12. Walks several steps alone	10–15 mo.	13 mo.

* Aldrich & Normal, *J. Ped. 29,* 304, 1946 (Modified and Simplified).

can sit without support and he will crawl before he can walk. Again, such charts will aid the physician to assess the development of the baby at a single visit. For example, if the physician is asked to evaluate a six-month-old child and notes that the infant does not lift his head from the prone position or respond to its mother's voice, he can be reasonably sure that this baby is retarded and will not achieve the other milestones until much later than the normal.

During the preschool years, the development of various motor and adaptive skills, speech development, and social behavior mark the transition from dependent infancy to the relatively independent five- or six-year-old school child. The child shows gradually increasing co-ordination of large and small muscles as he learns to climb stairs, run, jump and then skip. From a clumsy tower of two cubes he stacks at fifteen months, he learns to build higher and more complex models with blocks. He learns also to use a pencil with some skill. At fifteen months of age he can draw a line, whereas by five years he is able to print his name and can copy several letters of the alphabet. Speech progressively evolves, first through imitation, then by spontaneous naming of familiar objects and people. By two years, phrases develop, and complete sentences are usually learned by three years. At four, he may tell about events that have occurred to him recently, or relate a story he has heard. Little by little enunciation becomes clearer, and "baby talk" is usually discarded by five or six.

In his social behavior, the wholly dependent infant gradually recognizes himself as an individual, apart from his mother, and during the second year he is concerned primarily with himself and strives for independence. In some premises he is successful, such as in learning to feed himself, but in areas such as trying to dress himself or tie his shoes, his immature motor system tends to frustration. During the third year he begins to enjoy playing with other children and learns the meaning of possessions and taking turns. Nevertheless, even into the fourth year his play tends to be parallel with that of other children, rather than co-operative. Thus, if you observe three-year-olds in a sandbox, you will note that each child is making his own sand pie, whereas the four- and five-year-olds will be building a giant castle together or digging to China. At five years, a child really attains what he was striving for at two years. He can now feed himself with some dexterity, dress, undress and do a pretty good job at bathing. He can go to the toilet himself, and rarely wets his pants during the day or at night. He has a keen interest in the outside world and is full of questions about his environment and the meaning of words.

During the school years which follow, the child's performance in school and his adjustment to his peer group offer the best guide in assessing his continuing development. If the child seems to fall behind his peers, the Stanford-Binet, Wechsler-Bellevue, and other psychometric tests will help to determine his specific disability.

Understanding a child's normal development makes it easy to decide the ideal time to wean an infant from the bottle or start toilet-training a baby, when to punish a child and when to spoil him a little. All of these questions are intimately associated with mental health and the development of a healthy personality. Unfortunately, a great diversity of opinion is found among the experts, and even they change their opinions occasionally. The time for weaning may vary from six to eighteen months; toilet training can start as early as nine months or as late as two years. Some authorities favor permissive child raising in a relaxed atmosphere and others feel more rigid rules and discipline lead to a more healthy personality in a child.

These theories will go unanswered here, for we believe that the solution must be tailored to the particular needs and personality of the mother, her child, their doctor and the cultural background of all three persons.

Failure to Thrive: What are some of the reasons why children fail to thrive? All too frequently, external factors are responsible. The diet may be inadequate, due either to ignorance or to inability of the family to buy the proper foods. The parents may be guilty of neglect and find it easier to give the baby a bottle of milk that he can hold himself, rather than take the time to feed him solid foods. This, as has been shown, can result in anemia and failure to thrive. Psychological deprivation may also be a deterrent. The child who is neglected and does not receive an adequate amount of tender, loving care can become just as listless and "sick" as the child who receives inadequate nourishment.

Certain illnesses in children can profoundly affect their growth and development. "Blue babies" with heart disease, or infants born with kidney ailments or abnormal brains may be considerably retarded. Certain hormonal disorders such as diabetes mellitus, pituitary dwarfism, or cretinism may cause stunting of growth. Diseases in which errors in metabolism occur, such as fibrocystic disease of the pancreas or galactosemia, result in improper utilization of food and failure to thrive.

Temporary cessation of growth may result from infection from bacteria, viruses or intestinal parasites. Frequently the first sign of cancer in children is loss of weight and a slowing down in development or in schoolwork.

A wide spectrum of entities of disease may induce failure to thrive. Therefore, the responsibility is the physician's. He must seek the underlying cause through careful history, examination of the child and appropriate laboratory investigations.

IMMUNIZATIONS

Of vital significance in the prevention of disease in children are the all too familiar "baby shots" or immunizations. In this area, too, such rapid advances are being made that any recommendations suggested today may well be changed tomorrow. The following chart is derived from the 1964 Red Book, published by the American Academy of Pediatrics and modified by the American Medical Association.

Three types of immunization are currently being modified and warrant discussion. First is the live measles vaccine, which is expected to be produced in a further attenuated strain in the near future so that a single dose can be administered to any child at about nine months of age, without fear of untoward reactions. This inoculation will obviate the need of either giving gamma globulin at the same time or of giving a series of killed vaccines before administering the live one.

Next, the efficacy and desirability of giving inoculations against influenza A and B are still a controversial issue. The problem, moreover, is threefold. First, not enough vaccine is being produced to recommend mass immunization such as is done with the vaccines for poliomyelitis. Second, it is difficult to incorporate the many different known strains of influenza A and B all into one vaccine, and, strange as it may seem, when an epidemic occurs, usually the cause is a new strain which makes the vaccine administered against it ineffective. Third, the influenza inoculation is painful and often causes unpleasant reactions, such as fever and malaise.

The latest immunization procedure is a new one being developed against German measles. Since this is usually a mild illness in children, it may be desirable for them to have the disease and develop natural immunity. The vaccine can be given to pregnant women who are exposed to German measles during the first trimester and sometimes, too, to young adult females who escaped rubella during childhood and desire protection before becoming pregnant.

Temporary immunity to certain infections can be achieved by the use of gamma globulin. If a child has been exposed to infectious hepatitis, a dose of gamma globulin may prevent this disease. A child who has not been immunized against measles (rubeola) may be given an

IMMUNIZATION SCHEDULE FOR CHILDREN

Diseases	Age at Time of First Dosage	Material (Antigen)	No. Doses	Interval	Age at Time of Booster (Recall) Doses
Diphtheria Tetanus Whooping Cough	1½ to 2 months	Triple Preparation	3	4 weeks	15 months and again at 4 years (on the advice of the family physician after 4 years)
	6 weeks to 3 months	Inactivated (Salk) vaccine	4	3 at 6-week intervals; 4th after 6 months or longer	Every 2 years after 4th dose
Poliomyelitis	6 weeks to 3 months	Oral (Sabin) vaccine Type I Type III Type II	1 dose each	6 weeks apart	After 6 months, Types I-II-III combined
Smallpox	6 to 12 months	Cowpox virus	1		Every 5 years or when exposed
Typhoid, Paratyphoid Fever	Only when needed	Typhoid–Paratyphoid vaccine	3	1–4 weeks	Upon advice of physician or public health authorities
Measles (4 Plans)	1 9 months	Live, attenuated vaccine	1		No recommendations; immunity may be permanent
	2 9 months	Live, attenuated vaccine, plus gamma globulin	1		
Choice rests with physician	3 9 months	Inactivated vaccine	3	Monthly	One or more booster doses; intervals undetermined; not for routine use
	4 9 months	Inactivated vaccine followed by live attenuated vaccine			Recommendations pending

inoculation of gamma globulin which may either modify or prevent this disease, depending on the size of the dose. Because of the usual mildness of German measles (rubella) it is inadvisable to try to modify or prevent this infection in children.

ILLNESSES

Some experience and judgment on the part of the parents is helpful in deciding when an illness is minor, needing only supportive home care, and when the child should have the services of a physician. When mild symptoms of illness develop, probably it is safe to wait twenty-four hours before calling the doctor. Try to keep the child at rest, warm but not overheated, and encourage it to drink fluids. Aspirin, one grain per year of life (up to five grains, one adult tablet), may be given every four hours if there is increased temperature or malaise. If symptoms of the common cold are present, phenyleprine hydrochloride, or other similar nose drops, will help to relieve nasal congestion. When a cough is associated with the indisposition, a mild cough medicine may be given and a vaporizer is often helpful to reduce the drying and secondary swelling of the delicate mucous membranes. If the fever continues more than twenty-four hours or the coughing persists, it is advisable to call the family physician. Under no circumstances should antibiotics be administered without his approval.

Childhood diseases such as measles, mumps, and chickenpox should always be reported for documentation in the child's health record and also to the child's physician. Mumps is often confused with swollen glands, and the rash of scarlet fever can be confused with measles. Scarlet fever is caused by beta-hemolytic streptococcus, and if this disease goes untreated, the child might develop rheumatic fever, severe illness known to follow infection with this organism. Swollen glands are often secondary to a throat infection which might be caused by the streptococcus organism or even by tuberculosis. However, this is a decision the doctor should make, not the parent.

Vomiting and diarrhea which occur in an infant under six months of age should be reported promptly to the physician because infants can become rapidly dehydrated and dangerously ill in a short time. In the older child, if there is no stomach ache, he may be treated by withholding oral feedings until vomiting ceases, then cautiously given sips of a cola drink until he has retained at least six ounces. Then other clear liquids such as water, ice chips, soft drinks, clear broth, tea and gelatin dessert may be given. If symptoms persist, if the diarrhea appears bloody, or if abdominal pain develops, a physician should be consulted promptly.

Rules regarding the illnesses of children that are more insidious in onset are difficult to set down. When a child is somewhat pale, seems to have less pep, or appears to be failing in his schoolwork, should you call the doctor? If you are concerned and perturbed, by all means check with your doctor even if the symptoms seem vague or trivial. It is for him, with his training and experience, to decide whether or not a child warrants a checkup and medical care.

ACCIDENTS AND INJURIES

More than one-third of all deaths in the age group from one to fourteen years are due to motor vehicle or other accidents. Although deaths from other causes are rapidly declining, accidental death is only slowly decreasing in incidence. The important factor in further reducing accidents is the education of parents and children to the prime hazards at different ages. In infancy, falls, inhaling foreign objects, and drowning are the major problems. In the toddler years, death due to falls, drowning, ingestion of poisons, and burns bear serious review. In school years, automobile and bicycle accidents are the greatest threat to life, and drowning is still a major cause of death. One must protect the infant by keeping the crib sides up, never leaving him alone on a table or in the bathtub, and keeping small objects out of his reach. The toddler must begin early to learn safety rules, such as not to run into the street and not to play with matches or electrical wires. Nevertheless, he still must be protected, so windows should be barred and poisons kept out of reach. By school age, the child should have learned what is safe or is not on his own. He should be taught to cross the street carefully and ride his bike cautiously. He should learn to swim as early as possible, at the same time learning the rules of water safety. At the proper age, he should be taught to drive a car skillfully, preferably through a driver education program.

All head injuries should be reported promptly to the doctor even if unusual symptoms are not immediately apparent. Important signs to watch for are drowsiness, vomiting, and inequality in the size of the pupils of the eyes. Convulsions or coma are indications for immediate medical attention.

Any ingestion of substances that are potentially poisonous should also be reported, particularly if a large or unknown quantity of the substance. Many physicians suggest that parents keep syrup of ipecac or other emetic on hand to induce vomiting in case of such an accident. It is advisable, however, to check with your physician, for he may prefer that emetics should not be used for certain poisonous petroleum products, since, in the process of vomiting, they might be aspirated into the lungs and cause pneumonia.

HYGIENE AND HABITS

Hygiene has come to mean cleanliness to many people, and "good hygiene" is reflected in that great American institution, the daily bath. In infancy, the frequent eructations and messy diapers make the daily bath a necessity. A mild soap, preferably one that includes the germicide hexachlorophene, is recommended. The use of baby oils, lotions, and powders is inadvisable during the first few months, since some infants develop rash due to the perfumes incorporated in these products. Plain mineral oil may be applied to lubricate dry skin. Corn starch is recommended to dry any moist or inflamed areas as in the diaper region. Protective ointments such as Vaseline or zinc oxide ointment may be necessary if the skin becomes excoriated.

During the toddler years, most children enjoy the daily bath if it is kept as a time for play. In addition, it offers an opportunity to overcome some children's fear of water. Later, when they are in school, they generally balk at the daily bath ritual, although most children enjoy it once the bath is underway. Probably two or three good cleansing baths a week are adequate if this is the only way to avoid a daily argument. However, hand washing before meals and after toileting should be established as a regular habit. Cleanliness assumes greater importance again in adolescence, when skin problems such as acne, body odor, and greasy hair make their ugly appearances, along with a shift in hormones. Once again, the daily bath becomes a necessity for good hygiene.

The three main rules for keeping teeth healthy and free of decay are: first, supplementing the diet with sodium fluoride if the local water supply is not fluoridated, or including it in the vitamins; second, brushing the teeth regularly with a dentifrice containing stannous fluoride; and third, eating few sweets. Fluoride can be given to the pregnant mother to help avoid decay in her baby's teeth, and this medicine should be continued for twelve or thirteen years after birth. It is wise to start brushing a child's teeth at about eighteen months, or when he has sixteen teeth. Ideally, a child's teeth should be brushed after each meal, but if this is not convenient, once or twice a day is probably enough. Regular visits to a dentist should begin at three and a half years.

Adequate sleep is important at all ages. Hard and fast rules about the number of hours required at different age levels are difficult to make since children vary in their needs for rest. As a general rule, children should be given adequate opportunities to sleep. If you have to wake up your eight-year-old repeatedly in the morning and prod him through breakfast so that he catches the school bus, he is probably not getting enough sleep at night, and you should try putting him to bed earlier. The newborn infant generally sleeps sixteen to twenty hours out of twenty-four. As he grows older, his wakeful periods get longer, and by the second half of the first year he is taking two long naps during the day in addition to about twelve hours of sleep at night. Sometime between twelve and eighteen months, the morning nap is given up and an afternoon nap of one to three hours is all that is required, in addition to his twelve hours at night. At four or five years of age, the nap is also discontinued, and as the school years progress the night sleep is shortened to ten hours. In adolescence, the eight- to ten-hour rule should prevail. Occasional relaxation of the retiring hour should be permitted but is generally made up by a nap the next day or an earlier bed hour the following night.

Fresh air and exercise are essential factors in the maintenance of good health in the growing child.

During the first few weeks, it is probably sufficient to air the baby's room for ten minutes daily, and then maintain a fairly constant room temperature of 70° to 75° F. In clear weather, babies can be left outdoors for long nap periods if there is a safe and suitable place to leave them. Otherwise, a stroll in a coach or mother's arms for ten minutes or more is adequate. However, the baby's room with sunlight, change of air, and proper temperature is not to be disregarded.

The toddler enjoys a daily walk with mother too, although he may be left to play by himself if there is a safe, fenced-in area which can be viewed from the house for frequent checking on his activities. The school child, of course, must be permitted to go off on his own. Bicycle riding is a popular form of outdoor exercise during these years and should be encouraged if the child knows the safety rules and can be relied on to follow them. Ball games, roller skating, jumping rope, and similar games appeal to children of all ages and should be included in a child's curriculum just as much as schoolwork and homework. However, hazardous sports or games should be vigorously opposed.

Work is important, both physical and mental. Even by two or three years of age, children are capable of doing small tasks at home and enjoy the feeling of helping and being trusted by mother. As they get older, regular chores which are not too time-consuming should be allotted to children, and they should be allowed some choice in when and how their jobs are done. At the appropriate age, that is, about the time they are able to count money and make change, children should be started on an allowance. It is best for parent and child to sit down and estimate the child's expenses for the week, such as school lunches, church donation, savings, and a little extra for spending. At first, the allowance money will require supervision so that it is not lost or all squandered the first day on a new toy. As the child begins to understand what is expected of him and his money, he will take pride in being able to do this on his own, and this experience will serve him well in later years, both as a teen-ager and as the head of a household.

"Play is the work of children." In the toddler years this is quite appropriate. Children need little in the way of toys to stimulate their imagination, and they will "work" many hours building with blocks or digging in sand. In school, their real work begins, and if their early experiences have been rich with imagination of play and books, their motivation and performance in school are more likely to be good.

Good study habits in school and at home should be encouraged early so that these habits will carry over to the high-school years, when parental authority carries less influence. Juvenile delinquency and the increasing problem of school dropout certainly can be combatted by better guidance of children by their parents early in their school career.

We have endeavored to outline in broad terms what to expect from your child and how to manage different stages of his growth so that he will develop a strong, healthy body and mind. However, the most important contribution any mother can make to her child is not learned from books. This faculty is that strong, secure feeling she gives him of being wanted, needed, and loved beyond all bounds.

Chapter II

COMING OF AGE
Ida Nakashima Schneck, M.D.

With the advent of her first menstrual period, the young girl crosses the threshold from girlhood to womanhood. Her destiny as a woman is thus affirmed, and she is irrevocably committed to the physiological and biological life of a female. Rounded bosom and hips, as well as added height, have given her a new look; in addition, she has acquired the novel power of attracting boys. Proud, but often confused by her new contours, delighted, but frequently fearful of her attractiveness to boys, this young girl will need much guidance, reassurance, and wise supervision before she emerges as a confident young woman, secure and happy in her femininity.

In the two or three years preceding the onset of menstruation, the little girl's body undergoes striking changes. Responding to a series of metabolic events known as the prepubertal growth spurt, her height and weight increase sharply so that she often towers above many of the boys in her school class. Her body no longer seems familiar to her, for her hips broaden, her waist becomes a definite indentation, and her breasts soon enlarge enough to require the support of a brassiere. Pubic and axillary hair also make their appearance. The flawless complexion of childhood may become disfigured with the blackheads and pimples of acne.

Most adolescent girls have ambivalent or contrary feelings about their strange new bodies. They are proud of growing up and are particularly reassured that they are reaching physical maturity just as did their girl friends. At the same time, most are uneasy about their new shapes and unsure of handling themselves. No longer an engaging, self-assured little girl, the teen-ager is an awkward and self-conscious adolescent groping her way toward a new maturity. Because she needs the support of knowing that she is exactly like everyone else, even minor physical aberrations, like acne or moderate overweight, take on the proportions of a major catastrophe. Narcissistic preoccupation with physical appearance is characteristic of this period, a fact that is well recognized by manufacturers of cosmetic and hair preparations.

THE FEMININE IDENTIFICATION

The most consistent model of femininity for the young girl is, usually, her mother. If, during her early years, the little girl has received the warm and loving guidance of a mother who has found pleasure in motherhood and happiness in a womanly role, she has been provided with an ideal. However, not all girls are so fortunate. Some mothers are bitterly resigned to being the household drudge and the slave of an indifferent master. They find motherhood a burden and marriage a trap. Others feel that they have sacrificed intellectual growth and surrendered their potential talents to the demands of husband and children. They harp constantly upon the dissatisfactions and disappointments of their martyred lives. Identification with such a mother inevitably creates much struggle and conflict for the developing girl, so that she may emerge with a distorted concept of the feminine role. She may repudiate it altogether or attempt to find satisfaction in intellectual achievements alone, because the biological expression of femininity seems to her so barren of satisfaction.

The young girl's reaction to her first menstrual period reveals much about her feelings concerning her female role. Surprisingly, for such a singular and significant event, many teen-agers seemingly do not remember anything about it. If the mother's reply to her daughter's questions regarding menstruation was a curt, "Don't talk to me about such dirty things," the girl's reaction is likely to be one of dismay and disgust. Menstruation will mean for her a messy, frequently painful and unpleasant event to be endured, and, in addition, a periodic reminder of a state of sexuality that she fears and repudiates. Conversely, if the knowledge of the process of sexual maturation has been a gradual assimilation of facts in a relaxed and open atmosphere, the girl's feeling about her first menses may be one of pleased surprise.

An adverse reaction to the first menstrual period does not imply that the menses will always be regarded as a repulsive reminder of unwanted maturity or that subsequent adjustment as a female will be poor. If the girl's compliance in other areas is good, and she has further reassuring experiences regarding the desirability of being female, she can certainly come to understand, accept, and enjoy her newfound femininity.

CONFLICTS OF ADOLESCENCE

Little wonder, then, that adolescence is considered an era of major adjustment. Not only must the young girl learn to cope with her new body, but she is also struggling for emancipation from her parents. This period is a time of rebellion, of testing the limits of parental discipline, and of trying out her own ideas. Nevertheless, as much as this fledgling woman strives for complete freedom, and as much as she resents parental restriction, she still has moments of childish dependence. Frightened by the strength of her own impulses and afraid that she cannot handle them, she wants her parents to help her and tell her what to do. She needs them to give her support and security, even while she is attempting to break away from them. An adolescent girl expressed this ambivalence well when she said:

"I know my mother's right when she tells me I have to be in by a certain time from a date, and I'm glad she says so, but I still resent it."

Adolescence is a series of quick advances and hurried retreats. The girl may accept the refusal of the use of the family car with adult grace and understanding one day, and on the very next day she may go into a rage when denied it. Certainly this transition is also a difficult time for parents as they attempt to deal with a maturing child of shifting moods and bewildering, contradictory behavior which reflects her inner confusion and conflict.

In the girl's striving to find herself, she is particularly involved in entanglements with her mother. Early in life, she wishes to supplant her mother in the affections of her father, despite loving and depending on her. This potentially dangerous situation is usually resolved when the child identifies her relationship with her mother and then, as though she said to herself, "If I cannot replace her, I will be like her." The heightened sexual drives of adolescence reactivate the family triangle, and the mother is again the rival, and the father is the ideal, but forbidden, love object. The father has given her the standards by which most men are judged in later life. As Irene Josselyn outlines the conflict:

". . . She does not dare to be like her mother; she must deny her mother's virtues in order to assure herself of her own superiority to her mother. Yet her clearest definition of femininity is that with which her mother has acquainted her, and which she has accepted as a model for herself. She vacillates between contempt for her mother and father, idealization of her mother and father. . . ." She must prove to herself that "her mother is a hag, her father a nincompoop."

PEER GROUP

The group of her peers attains increasing distinction for the adolescent girl as she begins to break away from parental influence. She accepts the group's standards of dress and behavior, and adopts their attitudes toward authority and education. Membership in a particular group is determined partly by chronological age and by intellectual ability, but, at a deeper level, by the mutual emotional empathy that exists. The peer group is composed of individuals who are approximately at the same emotional level of development.

Adolescents and pre-adolescents apparently fall into sharply divided groups as early as the sixth grade. Depending on the socio-economic level, they vary all the way from the socially successful, college-motivated group, who maintain high grade averages and hold school offices, to the group, who, with precarious academic records and marginal attendance, have little interest in staying in school, and are characterized by an attitude of defiance toward all authority. This group, to a large extent, appeals to those teen-agers who not only have little control over their own impulses, but have great difficulty accepting authority. Many subgroups fall between these two extremes. Strict regulations of dress are enforced, depending on the various sections of the country.

DATING

Dating, and its more advanced form, courtship, has become much more complicated than it was even a few generations ago. Foremost among the changes that have occurred are the freedom and lack of supervision now enjoyed by the teen-ager. Not only are the rules that govern dating behavior much less clearly defined than they were formerly, but a greater part of social activity now takes place outside the home. Chaperones are rarely seen, except for school and church affairs. The affluence of the teen-ager in this age of relative prosperity has been another inordinate contributing factor to this change. What was not financially accessible to his father is often easily available to the adolescent boy of today. Finally, the pattern of dating has been revolutionized by the automobile. Boys and girls who live across town or are separated by long distances can now date each other easily, making it still more difficult for their parents to know anything about their respective dates. The automobile gives a young couple great mobility and affords them an opportunity for privacy and intimacy that may prove irresistible to susceptible young people. Certainly this kind of freedom of movement and action places a great burden for responsible behavior upon the individual who is often immature.

GOING STEADY

Another major distinctive social change that has developed recently is the great increase in couples who are "going steady" at an unusually young age. In response to social pressures, children in early puberty may be pushed into dating when they have little interest in the opposite sex and certainly little understanding of the complexities of going together. The practice of "going steady" may begin as early as twelve or thirteen years of age. Usually when it occurs in the younger age group, however, this implies a temporary commitment for only a few weeks, but it can stretch out to months or years in the later teens.

Mutual pleasure and security may be found in the steady company of someone congenial and attractive. However, in some communities, social activities are so tightly organized around "steady" couples that a single boy or girl feels excluded from social contacts. Evelyn M. Duvall asserts, "It is unfortunate that this pattern of almost compulsory going steady has become so widely accepted among teen-agers, because it means that many young people have been forced into it in order to enjoy any social life at all."

However, going steady is not wise when begun too early, for it necessarily prevents a girl from obtaining the experience of having contacts with many different kinds of boys whose friendship she can enjoy without committing herself to them. In this way, she can evaluate her own likes and dislikes and can develop poise and self-confidence which will be valuable in later years. Couples who date each other exclusively also run the risk of deep emotional involvement. Occasionally, depending on the young people, this may form the basis of a mature and happy marriage. But at this age, it can also become all-encompassing and all-absorbing, to the exclusion of normal interests and activities. Close companionship of this kind can also lead to physical stimulation and excitation so intense that it becomes difficult to control. Sometimes the affection is one-sided and the frustrated partner may make frantic efforts to continue the relationship.

During this dating period, one of the major concerns of the girl is petting. While for the married woman such behavior is the logical prelude to a valid climax, sexual intercourse, this is not usual for the unmarried female adolescent. Habitual indulgence in heavy petting, short of intercourse, may leave her so tense and irritated that she may eventually consent to the completion of the act or, alternatively, may break up the relationship in an atmosphere of frustration and resentment. Participation in heavy petting can arouse intense anxiety in a girl, for although she may find these caresses pleasurable and exciting, at the same time she may become quite frightened by her own response. Some girls are burdened with a sense of great guilt and wrongdoing, believing that they have engaged in a shameful and forbidden activity.

Traditionally, in our culture, the responsibility of setting limits on the relationship between the sexes belongs to the girl. Her sexual responses are slower and she can stop lovemaking more easily than can the average male. Both this physiological fact and custom place her in the role of the arbiter, and if she and the boy forget the rules, unfortunately she is held responsible.

Couples who progress from petting to sexual intercourse are motivated by a number of reasons, usually egotistical. The boy, with the urgent sexual drive of this period in life, may do so for the pleasure it provides him, or to prove himself a man. An adolescent girl remarked of a former boy friend, "He's not so much interested in the act as in the conquest." Often a cruel and vindictive quality attends his assault on the girl's resistance and he may have little regard for her feelings.

The girl may engage in sexual intercourse experimentally, "because it's supposed to be so great." Frequently, such behavior is acceptable for members of her particular peer group, or she may have been reared in an atmosphere of promiscuity by which casual sexual relationships with men are taken for granted. The undisciplined, impetuous girl may succumb to the impulses of the moment. Seeking primarily warmth and affection, the love-starved girl may turn to men to fill her need to be loved, and use sex as a means of holding a man's attentions. Surprising though it may seem, there are still girls who, because of limited intellect or sheer ignorance, simply do not understand the sexual act or its possible consequences. Sometimes a girl becomes promiscuous out of a neurotic need to debase and punish herself, desiring to revenge herself on a perfectionistic, puritanical mother, or to act out the unconscious wishes of a disturbed parent.

The inability of young people to face, frankly, what part sexual expression should play in their dating may produce other problems. Many couples engage in intercourse and later break up, without ever being able to discuss their feelings about it. A sense of having been exploited almost certainly arises from such experiences.

For the girl, the danger of pregnancy is always present and, because of this, she takes the greater risk in having sexual intercourse. If the sexual relationship has occurred without any real foundation for companionship or affection, the girl may find herself rejected by the boy although he is equally or more responsible than is she. Faced with an unwanted and unexpected pregnancy, she may seek illegal means of abortion with all its attendant risks of infection or hemorrhage. She may, however, choose the alternative of bearing the child to release it for adoption or to care for it herself. Certainly, few girls emerge from such a deeply disturbing experience without having their ideas and attitudes about sex seriously damaged.

Marriage is not always the best solution for such situations. While a marriage ceremony may solve the immediate problem of giving the child a more acceptable social standing, the result may be mismating of two unhappy people. This is particularly true if they never had any intentions of marriage, and such a poor union has every likelihood of ending in divorce. Sometimes the girl refuses to marry the father of her child and wishes to have nothing to do with him. Professional counseling can probably offer the most effective aid to such a couple and help them to work out a solution best suited to their particular circumstances.

Sexual experience before marriage is not an assurance that a person can adjust satisfactorily to marriage. A happy sexual adjustment in marriage does not depend on previous sexual experience but on the partners' wholesome attitudes toward sex, on a real understanding of each other, and on their appreciation of each other as persons.

HOMOSEXUALITY

Intense attachments to an older girl occur frequently, particularly in the early teens, when sexual identification is still unstable and uncertain. When such devotion involves a mature woman, a teacher or camp counselor, for example, the girl may be re-experiencing the same kind of childish love she gave earlier to her mother, now displaced to a substitute love object, but tinged with a sexual feeling. These attachments are generally fleeting and forgotten as the girl matures and develops other interests and relationships. Conflicts of sexual identity are part of adolescent development, and most of these tendencies subside in the course of normal emotional growth. Ardent homosexual feelings that persist into late adolescence have a graver significance, however, and competent professional counseling may be necessary for such a person.

MASTURBATION

While 80 to 90 per cent of adolescent boys are reported to masturbate at one time or another, somewhat fewer girls engage in similar practices. Probably the greatest hazard of masturbation is the intense guilt and anxiety that it arouses in those who practice it. Satisfactory adjustment to marriage may be more difficult for the girl who has habitually brought herself to orgasm by self-stimulation, and may require the same type of excitation from her husband. The shy, retiring girl who masturbates may become even more withdrawn. Unlike homosexuality, promiscuity, or premarital sexual relationships, masturbation involves only the person who indulges in it, and is the only physical outlet for sexual tension that is without social consequences. As Evelyn M. Duvall states, "One finds it hard to say that masturbation . . . is right or wrong, harmless or harmful; it all depends upon the many interrelated factors in the individual involved."

CHOOSING A MATE

The experience of dating should help the young girl toward a better understanding of herself and also aid her to clarify her ideas about the kind of man she would like to marry. Hopefully she has acquired from her past experiences a mature concept of married love. If this love is based on companionship, a sharing of many common interests and enthusiasms, if the couple appreciate each other's talents and intelligence, and if they respect their individual attitudes and opinions and can talk freely and easily to each other, if they have reciprocal sexual attraction, they will have a good foundation for an enduring union. This, of course, does not constitute love. A unique excitement and pleasure must be aroused in each other's company so that this person alone becomes the total focus of all the other one's affection and regard and the most important person in the world. At the real core of the relationship is the fact that consciously or unconsciously this person meets the other's deepest needs.

Occasionally in the quest for true love, a girl finds herself caught in an incendiary infatuation that burns violently. Usually, based on intense sexual attraction, such affairs rarely survive the tests of time or separation unless the two people involved have much in common.

Once a couple has decided that they love one another, the practice of going steady and the more formal commitment of an engagement will help to test both their affections and their intentions. The more immature the couple, the less sure they are of their feelings, and the more helpful they will find this period, as they come to know each other better through constant companionship. In our culture, two people who are dating tend to see each other at their best, in a pleasure-oriented setting, and the period of betrothal may be the first time that the young couple actually see one another at less than exalted appearance and behavior.

While love in our culture is considered the best and most acceptable motivation for marriage, people may enter into this relationship for a number of other reasons of which they may or may not be aware. Some girls say frankly that they would marry anyone to escape from an intolerable home situation. Others marry in rebellion against too-controlling parents, often to obviously unsuitable partners. The more calculating young women marry for social prestige or money. Unhappy people may feel that marriage will solve all their problems. Social pressures may also persist, and persuade people to marry "because everyone else is doing it." The present emphasis on the satisfactions of marriage and family life, embodied in "togetherness," may push a hesitant couple into marrying. Too often, because the participants are young and immature, the marriage is unwise. Little thought has been given to the demands that such an alliance makes on each partner, or to the responsibilities that they will have for future children.

To achieve a happy marriage, people need first to be given a clear idea what to expect from married life. Happiness in marriage is not a gift handed to a couple on their wedding day, but an achievement resulting from hard, daily work and effort. Successful marriage signifies the ability to compromise, to make adjustments to another personality, to learn to accept some undesirable qualities as well as the attractive ones. In marriage, each participant learns to survive the day-to-day intimacy of living in close physical quarters with another human being. A woman, who found this aspect of marriage extremely distasteful, said that she thought the ideal marriage would be one in which she met her husband only on weekends. A good marriage involves close communication between the partners, talking over the problems of the day from minor irritations to major emotional upheavals, and being able to make a happy and satisfactory sexual adjustment.

Young people are notoriously optimistic about "beating the odds" against a successful marriage, now about one in three. If they are

firm in their decision and feel ready to take on the challenge and responsibilities of matrimony, they will find that premarital examination
and counseling can offer them much help and reassurance.

The girl approaching marriage will want to know that she is free
from physical defects, and that, from an anatomical point of view,
she can bear children normally. The physical examination will be much
like any other physical study she has had, except that it will include a
pelvic examination. The doctor will check for developmental defects,
for immature sexual organs, for any abnormalities of the bony pelvis,
which might affect the sexual act or the reproductive function. He will
look for any vaginal discharge which may aggravate coital distress and
determine whether or not there might be any malformation of the
hymen which could interfere with the consummation of the marriage.

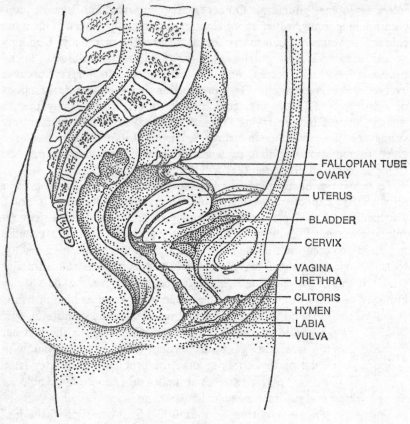

FALLOPIAN TUBE
OVARY
UTERUS
BLADDER
CERVIX
VAGINA
URETHRA
CLITORIS
HYMEN
LABIA
VULVA

Fig. 4. The female organs.

A blood count, urinalysis, chest X-ray and Papanicolaou smear may also be included, in addition to a careful investigation of past illnesses, particularly of those involving thyroid or endocrine dysfunction or of chronic debilitating diseases. The doctor will also take a careful gynecological history.

Many couples who come for premarital counseling often are quite concerned about previous sexual activity. Some have feelings of guilt and embarrassment about masturbation, about homosexual episodes or past promiscuity, and feel that normal sex life is impossible for them. Often the fear of sex itself can interfere with good sexual adjustment. The opportunity to talk about these experiences and impressions with a sympathetic and understanding physician will help to alleviate much of the person's anxiety.

A discussion of the young couple's plans for a family might also be included in premarital counseling. Most couples desire contraceptive advice, and an explanation and evaluation of the different methods available can aid them in choosing the one that they feel is most satisfying, according to preference and pocketbook.

Another myth of romantic love would have us believe that the honeymoon is a time of blissful happiness, when a couple may ecstatically consummate their marriage. Actually, weeks of taxing preparation culminating in a tense wedding ceremony, followed by a long trip, is certainly not the most relaxing way to begin married life. Temporary frigidity and impotence may result from such nervous beginnings, and while not uncommon and not serious, they may become grave if the cause is not understood. In addition, many young women are worried about what is "normal" lovemaking and what is deviant.

All questions of doubt pertaining to the marriage can be discussed in the counseling session by a skilled and sympathetic physician. Sometimes, the couple is so weighed down with anxiety that they are not receptive to too much advice, and a second session, when they are more relaxed and at ease, may be more valuable and more meaningful to them.

The young woman stands now at another threshold, this one leading to marriage and motherhood. The happiness and fulfillment that she finds in her husband, home, and children will depend upon the joy and satisfaction that she finds in being a woman, and in her own confidence in herself, as a secure and independent person who is able to give generously and to take graciously.

Chapter III

FORM AND FUNCTION OF WOMEN
Esther M. Greisheimer, M.D.

ANATOMY AND PHYSIOLOGY

The female organs concerned in conception and giving birth include sex glands, or ovaries; the tubes and the uterus, or womb; the vagina, with its associated structures, the external genitals, or sex organs, called the vulva; and the mammary glands, or breasts.

The determination of the baby's sex is governed by the sex-determining genes—the hereditary factors which are on the X and Y chromosomes. Chromosomes, integral parts of each cell, forty-six in each cell, twenty-three from each parent, carry the genes that convey hereditary characteristics. As the ovaries grow, they are, in turn, mostly responsible for the development of the tissues which are involved in childbirth.

By the time that the embryo, or fetus (the first stages of an unborn baby), is about seven weeks old, the ovaries are developing and the process is usually completed by the eighth week. Identification of the outer cells and inner portion of the ovaries is possible at twelve weeks. At the time of the infant's birth, the ovaries contain more than 430,000 primary follicles (egg cells) which, if fertilized by the male cell during the fertile period of the mature female's life, may result in a new pregnancy. Soon after birth, the number begins to diminish and from that time on, decreases progressively throughout the child's life.

After the sixth to seventh week of life, within the mother's uterus, genetic factors no longer control the growth of the tissues concerned in childbirth. From this time on, the development is controlled by the hormones which are produced by sex cells in the rudimentary or initial ovaries.

The primitive structures which are to shape the uterus, fuse to form it in the third month. About the seventh month of life, before the baby is born, a noticeable increase occurs in the rate of growth of the baby's uterus. The vagina of the baby becomes greatly enlarged during the latter part of intrauterine life.

At six weeks of age in the mother's womb, the embryo manifests the first differentiation in the cells that are to lead to the formation of

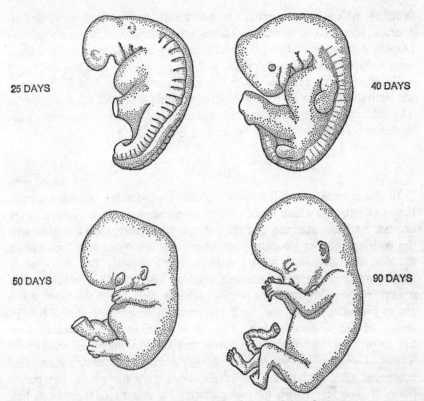

25 DAYS

40 DAYS

50 DAYS

90 DAYS

Fig. 5. The development of the fetus in its early stages.

the breasts or mammary glands. At birth, the mammary glands of the infant may be distended with a serous fluid, called witch's milk. This may be due to the sudden removal, at the time of delivery, of the usual influences of the mother's glands of internal secretion.

The ovaries of the girl remain small throughout childhood. The size of the uterus decreases shortly after birth, probably because of the loss of placental hormones. However, within two weeks after birth, the uterus is the same size as it is in an eleven-year-old girl. The vaginal wall becomes quite thin within a few days after birth, and remains so until the age of puberty, when menstruation begins. The vaginal secretions are scant. Both white blood cells and bacteria are present in the smears.

The amount of estrogenic hormones (specific chemical products found in the ovaries and in some other organs which stimulate the accessory sex structures and the secondary sex characteristics in the female), which is too small to be measured by the usual methods, increases just before puberty. During the stage before puberty, the trophic hormones of the pituitary gland—which influence the ovaries—are produced in small amounts.

Trophic hormones are those chemical substances which influence the activities of the thyroid, mammary glands, sex and adrenal glands. The adrenal glands lie above the kidneys and secrete hormones, particularly cortisone and adrenaline.

PUBERTY

In the normal girl, full function of the reproductive organs is established at puberty, which usually occurs between eleven and fifteen years of age. At this time, the ovaries enlarge with more blood vessels and the ovarian follicles develop in greater numbers. With this increase in follicles, the secondary sexual characteristics appear. The body takes on the adult contour of hips and breasts. The accessory reproductive organs reach maturity. The rapid physical growth of the adolescent girl is probably due to androgen (the male hormone) produced by the cortex of her adrenal glands. This same hormone seems essential to the growth of hair under the arms and on the pubis, or mount of Venus. The mons pubis, or mount of Venus, is a rounded elevation, composed of a pad of fat under the skin, over the pubis, the pubic bone. It is covered with hair at puberty. By this time, the uterus has descended into the pelvis.

A most significant change in glandular functions occurs at the age of puberty. Now the hypothalamus, a structure in the brain, and the hypophysis, or pituitary gland, which it controls, appear to be less concerned with growth of the body than they are with the secretion of the sex hormones. The hormones from the pituitary gland control secretions of the sex glands, also the secretions of thyroid, the adrenals, and the breasts. The resulting increase in generation of ovarian hormones is essential to the normal development of the secondary sexual characteristics.

The tissues of the mammary glands increase. Fat begins to accumulate. The production of estrogen by the ovaries is responsible for the growth of the ducts in the breasts.

Puberty may be delayed by decreased function of either the thyroid gland or the hypophysis. Sometimes, precocious sexual maturity develops in children who have tumors of the adrenal glands.

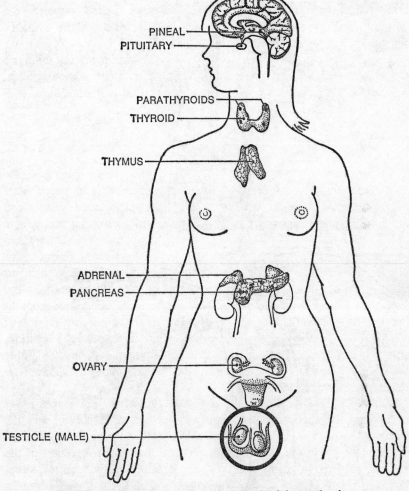

Fig. 6. The Glands—regulators of the body's mechanism.

ADULT FEMALE REPRODUCTIVE SYSTEM

The ovaries are small bodies that lie near the side walls of the pelvis. The cortex, or outer portion of the ovary, contains the egg cells which when ripened are enclosed in follicles. Several hundred thousand primary follicles are present at birth and the number decreases progressively throughout life. During a woman's reproductive lifetime, only 400 to 500 secondary oocytes, egg cells, reach the stage at which they

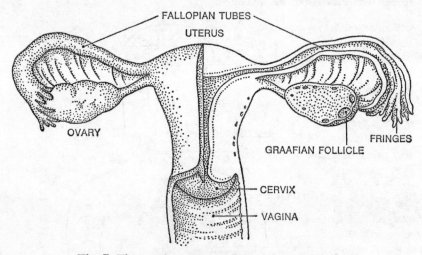

Fig. 7. The ovaries and the organs of reproduction.

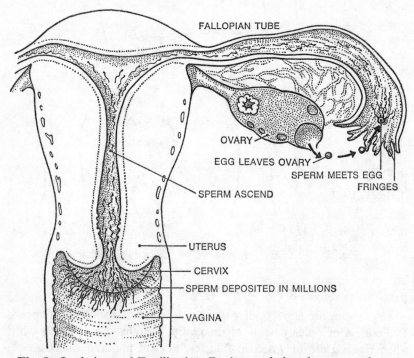

Fig. 8. Ovulation and Fertilization. During ovulation the ovary releases an egg which is picked up by the end of the Fallopian tube and carried downward to the uterus. Fertilization occurs if the egg is impregnated by male sperm cells.

are released from the ovaries. The remainder gradually are absorbed and disappear.

The release of the egg cells from the ovary is called ovulation. The rupture of the follicle usually occurs in the middle of the menstrual cycle, but it may happen at unusual times, even during menstruation.

After ovulation, the ruptured follicle collapses, and the edges of the space approach each other. The remaining follicular cells are thrown into folds. Now the follicular cells and surrounding tissue develop yellow pigment, called lutein cells. Still other changes occur, and the structure becomes a corpus luteum, a mass of yellow tissue formed in the ovary when the ovum (egg cell) is discharged. The lutein cells produce the ovarian hormone, called progesterone. If the egg cell is fertilized and pregnancy follows, the corpus luteum will continue to function for a month or more, then regress. If fertilization does not occur, the corpus luteum regresses sooner, even before the next menses.

The egg cell, after its release from the ovary, enters the uterine tube, and is moved along toward the uterus by successive waves of contractions. If the egg cell is not fertilized, it will not become a mature ovum, but will disintegrate before the next menses. If the egg cell is fertilized in the tube, it starts to divide immediately, giving rise to a mature fertilized ovum. Pregnancy follows the fertilization process, or union with the spermatozoon, the mature male germ cell.

Each ovary is attached to the posterior layer of the broad ligament of the uterus, a little below its upper border. The ovaries are in close relationship to the free ends of the uterine tubes. The suspensory ligaments contain the vessels and nerves passing to and from the ovaries.

The uterine tubes are known also as the Fallopian tubes. The function of the tubes is to furnish a place for fertilization to occur, and then to conduct the fertilized ovum or the unfertilized disintegrating cell to the uterus. The uterine opening of the tube is small and can admit an object the size of a bristle. The free end of the tube is trumpet-shaped, infundibulum, and its margins show a fringe known as the fimbria. The fimbria surround the abdominal opening of the tube, like little fingers ready to grasp the ovum. The journey of the cell through the tube takes three to six days.

The uterus is a hollow, muscular, pear-shaped organ. The lower portion is embedded in the pelvic floor, between the urinary bladder and the rectum. The upper portion of the uterus is free and movable, and rests on the upper surface of the urinary bladder. The uterus is connected to the surrounding structures and to the walls of the pelvis by means of ligaments.

In the standing position, the uterus is tilted forward, with the upper portion resting on the upper surface of the urinary bladder, anteversion. The position of the uterus changes with the size of the bladder. When the bladder is distended, the uterus may be tilted backward—known as retroversion.

The uterus consists of two portions: the upper part, called the body, and the lower section, the cervix. The portion of the body above the entrance of the uterine tubes is the fundus. The end of the cervix terminates in thick, prominent lips that surround the external opening of the uterus, the external os. The uterus has three openings: those of the two tubes, on the sides, and the opening into the vagina below.

The cervix dilates widely and almost disappears during childbirth. The mucous membrane of the cervix includes large mucus-secreting

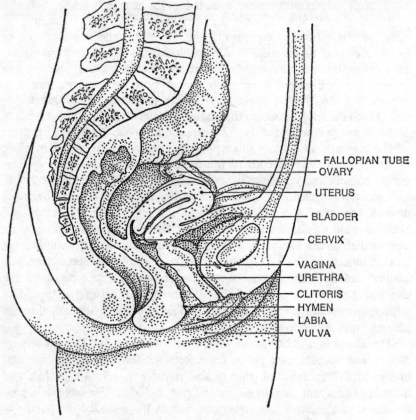

Fig. 9. A side view of the female organs.

glands. The secretion from these glands is increased at the time of ovulation.

The endometrium, or inner lining of the uterus, consists of cells that lie on a layer of tissue. The tissue is filled with glands and is continuous with the underlying muscle.

In a non-pregnant woman, from puberty to menopause, the functional layer of the uterine lining undergoes cyclic changes, called menstrual cycles, that are closely related to changes in the ovaries. The cycles normally recur at intervals of twenty-five to thirty-five days. Menstruation is the discharge of blood, associated with the shedding of the functional layer of the uterine lining. Menstrual blood does not coagulate. The menstrual flow, ordinarily, lasts from one to five days. Before it begins, the surface of the endometrium appears pale, which indicates a decrease in its blood supply.

If the entire endometrium were involved at one time, an uncontrollable and severe hemorrhage would develop. Normally, between 10 and 200 ml., from a spoonful to about a fifth of a quart, of blood is lost, with an average of 35 ml. The uterine glands discharge their secretions and then collapse. The fluid that has accumulated is lost. Now the lining of the uterus is extremely thin, since only the bottom layer of cells remains. This basal layer is responsible for the generation of a new functional or superficial layer of endometrium after each menstrual flow.

Even before the menstrual flow ceases, repair begins. The ensuing phase of the cycle is called, by various authors, the reparative, the estrogenic, the follicular, the proliferative, the postmenstrual, or the preovulatory phase.

The covering epithelium is regenerated first, and then the superficial layer grows until it becomes at least three times as thick as the basilar layer. The estrogenic phase is associated with a rapidly growing ovarian follicle, and lasts from seven to ten days, from the fifth to the fourteenth day of the cycle. At the end of this phase, ovulation may occur.

The ovaries are responsible for the cyclical changes of the uterine mucosa, mucous membrane, and for the preparation, essential to the maintenance and growth of the embryo, in the early period of pregnancy. The ovaries, in turn, are controlled by the hypophysis in the brain. The secretions of the follicle-stimulating hormone and the luteinizing hormone are entirely dependent on control from the brain. A vastly intricate relationship exists between nerve fibers from the hypothalamus in the brain and from the blood supply of these fibers and the pituitary gland. Evidently, when the concentration of a particular hormone, such as estrogen, rises in the blood, the hypothalamus can inhibit the release of the follicle-stimulating hormone from the hypophysis. When the concentration of estrogen in the blood falls below a critical level, the hypothalamus permits the release of the follicle-stimulating hormone, and the cycle is repeated.

The uterine lining is prepared periodically for pregnancy. If fertilization does not occur, hormone support of estrogen and progesterone is withdrawn, and a decrease occurs in the blood supply to the functional layer of the lining with subsequent sloughing and menstrual flow.

The definite functions of the uterus are to implant and permit growth and development of the embryo for the first two months, and for the fetus beginning with third month to term, and to expel the fetus and the placenta at the end of pregnancy.

The vagina is a muscular tube about 8 cm. (3½ inches) long. It lies in front of the urinary bladder and the urethra with the rectum behind it. The vagina extends from the uterus to the external opening in the vestibule and is attached to the cervix a short distance above the lips. In the virgin, the external opening is partially closed by a fold of mucous membrane, called the hymen.

The mucous membrane of the vagina undergoes cyclical changes with the menstrual cycle. The time of the cycle can be determined by examining the vaginal "smears." Vaginal smears are useful in testing for the presence of cancer of the body of the uterus, or of the cervix. A characteristic type of cell is present when cancer occurs in the genital tract.

The labia majora, or large lips, are two folds of skin that pass from the mons pubis backward, to join each other over the ridge, formed by the body of the clitoris, a sensitive erectile organ, and to unite again behind the opening of the vagina, in the region known as the perineum. Both surfaces of the folds are covered with skin. The epidermis of the skin, covering the outer surface, is pigmented and covered with hair; it also contains sebaceous glands. The hairs on the epidermis (skin) of the inner surface are delicate. Sebaceous and sweat glands are also present.

The clitoris is located near the anterior end of the cleft between the labia majora.

The labia minora, or small inner lips, are two folds of delicate skin that arise just in front of the clitoris, pass over part of it, and then pass backward.

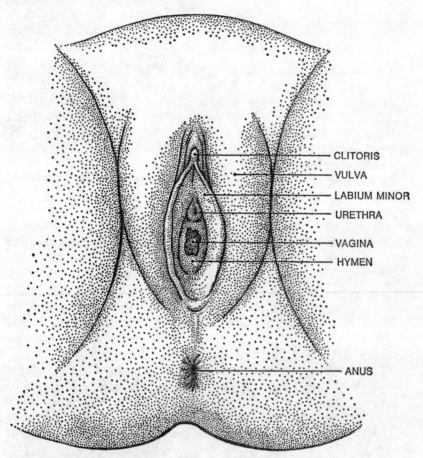

CLITORIS

VULVA

LABIUM MINOR

URETHRA

VAGINA

HYMEN

ANUS

Fig. 10. An external view of the female organs showing, above, the clitoris, or organ of sensation; just below that, the urethra through which urine is released; and then the entrance to the vagina; below this is the anus, or opening of the bowel.

The urethra and the vagina open into the vestibule. The major vestibular glands, Bartholin's, are located on either side of the vestibule, and the mucus they secrete drains into a duct that empties into the groove between the hymen and the small lips on each side.

The external genitalia are supplied with nerve fibers.

MAMMARY GLANDS

The mammary glands, the breasts, are located on the anterior surface of the chest, extending from the second to the sixth ribs, and from the breastbone to the anterior edge of the arm. The sizes are variable. At the center of the front surface is a nipple that has a rounded tip containing fifteen to twenty depressions into which ducts empty from the lobes of the gland. The nipple is surrounded by a pigmented area, called the areola.

Each mammary gland is composed of fifteen to twenty lobes, radiating from the nipple, and each lobe, in turn, consists of many lobules.

CHILDHOOD   ADULT   ADULT WITH MILK-SECRETING LOBULES

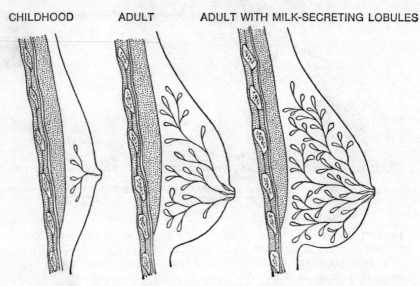

Fig. 11. The development of the breast from childhood.

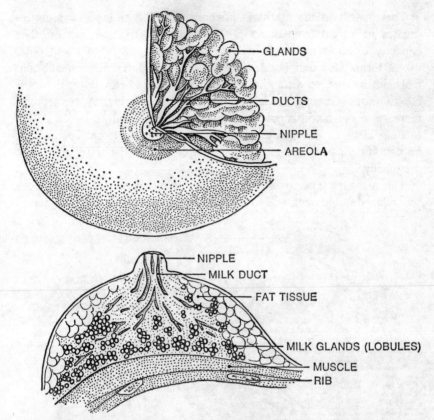

GLANDS

DUCTS

NIPPLE

AREOLA

NIPPLE

MILK DUCT

FAT TISSUE

MILK GLANDS (LOBULES)

MUSCLE

RIB

Fig. 12. Diagrammatic views of the breast in cross-section.

PREGNANCY

If a spermatozoon (male germ cell), which has succeeded in traversing the female genital tract, encounters a secondary egg cell, fertilization occurs. Thus begins the greatest miracle in human life.

The fertilized ovum, zygote, contains forty-six chromosomes, having received twenty-three from each parent. This is the beginning of life, of a new person, at the one-cell stage. As the ovum journeys to the uterus, it divides repeatedly, and by the time it reaches the destination, in three to six days, it consists of a large mass of cells. The uterine mucosa is prepared to receive the developing mass of cells, and implantation begins at once. This mass embeds in the superficial portion of the mucosa. The maternal blood must sustain life and provide for growth of the unborn child.

The growth in the uterus is phenomenal. The embryo or fetus increases in weight from about 60 grams to 1000 grams at term. The capacity increases from about 3 ml. before pregnancy to about 6000 ml. at term. This remarkable growth is due, in part, to hormonal control and, in part, to distention, which stretches and stimulates the muscle to grow. Growth in size of muscle fibers occurs. A tremendous increase in the blood supply to the uterus ensues, and an accumulation of fluid in its tissues also takes place. Uterine enlargement begins after implantation and continues until the beginning of the third quarter of pregnancy.

The placenta takes over the glandular function of the ovaries. Both follicular development and ovulation are inhibited during pregnancy.

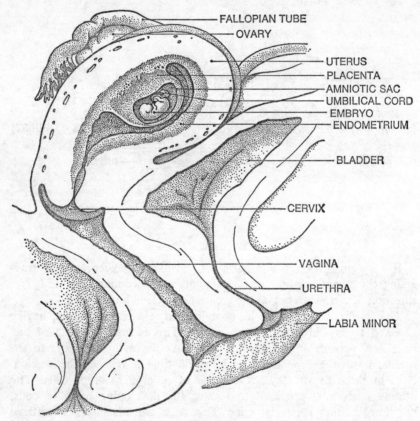

Fig. 13. The pregnant uterus showing the fetus lying within a sac and the beginning formation of the placenta.

The corpus luteum continues to produce progesterone for a time, until the placenta takes over. Estrogen production by the placenta increases during pregnancy, until the onset of labor. Progesterone formation increases for about five months, and then is sustained at a fairly high level, until just before labor, when it diminishes greatly. In addition to the secretion of estrogen and progesterone, the placenta produces a gonadotrophic hormone which influences the sex glands.

A progressive increase in the spontaneous contractility of the uterus occurs during pregnancy. This increase, during late pregnancy, is related to a rising estrogen level in the blood.

The maternal blood flow, through the placenta, near term, is 600 ml. per minute, which is about one tenth of the total cardiac output. The total blood flow through the uterus is about 750 ml. per minute.

An increase of 10 to 15 per cent in the blood volume appears as pregnancy advances, and also a simultaneous increase in fluid volume between the cells (interstitial).

The average expansion in the cardiac output (work of the heart) is approximately 30 per cent.

The mammary glands present a tremendous growth during pregnancy. Enlargement is apparent after the second month. The nipples also increase in size, and the areola, the pigmented portion surrounding the nipples, becomes larger and more deeply colored. Most of the extension of the duct system occurs during the first two-thirds of pregnancy. Thereafter, the changes involve the differentiation of the clumps of cells, as they are undergoing preparation for secretion of milk.

PLACENTA

The placenta, or afterbirth, consists of both fetal and maternal portions, and is the organ through which exchanges between mother and fetus take place. The mother must supply oxygen and food, and excrete carbon dioxide and waste for herself and her unborn child. The hormones essential to pregnancy are produced by the fetal portion of the placenta.

The waves of contraction of the uterus, during labor, have been studied in a large number of women. Rhythmic contractions of low intensity begin about the ninth week. A second, non-rhythmic type of contraction wave, of higher intensity, seldom occurs during the first eight months and increases in frequency as pregnancy progresses. It does not occur regularly until about two weeks before delivery.

The cause of the termination of normal pregnancy is unknown. The contractions of the uterus become fairly periodic and are forceful. The maximum pressure that can be developed by a contraction of the uterine muscle is a little more than three pounds per square inch. This is about three times the force required to dilate the cervix and rupture the membranes. In order to dilate the cervix, the contractions of the fundus must be strong and they should reach maximal force quickly. The contractions of the uterus decrease, in both intensity and duration, as they progress toward the cervix, and the lowest segment of the body of the uterus is inactive throughout the first stage of labor. This kind of activity seems essential to accomplish dilatation of the cervix.

During the delivery of the head of the fetus, the contractions of the muscles of the abdominal wall add immeasurably to the expulsive force of the uterine contractions.

After delivery of the placenta, the uterus decreases rapidly in size. Part of this is the result of elasticity, but much of it is due to the contraction of the muscle fibers of the uterus. This helps to close the open spaces of the endometrium or denuded inner walls of the uterus, and to prevent bleeding. A fatal hemorrhage could occur if the uterine muscle relaxed at this time.

The estrogen level falls rapidly to prepregnancy state, due to the removal of the placental source of the hormone. The level remains low during lactation, since the ovaries are quiescent during this time.

LACTATION

The activity of the mammary glands is integrated by the brain. The glands have been prepared during pregnancy by estrogen and progesterone. After this development, the hormone prolactin initiates and maintains lactation in the mammary glands.

The release of the lactogenic hormone, by the brain, is thought to be under nervous control. Impulses arise in response to the sucking stimulus. The greater part of the milk in the gland becomes available, only if it is forcibly expressed from the more distant areas into the larger ducts, by the reflex contraction of cells which form a network over the surface of the alveoli. A sudden rise in milk pressure appears in the gland, in response to stimulation of nerve endings in the nipple.

The termination of lactation is due to the removal of the sucking stimulus and to rising concentration of estrogen and progesterone. When lactation ends, the mammary glands regress and the alveoli are largely reabsorbed.

In bringing this chapter to a close, I would bring to the attention of the reader some things to "wonder" about. What is it about the so-called X chromosome of the father that determines that the new individual will be a female? How does this paternal chromosome influence the development of the gonads, primal cells, into ovaries? How do the embryonic ovaries direct the differentiation of embryonic structures into the female pattern? Why do the adrenal glands produce both male and female hormones? What initiates the changes, at the age of puberty, that suddenly transform a young girl into a woman? What really governs the strong complex hormonal relationships of the menstrual cycles and their associated anatomic changes? How does the hypothalamus become involved with the hormonal functions of the hypophysis? How do the germ cells reduce the number of chromosomes in one stage of their development? What power changes a one-celled product of conception to such a complex individual as you or me? These, and innumerable additional questions, may arouse a sense of wonder and appreciation. The bodies that we have been permitted to inhabit are truly beyond our comprehension.

Chapter IV

PREPARATION FOR MARRIAGE
Catherine L. Dobson, M.D.

By the time you read this—it is actually too late to begin preparing for marriage. Preparation for marriage begins in the cradle. From your parents you first learned about the day-to-day joys, disappointments, give and take, disagreements, fights—the fun of "making up," dull daily chores and the need for discipline. Your parents have loved you and protected you from danger, tried to help you develop good habits by their example, and equipped you with a good education so that when you leave the protection of the parental home, presumably you are ready for the challenge of life and a home of your own. They are happy over the engagement.

Not true?

Whatever the situation with your parents, they have probably done what they thought best for you—based on their own past experiences. So *do* be charitable.

You are likely to choose a man who is a reflection of your father. If you have had a good relationship with him, you have good prospects for enduring mature love with your future husband.

In these days of high divorce rate, you should take a long steady look at yourself and your fiancé. What are your ambitions and cultural interests? Do you run out of subjects to discuss? Do you enjoy doing things together? Can you spend a quiet evening at home with him without being bored? Are either of you jealous? Do you feel that he should account to you for all his activities while away from your side? Does he expect the same of you? Try to remember that marriage is a partnership—not an ownership.

To be objective about each other is sometimes difficult since a person in love projects his own ideal self onto the loved one and does not appreciate the other's true personality. In mutual love, both are blinded by their self love. This first flush of love is eventually replaced by some degree of reality. A cruel awakening may occur and the young person may find himself engaged to a stranger instead of the perfect mate. Unfortunately, this discovery usually occurs some time after marriage.

Do not rush into marriage. Give yourself plenty of time to know the various facets of your beau's personality, under many different circumstances. Be honest in your evaluation of him. Are you proud as he meets your family and friends, or do you make excuses for him, plan to improve or change him after marriage? Do not hope for change; it is difficult. I have several patients who have made the mistake of trying to reform their husbands after marriage. In all cases, it failed and the couple either divorced or continued a miserable life together. Therefore, if your fiancé is not fully acceptable *as he is*—do not marry him.

Remember, to marry takes only a few minutes, but divorce is a prolonged, expensive, traumatic experience. During the endless weeks or months before the final decree, you may be embroiled in a bitter war of words, and you both will be at your worst. A previously delightful relationship will have become intolerable, and you will wonder what you ever saw in him.

Suppose you are thirty years old, anxious to be married, and are engaged. A big wedding has been planned, the invitations have been mailed, gifts are arriving, and on the surface all is quite gay. But a nagging little voice deep inside keeps telling you the whole thing is a mistake; and you have a heavy heart. Should you go through with the wedding anyway? What will your family think—and your friends, too—if you back out now? Great strength will be necessary for the decision to cancel the ceremony. But is this not better than a marriage built on a foundation of sand?

In general, a happy marriage is more assured if the partners are of similar religion, from the same socio-economic background, have had the same amount of education, share mutual interests, and are about the same age.

Thirty to fifty years is a long time to live with the same person. One can become bored with the same face and the same habits, unless there is more to sustain the relationship than that interesting difference between male and female!

Marriage is not easy, and it is not successful without the diligent effort of both partners. Many brides take this most important step in their lives without thinking beyond the bridal gown and walk down the church aisle. After the honeymoon, the work begins. If you are prepared for these new duties, the work will be joyful. Suddenly, you must know how to budget for household expenses, how to take care of an apartment, how to cook and how to sew. And if you are working, you must also be an efficiency expert. The time to learn these tasks is during adolescence, while you are only dreaming of marriage to some knight in shining armor. After marriage is a bit late.

PREPARATION FOR MARRIAGE

While still in high school, take full care of your own room, polish the furniture and floor, clean the inside of the windows, the window frames and sills, vacuum the rug, change the bed linen weekly and learn to make a neat bed, without bumps. The top of your dresser should be neat and dust-free. The dresser drawers have a way of getting messed up—so plan to put them in order at least once a month. Keep your clothes clean and pressed. Assume the responsibility of taking your own clothes to coin-operated cleaning establishments and learn how to press without spoiling your garments. If a hem needs to be changed, learn to do it. When a button is about to fall off, learn how to sew it on correctly. And for further experience, sew a button on your father's coat or suit.

On Saturdays, clean the bathroom. Learn how to get a ring out of the tub and how to keep the toilet bowl clean. Shine the shelves in the medicine chest and arrange the contents neatly. Study ways of accomplishing these things with the least wasted time and motion.

Have your mother help you cook one dish for Sunday dinner. Learn to make many different casseroles; they are inexpensive, good, and nourishing. Then, you can save the budget for steak now and then. As your skill increases, cook a whole meal and invite your friends over to enjoy it. Entertaining them will help you later to function as a hostess in your own home. After the party, clean up the kitchen, wash the dishes, and put them away. Learn how to take care of the silver.

Regardless of income, many American families have a grossly inadequate diet. Breakfast is usually coffee and a sweet roll on the boss's time, a sandwich or pie and Coke for lunch, and a dinner which may contain meat. Adequate nutrition is essential to continued good health. To start your day without fuel for energy is foolish—so *learn* to eat breakfast at home. Get up five minutes earlier, so that your breakfast will not be rushed. Basically, your daily diet should include two citrus fruits, one other fruit, two to three glasses of milk, a raw green salad, yellow and green cooked vegetables, and meat or fish. Eggs are not a meat substitute and they are not a daily essential. Literature is available in your local library on the adequate diet, with many menu suggestions. Try planning menus for your family and endeavor to avoid monotony. Breakfast does not have to be the same day after day.

If you are working, you must have some idea of the value of money. To learn to buy groceries economically requires practice. Plan the menu for one week, make out a grocery list (don't be an impulsive buyer), and shop for the week in one trip. Keep an expense account. After you master efficient grocery shopping, learn about the other expenses of running a home. Gradually, take over the management of all the expenses of your home. Then, just for experience, see if you can manage on ten dollars less per month. Inability to budget the available money is the basis for some of the earliest arguments among newlyweds.

PREMARITAL EXAMINATION

Good health, essential in your new life, is a gift to be cherished and protected. You should have a complete physical examination, with complete blood count, annually, to detect any disorder in the earliest stage. The premarital examination is not just a blood test for syphilis but a careful pelvic examination as well. This should not be delayed until just before the ceremony, but should be done at least six to eight weeks prior to the wedding date. If you have a normal menstrual history and have never had any pelvic complications, the chances are that you will be found completely normal. Occasionally, a thick, inelastic hymen is encountered, which requires a simple operation. This slight complication looms large when discovered four or five days before the wedding. To operate before the wedding would mean a painful wound, incapacitating the bride for coitus on her honeymoon. Not to operate would probably mean painful, possibly fruitless attempts at penetration. Occasionally, the tough hymen will yield to the herculean efforts of the groom, and it may then bleed excessively and require hospitalization. In the past twenty years, I have hospitalized three brides on their honeymoons in Chicago, for suturing of torn, bleeding hymens.

Less often, the pelvic examination may reveal an ovarian tumor, which may require surgery because it is too large to be functional in origin. A fibroid tumor of the uterus may be discovered. It may be too small to indicate surgery, yet your fertility is at once threatened. Therefore, do not complicate your new life by delaying the all-essential visit to the gynecologist.

Remember these points in preparing for your visit to the gynecologist:

(1) Check your menstrual history and take the data with you.

What was the *first* day of your last period?
What was the first day of the preceding period?
How old were you when you first menstruated?
How often do you menstruate? Count from the first day of one

period to the first day of the next period. Many people incorrectly count from the *end* of one period to the beginning of the next, and think that they menstruate every three weeks.
How many days does your period last?
How many pads or tampons do you really need in twenty-four hours?
Do you have pain? At what time is it worst? What relieves the pain?

(2) Many patients want to be very clean for their examination, so they douche the morning of the appointment. Often a low-grade infection exists and the douche washes away the evidence, so that a diagnosis cannot be made. If a Papanicolaou smear for cancer is done, it will mean nothing if you have just washed away the cells. Therefore, do *not* douche for five days prior to the examination if you are in the habit of douching.

(3) If you have not had a bowel movement on the day of your appointment, take a cleansing enema. It is essential that the lower bowel be empty.

(4) You will be asked to empty your bladder just before the examination.

At the time of the premarital examination, you should not hesitate to ask the gynecologist any questions you may have about sexual intercourse. If you are interested in contraception, this is the time for a discussion of the various methods.

HYGIENE OF SEXUAL INTERCOURSE

An understanding of the anatomy of the reproductive organs is essential to full sexual enjoyment. This was reviewed in Chapter III. Figure 14 will re-emphasize a few significant facts. The clitoris is in the midline on the lower portion of the public bone, and is concealed by the labia. However, it can be seen by separating the labia minora, the smaller lips. The clitoris is the prime source of pleasurable stimuli leading to orgasm. For some reason, the word is almost always mispronounced as kli-tor'-is instead of correctly kli'-to-ris.

Immediately below the clitoris is the small opening of the urethra, which is the channel leading from the urinary bladder, in front of the vagina. Contrary to common belief, the bladder is not emptied through the vagina. The vaginal opening is below the urethra, medically called the meatus. The hymen, a fold of tissue at the lower end of the vagina, may vary greatly in width, thickness, and elasticity. Furthermore, the

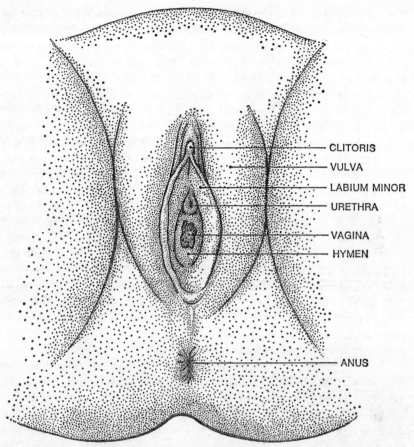

CLITORIS
VULVA
LABIUM MINOR
URETHRA
VAGINA
HYMEN

ANUS

Fig. 14. The external female sex organs.

hymen may be so elastic and shallow that it does not tear until the first child is born. Further back is the anus, from which the bowels are emptied.

Personal cleanliness is of paramount consideration in a sexual relationship. Daily bathing should include using soap and a washcloth between the labia minora and majora, where smegma accumulates. The anal area also should be carefully cleansed. Washing more than once a day is unnecessary and may lead to excessive dryness and itching, nor is routine douching required and may even be harmful. A daily change of underwear is urged, and if a panty girdle is worn, cotton panties should be worn underneath. After you have a bowel movement, cleanse

the anal area from front to rear, in a rearward motion. Be sure that the
area is thoroughly cleansed. Never wipe toilet tissue from the anal area
up over the vulva. The bacteria found in the bowel are not normally
present in the bladder, and to smear fecal material over the urethra
may lead to a bladder infection.

You may think that these suggestions and instructions are redun-
dant, but let me give you a few examples from personal observation
of private patients. The examining room reeks with body odor—even
before the patient's clothes are removed. This unpleasant smell is due
to soiled clothes, stale perspiration, and a dirty body. The patient may
be well dressed outwardly, but her underwear can be quite dirty from
weeks of wear. The crotch of her panties or panty girdle is occasionally
stiffened with old discharge. If not stiff, then stained a deep gray-
yellow. The pelvic examination often reveals an accumulation of
smegma, between the labia minora and majora, and about the clitoris.
Frequently this discharge is found in the daily bathers who neglect this
particular area. Smegma is a thick, cheesy, foul-smelling secretion
made up of cast-off skin cells, obviously of lengthy duration. In addition, pelvic examination reveals a ring of bowel movement about the
anus, or smeared up over the labia. Such carelessness is extremely
common but is easily corrected. Fecal matter, bowel movement, can be
extremely irritating to the skin.

The first sexual intercourse will be nothing like what is to follow.
You may be frightened, pull away, put your knees together and cry.
The groom may be clumsy, fail to have an erection, or, having succeeded with an erection, may spoil it all with a premature ejaculation,
discharge of semen. You can expect some discomfort with the first
penetration; it is pain mixed with pleasure and nothing to fear. The
hymen usually tears a little and may or may not bleed. The erected
penis may appear enormous, more than you can accommodate. However, the vagina is distensible and easily receives the penis. The shaft
of the penis is firm, but the head, the glans, is quite soft, highly sensitive, and will not injure you.

The hump, at the lower end of the vagina, separating it from the anal
canal, is the perineal body. After the hymenal ring has been stretched,
the perineal body offers the next resistance. Once the glans of the penis
has been introduced beyond the perineal body, further resistance to the
free, back-and-forth motion of sexual union ends.

Sexual excitation for the girl begins with kissing or caressing the lips,
back of the neck, and breasts. Kissing the nipples is perfectly normal,
but sucking is not advised, since breast infection may follow. The pulse

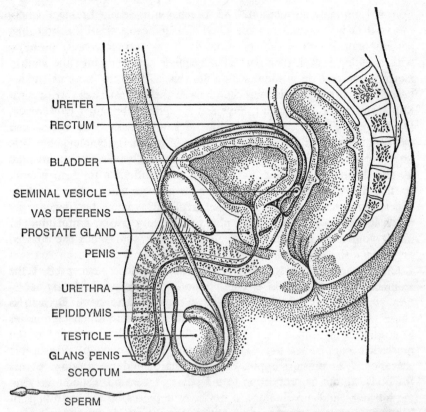

Fig. 15. The male sex organs showing the connection of the bladder with the urethra which passes downward through the penis; also the testicle with the tube (vas deferens) which carries the sperm into the urethra after ejaculation. At left, a greatly enlarged diagram of a sperm cell.

quickens, breathing is more rapid, and the nipples become erect. Vaginal secretion is increased. Contrary to past opinion, this secretion is not from the cervix or from the glands, but from the vaginal cells themselves.

As sexual excitement mounts, the husband seeks other erogenous areas, the inner aspect of the thighs, the labia minora, and finally the clitoris. The external genitalia become congested and the clitoris and labia minora are enlarged.

The wife need not be inert while experiencing this rapturous delight. She may caress his thighs, penis, and scrotum. Only experience will teach how much fondling the husband can enjoy without overstimulation and untimely ejaculation. The wife has now reached a stage where the void in her vagina must be filled. She indicates this by a little tug, getting herself into better position for easy entrance, and, perhaps, with a telling kiss. Either partner may guide the penis into the vagina. Entrance should be gradual with little, back-and-forth motions, taking care to touch the clitoris with the glans in the earliest phase. If lubrication seems to be insufficient, have some vaginal lubricating jelly handy. Do not use Vaseline, since it is too thick and sticky. The vagina and perineum become fully engorged. When insertion is complete, the wife does not lie in bed motionless, but joins her husband's rhythm with an up-and-down and circular motion. The husband tries to pace himself so that he will not have an orgasm before his wife does. The time necessary to reach an orgasm varies greatly in women, but is generally much longer than in men. Men always have an orgasm. Unfortunately, many women never achieve one. However, if a woman has experienced an orgasm, she knows it.

Orgasm is neuro-muscularly similar in both sexes, except that the woman does not have an ejaculate; she does have a lubricating secretion which begins in the first stage of sexual excitement. Orgasm is characterized by a mounting tension and excitement which culminates in a burst of joy, involving the whole being. A spastic contraction of the muscles occurs about the vagina with a pelvic spread of pleasurable sensation. The pulse is rapid, breathing hard, and perspiration covers the body, all out of proportion to the physical exertion. Pseudo-weeping may occur, and involuntary aggressive impulses, such as biting or beating. Certainly privacy is of utmost import, so doors and windows should be closed beforehand to permit a wonderful, uninhibited time.

Immediately following the orgasm, relaxation is profound. Contrary to popular custom, this is not the time to get up, go to the bathroom, wash and douche. Kleenex and a wastebasket should be kept handy so that the excess discharge can be wiped off, and you can remain quiet in each other's arms. Sleep will soon follow.

Suppose the wife does not have an orgasm. The thoughtful husband will gently stimulate her clitoris until he has brought his mate to a satisfactory climax. To be repeatedly stimulated sexually but not satisfied will render the girl nervous, irritable, and sleepless. She will soon develop a distaste for intercourse and will find excuses to discourage her husband's desire. The wise husband will be patient, tender, and reduce the frequency of union to two or three times a week. He will come to the marriage bed immaculately clean, since odors are particularly significant in this intimate relationship. He should check his armpits for possible unpleasant odor, since his wife's sense of smell cannot escape this area. He will indulge in a preferably prolonged period of preliminary caressing and gentle stimulation of the clitoris. If the mate can be brought close to a climax in this way, successful coitus may follow.

If a manual orgasm for the girl is followed by intercourse, she may feel nothing pleasurable. The erogenous or sexually exciting zones are temporarily dulled. The husband's performance may bore her and she may find herself wondering, *"When* is he going to get through?" Couples vary greatly in their needs and tastes, and each will gradually work out a program best suited to them both.

A simultaneous orgasm or "coming together" is difficult to achieve. This climax is not as significant as it has been thought to be. Worrying about such timing leads to a loss of spontaneity. Often a wife, anxious to please her husband, will feign the orgasm, while he is throbbing away, oblivious to her plight. If the wife is capable of orgasm, the husband will be happy to co-operate either by manual stimulation or with second coitus, after a little rest.

Some girls are incapable of an orgasm, despite the best efforts of the partners. Frequently they seek professional advice, hoping to find a physical defect which can be easily corrected. The problem is emotional, however, and may require expert psychiatric help. The reasons for inability to enjoy coitus are many. For example, the girl may have been brought up in a rigid atmosphere in which sex was considered disgusting and dirty, to be endured but not enjoyed. Or the girl may have had premarital sexual experiences associated with deep guilt. Now she cannot accept socially acceptable sex because of guilt.

The husband is often a factor in his wife's lack of sexual response. He may have been brutal on the wedding night. He may be selfish or uninformed, thinking only of his own pleasure. He may skip the preliminary loving, mount his wife, pump away, get release, and withdraw, leaving her in a confused, angry condition. She, indeed, has been "used." In addition, he may insist on this performance nightly and occasionally more often. At times she may be getting dinner for guests when he insists on a matinee. Of course, she would hardly be in a receptive mood under these circumstances. She may be shy, and he may insist on having her walk around the bedroom nude. Excessive shyness prevents the girl from being spontaneous and from fully enjoying the relationship. The husband may sit on their new sofa naked after coitus, or he may indulge in sexual practices that frighten her. He may deem it advisable to consult a marriage counselor and if he fails to benefit from this, he may seek the help of a psychiatrist.

Nothing in married life should be permitted to be monotonous or dull. Variety in coitus will add vitality to the relationship. Variation of sexual positions, using the floor or a chair instead of the bed and copulation at no fixed time of day are not out of order. No sexual position is "wrong." Some require less energy and some give more clitoral stimulation than others. Some of the more common positions are:

(1) Man above.
- (a) The wife lies on her back, her thighs are flexed, her knees apart. If the man's body is moved nearer the head of the bed, so that his pubic bone is in close contact with hers, she will receive clitoral stimulation from the shaft of the penis.
- (b) The wife puts her legs over her husband's shoulders. This rotates the pelvis so that chance for clitoral stimulation is better.

(2) Wife above. This also provides for good clitoral stimulation. The wife is more active in the body rhythm and she sets the pace.

(3) Side to side—facing one another. This position prevents deep penetration and seems difficult.

(4) From the rear. This position does not give the wife any clitoral stimulation and is not, therefore, much fun. Occasionally, this position is recommended to facilitate pregnancy, when the uterus is retroverted.

(5) On a chair. The husband sits on the chair. The wife straddles the chair, facing her husband. The wife sits on the husband's lap as the penis glides into her vagina. This posture gives good clitoral contact. This position is not a guarantee against pregnancy but conception is least likely, since the semen is almost immediately lost.

If the wife is capable of vaginal orgasm, clitoral stimulation becomes less urgent. However, most women have clitoral orgasm. If the husband finds that he cannot "hold out" and his wife does not seem quite ready for orgasm, he may resort to manual stimulation of the clitoris while intercourse is in progress.

Newlyweds usually have sexual intercourse daily. During this period of frequent pelvic congestion, the wife may develop a bladder infection known as "honeymoon cystitis." She should consult a gynecologist promptly for a pelvic examination, urinalysis, and treatment. Part of the therapy probably will be more gentle, less frequent intercourse.

By the time the honeymoon is over and the couple settle down in their new home, the frequency of intercourse tapers off a little. Couples vary greatly in their need for sexual expression, but generally two to three times a week suffices. Occasionally, the wife will make the overtures, to the delight of her husband. Overindulgence in this, as in any other field, leads to diminished appreciation. If you strive for quality rather than quantity you usually will reap rich rewards.

CONTRACEPTION

Until the couple is thoroughly adjusted to one another and sure that their marriage is stable, they are wise to postpone conception. Divorce is always a tragedy for children, but so is the home that is filled with tension and insecurity.

The ejaculate which is deposited in the vagina during orgasm contains many millions of sperm cells. The number varies, depending on the frequency of coitus and the health of the husband. If the penis is quite close to the mouth of the womb, the cervix, during ejaculation, some sperm may be deposited at the opening of the cervix. The normal sperm cells have remarkable motility and this is a significant factor in sperm transport through the uterus and out into the tube. Douching immediately after intercourse is one of the most ineffective means of contraception. By the time that the douche is given, the sperms are already beyond reach.

The purpose of contraception is to prevent the meeting of the sperm and the egg. Usually only one egg is available during the month. Ordinarily this occurs about 14 ± 2 days before the onset of the next menses. The unfertilized egg is extremely delicate and does not survive more than twenty-four hours. To complicate what should be simple, however, women with cycles "regular as the clock" may experience an irregularity at any time. They may ovulate earlier than usual, but more frequently ovulation will be delayed due to some mental stress, which, naturally, is inescapable in daily living. For this reason, constant, consistent practice of contraception is recommended not only during the supposed fertile period but during the "safe" period too. Many an unwanted pregnancy is the result of such timing.

One of the oldest methods of contraception is the condom, or "rubber," used by the male. The condom is safe, harmless, and easily obtainable. However, it may break during intercourse and can slip off afterward, permitting the semen to spill into the vagina. The additional disadvantage of having to place the condom on the fully erected penis, when the husband is at the height of sexual excitement, may mar the spontaneity of the union. To be effective, it must be donned before the first penetration. To use the condom for ejaculation only is unsafe and might necessitate withdrawal just when the wife is beginning the climactic phase, and in need of the closest contact with her lover. To prevent the condom from slipping off, he should hold it during withdrawal of the penis from the vagina. After removal, the condom should be tested for tears. If it is torn, the wife should place contraceptive jelly immediately into the vagina. This procedure will not reach the sperm that have already made their way into the uterus, and therefore is not completely effective. The torn condom should be then abandoned. To prevent tears and to give added protection, the wife may place contraceptive jelly into the vagina prior to intercourse. The objection to this extra precaution is the excess lubrication.

Withdrawal is another means of contraception used by men. The method is not safe and spoils the spontaneity of coitus. If the husband is not nervous, the wife is, lest withdrawal be too late. Joy and abandon, with eventual climax, are impossible for the wife under these circumstances. In addition, some sperm cells may find their way into the vagina prior to orgasm.

Another time-honored method of child spacing is the diaphragm, used by the woman. This is made of soft rubber, is dome-shaped, and has a flexible rubber-covered metal spring about the edge. The diaphragm is harmless. This gadget fits between the upper back part of the vagina, in the little niche under the pubic bone in front, and covers the cervix. The distance covered by the diaphragm varies greatly in each woman and requires measurement by a doctor thoroughly versed on this subject. The diaphragm can be obtained from the doctor or on prescription at a pharmacy. A diaphragm that fits is not enough. The woman must be shown how to place it and how to insert it correctly. The best place to learn is in the doctor's office or clinic.

The diaphragm is used with a contraceptive jelly. Many patients think that the diaphragm alone prevents pregnancy; this is not true. Millions of sperm, too small to be seen with the naked eye, are involved, and these lodge around the edge of the diaphragm and up onto the uterus. The purpose of the diaphragm is to hold the jelly in the correct place because the *jelly kills the sperm*. Why not, then, use the jelly alone? The act of intercourse can displace the jelly from the mouth of the womb, thereby permit access of the sperm to the uterus. The

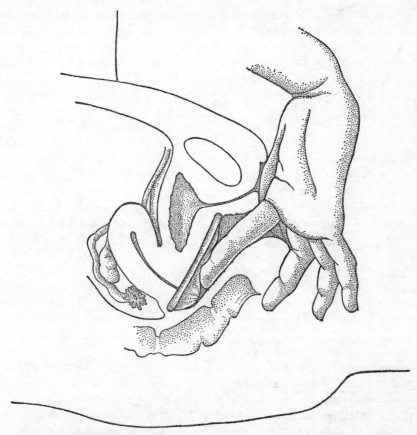

Fig. 16. The placement of a diaphragm, closing the opening of the cervix into the uterus.

type of jelly used is salient. It must be a contraceptive jelly, and *not* Vaseline or any other handy lubricant.

Diaphragm failures are known, although both the diaphragm and the correct jelly are used. Perhaps too little jelly was used, or it may have been lost in placement of the diaphragm. Since jelly should be around the cervix and also held by the diaphragm, I have varied the technique of applying the jelly for more favorable success. I advise patients to place the dome side of the diaphragm next to the cervix, using contraceptive jelly on the diaphragm rim before placement. When the diaphragm is in place and the patient has felt her cervix, through rubber, thereby making sure of correct placement, I teach her to depress the lower part of the diaphragm, place an applicator full of jelly on

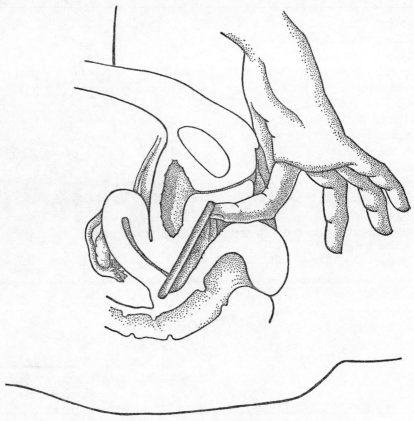

Fig. 17. The diaphragm being correctly placed.

top of the diaphragm and between it and the cervix, depositing the jelly deep into the vagina near the cervix. Instead of having jelly all over the patient's thighs and vulva, it will be spread where it is effective. The patient need not add additional jelly to the vagina if intercourse should be repeated. Although it is known that motile sperms do not survive in the vagina more than two or three hours, I have continued the current teaching of leaving the diaphragm in place until six hours after the last ejaculation. A douche is not necessary when the diaphragm is removed. I have recommended this method for fourteen years without any failures. Patients report that the husbands are delighted with the lack of excessive jelly and excess lubrication.

Another method employed by women is the introduction of jellies, creams, or foams, used without a mechanical device such as a diaphragm. These are designed so that they stay in place without any device. They can be obtained without a prescription at most drugstores. Furthermore, the woman does not need a pelvic examination by a physician. Harmless chemicals, which kill or immobilize the sperm, are the active principles in these substances. Each tube of such contraceptive ointment is supplied with an applicator, which measures the right amount to be used. Not more than one hour prior to intercourse, the material is deposited deep into the vagina. If coitus is repeated, another application must be inserted. Douching is not recommended, and, in any case, must not be done under six hours after the last ejaculation.

Vaginal tablets, different from suppositories, are also obtainable at the drugstore without prescription. This method requires that a moistened tablet be placed high in the vagina before each coitus. The vaginal suppositories, not the tablets, on the market today are not too reliable.

Rhythm is the method sanctioned by the Roman Catholic Church. In this method, intercourse is avoided during the fertile period. Since the unfertilized egg survives only twenty-four hours and the sperm a maximum of forty-eight hours in the cervical mucus, this should not present a great problem, and, indeed, for many women it has proved highly satisfactory. The difficulty is figuring out exactly when ovulation will occur in a specific woman. If she has kept the exact dates of the onset of menses for six to twelve months and, in addition, has kept a basal body temperature record for this same period, her gynecologist can help her to figure out a fertile time chart.

The basal body temperature curve is obtained by taking the temperature on awakening, before talking to or even kissing your husband, before getting out of bed, and at the same time of day. Although a thermal shift occurs with ovulation, the shift does not pinpoint ovulation. The temperature curve is low in the first half of the cycle and elevated in the last half. The temperature remains high until the day before or the day of the onset of menses, when, usually, a sharp drop occurs. If the woman is interested in keeping a temperature curve, she may obtain graphs and instructions from her gynecologist. She must know how to read a thermometer accurately and how to shake it down after the reading. After the temperature has been up for three or four days, the woman may be sure that she has ovulated and that the fertile period is over.

Many girls, using the rhythm method, have conceived when having coitus just once, at the end of a period. Was this caused by an early, unexpected ovulation or do the doctors have much more to learn about

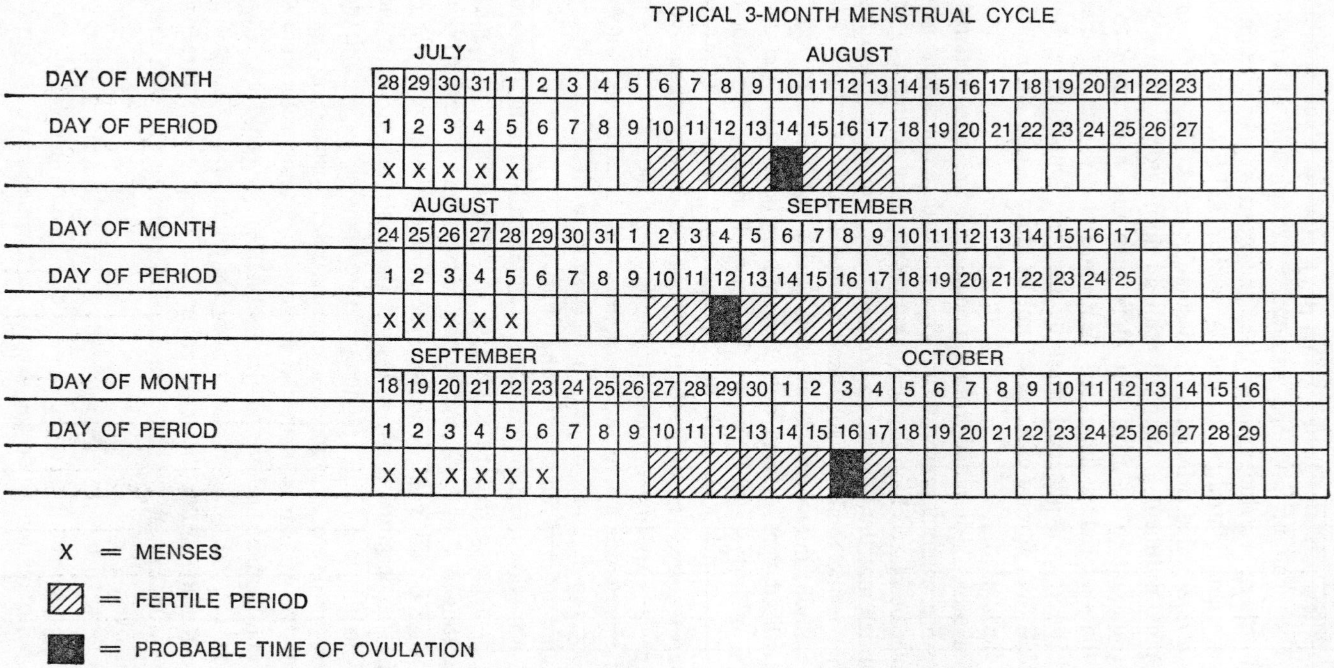

TYPICAL 3-MONTH MENSTRUAL CYCLE

Fig. 18. A chart of a typical three-month menstrual cycle.

X = MENSES

▨ = FERTILE PERIOD

■ = PROBABLE TIME OF OVULATION

SAMPLE RHYTHM METHOD CHART

JULY / AUGUST

DAY OF MONTH	JULY				AUGUST																						
DAY OF MONTH	28	29	30	31	1	2	3	4	5	6	7	8	9	10	11	12	13	14	15	16	17	18	19	20	21	22	23
DAY OF PERIOD	1	2	3	4	5	6	7	8	9	10	11	12	13	14	15	16	17	18	19	20	21	22	23	24	25	26	27
	X	X	X	X	X	X	S	S				▨	▨	■	S	S	S	S	S	S	S	S	S				

AUGUST / SEPTEMBER

DAY OF MONTH	AUGUST								SEPTEMBER																
DAY OF MONTH	24	25	26	27	28	29	30	31	1	2	3	4	5	6	7	8	9	10	11	12	13	14	15	16	17
DAY OF PERIOD	1	2	3	4	5	6	7	8	9	10	11	12	13	14	15	16	17	18	19	20	21	22	23	24	25
	X	X	X	X	X	X	S	S	S			▨	▨	■	S	S	S	S	S	S	S	S	S	S	S

SEPTEMBER / OCTOBER

DAY OF MONTH	SEPTEMBER													OCTOBER															
DAY OF MONTH	18	19	20	21	22	23	24	25	26	27	28	29	30	1	2	3	4	5	6	7	8	9	10	11	12	13	14	15	16
DAY OF PERIOD	1	2	3	4	5	6	7	8	9	10	11	12	13	14	15	16	17	18	19	20	21	22	23	24	25	26	27	28	29
	X	X	X	X	X	X	S	S	S			▨	▨	■	S	S	S	S	S	S	S	S	S	S	S	S	S	S	S

X = MENSES

▨ = FERTILE PERIOD

■ = PROBABLE TIME OF OVULATION

S = SAFE DAYS

░ = SAFETY FACTOR

Fig. 19. A sample chart for the Rhythm Method of birth control. This chart is based on a history of monthly cycles that vary between 25 and 29 days. The safety factor is necessary because of the ±2 day variation in ovulation, which occurs 14 days (±2) before onset of next menses; and also because the life of the male sperm is approximately 48 hours.

sperm survival in such fertile girls? When a patient, using rhythm, is particularly anxious not to conceive, I instruct her to defer coitus until well after ovulation, as indicated by a basal body temperature rise, for three days. Elevation of temperature due to an infection, lack of sleep, or sleeping late in the day, and alcohol intake, nullifies the significance of the temperature curve.

If a woman has a regular twenty-eight-day cycle, then she will probably ovulate on the fourteenth day. Allowing for the egg and sperm survival, one should avoid the sexual act for three days before and three days after ovulation, that is from the eleventh *through* the seventeenth days. Barring an unexpected delayed ovulation, the woman should be definitely safe after the seventeenth day. However, it must be remembered that the period before the eleventh day is not so safe for the reasons already given.

Practically everyone has heard about the PILL by now. The pill is an oral contraceptive aimed at inhibiting ovulation. Several products now are on the market, and as yet they are relatively expensive. This oral contraceptive is obtained on prescription only and is not prescribed until after a careful gynecological examination. The pill is taken for twenty days, at the *same time* of the day, beginning on the fifth day of the menstrual period. If the period lasts only three days, the woman still starts on the fifth day, counting the first day of the period as day number 1. If one starts on day number 6 or forgets to take the pill for one day, the chance of accidental pregnancy is increased. If bleeding occurs while she is taking the pill, this is not menstruation but "breakthrough" bleeding. The pill must not be stopped, but the dose increased, according to the instructions of the gynecologist. Menstruation begins two to three days after taking the last pill.

Initially, nausea and other subjective symptoms of pregnancy may ensue, but usually these do not persist. The weight gain and salt retention noted with the first pills are less common today with the newer, improved tablets.

Many patients worry that they are not "safe" on the two to three days, just prior to a period, when they do not take the pill. Apparently they feel that the pill protects them for the day, and without the pill there is no safety. One must remember that the whole purpose in taking the pill is to prevent the release of an egg, and that an egg is not available when this medication is taken correctly. Therefore, such anxiety is unnecessary. Without an available egg, pregnancy is impossible.

The intrauterine contraceptive devices offer new freedom to the woman. She does not have to remember to take a pill, fuss with placement of a contraceptive device, or consult the calendar. She is completely free and always ready. Various types of intrauterine devices are made, most of which are constructed of plastic and are non-irritating. The device fits into the uterine cavity. Once the device is placed, it remains in the uterus until removal by the doctor. The usual reason for removal is a wish for conception.

The mechanism by which pregnancy is prevented with the intrauterine device is still not perfectly understood. Much research is going on at this time. However, it has been established that ovulation is not suppressed. Those patients who have been fitted with the intrauterine device seem most grateful.

Chapter V

BIRTH OF THE FIRST BABY
Charlotte H. Kerr, M.D.

How exciting it is to have children, and especially the first one, since everything is so new and strange to the uninitiated: No matter how many children one has and no matter how many babies a physician has delivered, the miracle of pregnancy and birth never cease to bring joy both to the mother and to her doctor, but the first born is particularly special.

How long should you wait after marriage before having children? How will you know that you are pregnant? What should you do if you have difficulty conceiving? These and many more questions race through the mind of a new bride anxious to begin her family.

Each newly married couple has special needs which will influence their feelings about when to have children. In general, marriage requires adjustments. It is a good idea to allow time for the new husband and wife to learn to know each other in a day-to-day living situation and to enjoy each other before the onset of pregnancy. Regardless of how smoothly a woman goes through pregnancy, some adjustments must be made because of a change in her physiological processes. These are more easily met if she is "over the hump" in making the initial adjustment in marriage. Such adaptation is equally true for the husband. His problems involve not only emotional difficulties, adjustment to living with his new wife, but also economic challenges besetting the family breadwinner. Ideally then, the new couple would have sufficient time to live alone, to become adjusted to each other, and to have a minimum of financial security before the first baby comes. We hasten to add that it is inadvisable to defer pregnancy too long, because a couple may become accustomed to think only of themselves. When children do come, the parents often find that it is difficult to make the adjustment and the many sacrifices that are necessary. As can be readily understood, the most fertile years are before thirty. Therefore, the older couple would have greater urgency in having the first child.

In a normal, healthy young couple having regular marital relations, an average of three to six months may elapse before the wanted conception occurs. Certainly a tremendous variation may be noted in the

DAY OF PERIOD

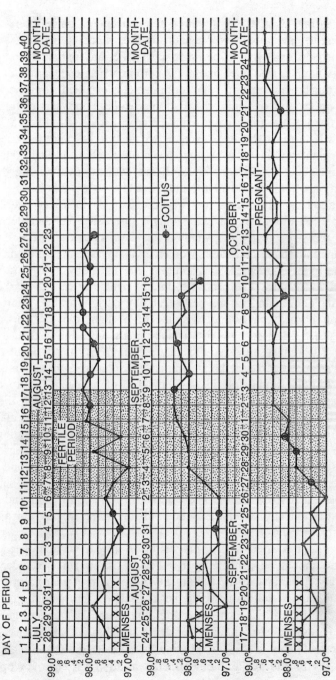

Fig. 20. A basal temperature record covering three months.

length of time of marriage required for conception, since many brides will attest to having become pregnant on their wedding night. Assuming both husband and wife to be normally fertile, approximately only one thirty-six-hour period each month is certain when conception can occur. At this special time of ovulation, the egg is expelled from the ovary, picked up by the oviducts, the Fallopian tubes, and carried into the middle third of the tube. Here, if intercourse has occurred recently, the sperm will fertilize the egg, carry it to the uterus, and there embed itself, beginning a new life. The egg has a life of about twelve hours and the sperm about twenty-four hours; hence with the overlap, we deduce the thirty-six-hour period of monthly fertility.

Ovulation usually occurs two weeks before the onset of each menstrual period, but much variation may be obtained. In the theoretical normal menstrual cycle of twenty-eight days, ovulation occurs about the fourteenth day, but some women ovulate as early as eight days after the onset of menses, and some as late as a day before the menstrual period begins. The probable time of ovulation can be established by taking one's temperature before arising each morning, charting it on graph paper, and noting the time of a slight dip in temperature which is then followed by a rise, which persists until the next menstrual period. This chart may require interpretation by a physician, since minor variations in basal body temperature may appear and are confusing. Another home test involves the use of a special kit to check the presence of glucose in the cervical secretions. In this test, the glucose will be noted high at ovulation and also it turns a special test paper from blue to pink. Other methods of determining ovulation can only be done in the physician's office and involve vaginal smear tests, biopsies of the endometrium, the inside lining of the uterus, and daily measurements of the length of cervical mucus, when drawn between two glass microscope slides. These tests are time-consuming and more difficult, technically, than basal body temperature graphs, so are reserved for problem cases.

If a wife has tried to get pregnant for a year without success, a physician should be consulted. If either marital partner is older than commonly customary at the time of marriage, more urgency is probably indicated and consultation would be advisable after only three to six months of infertility. Particular attention then will undoubtedly be given to possible abnormalities of the vaginal tract which may have been present from birth, but previously undetected. Occasionally, the hymen, the fibromuscular tissue which partially surrounds the opening of the vagina, is found to be intact. Successful coitus, intercourse, may never have occurred.

In order to achieve pregnancy, not only must a woman ovulate, but her Fallopian tubes must be patent, or open. The Rubin test may be done in the physician's office to determine tubal patency. For this test, carbon dioxide gas is introduced into the tubes by way of the cervical opening in the uterus through the vagina. The physician confirms patency by using a stethoscope on the lower abdomen and listening to the gas bubbles come through the tubes.

In selected cases of infertility or frequent miscarriage, the physician may suggest that an X-ray be made of the patient's uterus and tubes. This procedure, called a hysterosalpingogram, is usually done in the office of a radiologist, an X-ray specialist, or in the X-ray department of a hospital. Radiopaque dye is inserted into the uterus with the same technique with which carbon dioxide is introduced in the Rubin test. The radiologist follows the path of the dye through the uterus and tubes, and X-rays are then made so that a permanent record is obtained. In some cases in which the tubes have been partially closed, the pressure of the radiopaque dye has actually opened them.

In about 40 per cent of infertile couples, the man is partially or wholly responsible. Referral of the husband to a urologist is advisable. The doctor will not only examine the sperm but also evaluate the male organs of reproduction and the husband's sexual habits. Men seem more reluctant than women to be examined. The wife must, therefore, encourage her husband to participate if so requested by her doctor.

SIGNS OF PREGNANCY

Although twenty-eight days is the theoretical normal cycle, only a few women are this regular. Some delay in menses may occur with excitement, on moving to a new climate, or by just being anxious to get pregnant. A physician can make a fairly definite diagnosis of pregnancy more easily if the woman will wait until she has missed her menstrual period by two or three weeks. Diagnosis is made on the basis of increased size and softness of the uterus, the bluish discoloration of the cervix, and the increased glandularity of the breasts, along with the history of amenorrhea, the missed menses. In some cases of uncertainty the patient may be asked to take a urine specimen to the laboratory or to the physician's office for a pregnancy test. The test most frequently used is one which detects chorionic gonadotrophin, a substance formed by the newly developing embryo and its placenta, the afterbirth.

Positive diagnosis of pregnancy should be made as soon as feasible so that the woman may take suitable precautions to protect her unborn child against drugs and disease. Many new drugs are being marketed each year and because their effects on pregnancy are not always known, a woman who might be pregnant should avoid unnecessary drugs and inform her physician as soon as possible of her probable pregnancy. Although pregnant women may have necessary X-rays of their chest, teeth, and fractured bones, if possible they should avoid abdominal X-rays during early pregnancy. The fetus is probably not injured by minimal X-ray exposure, but prolonged exposure as from a barium meal and barium enema given for detection of abnormalities of the stomach and bowel might cause abnormalities in the baby. The pregnant woman should make a conscious effort to avoid all infections by staying away from friends who have sick children and by shunning large crowds of people. In a small percentage of cases any virus infection in a pregnant woman might cause a problem with the baby. Particular caution, however, should be taken to avoid German measles, the so-called "three-day measles" and medically termed rubella. Generally, if a girl has had rubella once, she will not get it again; hence some authorities recommend that young girls be exposed to the disease so they will be immune to it when they marry and have children. The incidence of abnormal babies born to mothers who have had German measles during pregnancy is variably reported from 20 to 60 per cent, depending on where and how the study was conducted. Congenital heart disease, blindness, and deafness are among the abnormalities noted. The greatest danger of German measles to the pregnant woman is in the first three months when the new baby organs are being formed. Minor abnormalities in the baby may develop if measles occurs in the fifth or sixth month. After the sixth month, danger to either the baby or mother is almost nil.

In the past, if a pregnant woman was exposed to German measles and never had the disease, physicians frequently gave her immune gamma globulin by injection. The American College of Obstetricians and Gynecologists has recently issued a statement that their research committees have not found any benefit from the administration of gamma globulin and, therefore, they are no longer recommending it.

In some non-Catholic hospitals, a positive diagnosis of rubella in the first three months of pregnancy is considered an indication for therapeutic abortion; that is, terminating the pregnancy surgically, if this procedure is so desired by the husband and wife and agreed to by the consultation committee of the hospital.

The incidence of poliomyelitis has dramatically decreased since the discovery of the Salk, and now of the oral Sabin, vaccine. However, the young married woman must continue to be protected against polio, preferably before she gets pregnant. Her obstetrician, internist, or family physician should be consulted to decide whether or not booster immunization is indicated. Polio during pregnancy is uncommon but poses additional serious problems to the mother and baby when it does occur.

THE FIRST MONTHS

An early diagnosis of pregnancy helps the doctor advise his patient about her diet and her changing food requirements for proper fetal and maternal well-being. Increased amounts of protein, as found in meat, fish, chicken, and eggs are essential, as well as increased amounts of minerals, especially calcium which is supplied by milk, and iron, which is furnished by meat and certain vegetables. A pregnant woman's requirement for calcium is provided by one quart of milk daily during pregnancy and by one and a half quarts daily when she is breast feeding. For patients who are unable to drink milk, calcium supplements are prescribed.

Depending on the size of the patient and her body build, between fifteen and twenty pounds total weight gain during pregnancy is considered ideal. Early in pregnancy some women lose their appetites and a few have nausea before meals, characteristically in the morning; hence the term "morning sickness." If the pregnant woman seeks medical aid early, the physician can recommend a special diet to minimize this discomfort and he can prescribe medication to be taken at bedtime which often prevents nausea. Eating small amounts of bland food at two-hour intervals along with temporarily decreasing fluid intake often will curb nausea. Crackers or vanilla wafers kept at the bedside to be eaten as soon as the prospective mother awakens in the morning, before she prepares her husband's breakfast, frequently is helpful too. The pregnant woman should avoid cooking bacon, sausage, or strong-smelling foods early in the morning. Furthermore, she should delay eating her fruit or drinking juice until after she has eaten her cereal or toast and until after her stomach feels "settled." This problem is much like seasickness. Getting out-of-doors and keeping busy along with eating small amounts of food frequently will help the uncomfortable young woman much more than languishing in bed and having someone wait on her. No doubt, a physiological basis, a low blood sugar in the morning, is the cause of such nausea. This condition is due, no doubt, to the long night of fasting and to the changes in the pancreatic and other hormonal secretions caused by the pregnancy itself. Furthermore, the condition assuredly can be minimized by the measures described here or they can be made worse by failure to follow the suggestions. Although we do not feel that nausea in pregnancy is psychological in origin, tensions within the mother relating to the pregnancy itself, or conflicts with her family or with her job, can make the conditions worse.

Moderate amounts of physical exercise are encouraged during pregnancy, and will aid the mother-to-be in maintaining good body tone. Mild sports, such as golf, bowling, volley ball, and badminton, can be continued until the patient becomes awkward because of her protruding uterus. Swimming in water of comfortable temperature is not harmful, even in the last month. Sports involving violent motions or sudden stops including diving, horseback riding, and water and snow skiing should be abandoned until after delivery.

Specific exercises in preparation for childbirth are of proved value. Some are intended to aid relaxation during labor and others to keep muscles in tone so that the new mother again will have a good figure. Of particular interest is the book *Have Your Baby, Keep Your Figure* by M. Edward Davis, M.D. and Edward Maisel, published by Stein and Day, New York, and the pamphlet entitled "Rest, Relaxation, Controlled Breathing and Exercise During and After Pregnancy," published by the Maternity Center Association of New York.

How fortunate is the prospective mother today in her choice of clothing during pregnancy! Infinite variety of maternity wear is available for all occasions. Girdles are an elective item, but most patients are more comfortable, especially in the last trimester with a two-way stretch girdle which allows room for growth. Such a garment lends support to the pendulous abdomen, helps prevent backache, and decreases abdominal discomfort. Many girls complain of pain on one or both sides of the lower abdomen. This discomfort is due to the stretching of the round ligaments which support the uterus at the top. By wearing a girdle, the mother-to-be can take some of the pressure off these ligaments.

Generally, the legs will ache during pregnancy, due partly to the increased weight and partly to varicose veins in some patients. Elastic-type hose will minimize such leg discomfort. In order to get the maximum benefit from these hose, the patient should put them on before getting out of bed. Thus, the blood is drained out of the superficial vessels that form the varicose veins which are to be compressed with the elastic hose. If the hose are slipped on in the usual position, with the patient seated and her legs hanging down, the hose will give little relief.

Choice of shoes during pregnancy should be governed by comfort and stability. Spiked heels should not be worn even for dress-up occasions since they can easily cause falls when advancing pregnancy throws the body off balance.

Formerly, many physicians felt that tub baths should be discontinued six weeks or so before delivery but this point of view is now changing. With the average patient, falling while getting in or out of the tub would be the only danger. Most obstetricians believe that douches are contraindicated during pregnancy and that during the non-pregnant state, they are needed only rarely for specific vaginal ailments. Most physicians believe it is advisable that the pregnant woman abstain from intercourse during the last four to six weeks of gestation.

PHYSICAL EXAMINATIONS

After the diagnosis of pregnancy has been made, a complete physical examination is desirable. This includes a pelvic examination, inspection of the vagina and cervix, and palpation of the uterus, tubes, and ovaries for abnormalities. To feel reticent about having pelvic examinations is normal but patients must realize that doctors work objectively and do not feel any differently about this than they would in checking blood pressure.

In selected cases, depending on the patient's age, history, and on the appearance of the cervix, a Papanicolaou smear test of the cervix for cancer cells will be taken. However, more and more physicians now take these on all patients; others, only after a woman has had one or more children or is in a certain age group. The physician also evaluates the pelvis for normal bony structure and estimates the size of the various diameters through which the baby must pass in delivery. Mentally, the doctor will make an assessment of the entire bony and soft tissue structure of the pelvis in order to estimate whether or not a normal-sized baby can be delivered vaginally. If the physician observes any bony deformities or any abnormal measurements, he will plan for X-ray pelvimetry, measurements of the pelvis and the baby's head, in the third trimester.

A blood specimen is taken either in the physician's office or in a laboratory and tested for anemia. A blood test for syphilis, serology, is required of pregnant women in most states, and, if positive, treatment is immediately instituted to protect the unborn baby from this disease.

Early in pregnancy the blood type and Rh factor of the mother-to-be are also tested. Approximately 85 per cent of the population is Rh positive and only 15 per cent Rh negative. If an Rh negative woman has an Rh positive husband, then the physician is alerted to the fact that antibodies may form in the mother's blood. These reach the baby and cause some degree of breakdown in the baby's hemoglobin, thus causing the baby to become anemic and jaundiced, to become an "erythroblastotic baby." Fortunately, this almost never happens with a first pregnancy, because antibodies must be present in the mother's blood from a previous sensitization, as would occur if she were having her second or third pregnancy, or if she had received blood transfusions before 1940 when the Rh factor was discovered.

At each office visit, the pregnant woman's weight and blood pressure are recorded and a sample of morning urine is examined. A sudden rise in blood pressure indicates that the patient needs more rest, and

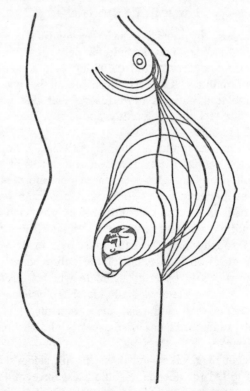

Fig. 21. A diagrammatic view of the development of the uterus and the enlargement of the breasts during pregnancy.

therefore the doctor might prescribe medication. If edema, swelling of the hands, legs, or face occurs, a lower salt intake is advised since the sodium in salt causes the tissues to retain water and swell. Sudden gain of weight can be a reflection of edema or of excessive food intake, both of which will require attention.

The urine is checked for the presence of glucose, sugar, which might suggest diabetes; it is also examined for albumin, a protein substance which appears when the kidneys are functioning abnormally.

Any unusual occurrences such as persistent headaches, bleeding, or vaginal itching should be reported to the doctor's office. Spotting of blood early in pregnancy might be a manifestation of the normal embryo becoming well established in the uterus, or it might indicate a threatened abortion, miscarriage. In the last trimester, spotting might be due to onset of labor, to the placenta or afterbirth lying in front of the baby's head, or to the abnormal separation of the placenta before labor begins.

Some increase in vaginal secretions is normal in pregnancy. This secretion if it is accompanied by itching may be due to Monilia (yeast) or Trichomonas (amoebae) vaginitis. Such infections are not serious and do not harm the baby, but they should be treated promptly for the patient's comfort.

Periodically, the patient is placed on the examining table and the size of the uterus is evaluated for enlargement. When the baby gets large enough, the doctor will determine the baby's position by palpating the abdomen. About the sixth month, the baby's heart can first be heard by the physician when he applies a stethoscope to the mother's abdomen. The mother usually notices "life" or fetal movement at about four and a half to five months. At first this is like a faint ripple in the breeze or the gentle flutter of butterfly wings, felt internally by the patient in the lower abdominal area. When first noticed, it seems more like gas, but when it persists, the patient realizes that this is the movement of her baby. It is well to note the first date of "life" and report this to the doctor as it will help him establish the probable date of delivery. Usually, to arrive at the due date, five calendar months are added to the date of "life."

Near the end of pregnancy, the physician may give the patient an internal examination, rectally or vaginally, to determine the position of the baby and the condition of the cervix, the opening of the uterus. By examining the cervix, the doctor will evaluate the amount of effacement, or shortening of the cervical canal, present and also the amount of dilatation, widening of the opening of the cervix, which has occurred. This information helps the doctor estimate approximately when the patient will be ready to go into labor.

ONSET OF LABOR

What is labor like when it begins? How will the mother-to-be know that she is in labor? Labor may begin in one of three ways. Most commonly the mild, irregular, painless contractions of the uterus which are felt throughout the last weeks of pregnancy change in character and the patient feels waves of tightening up of the uterus, properly called contractions, but sometimes called labor pains. These pains ordinarily occur at regular intervals and can be timed. Sometimes they begin at five-minute intervals, but more often the contractions are farther apart at the beginning of labor. In order to be considered labor pains, the contractions should occur at least every ten minutes.

Furthermore, labor may begin with leaking of the amniotic fluid, the bag of waters, or with a big flood of water, if the membranes rupture suddenly. Rupture of the membranes will actually facilitate labor and not delay it, as the saying that "a dry birth is a hard one" would lead

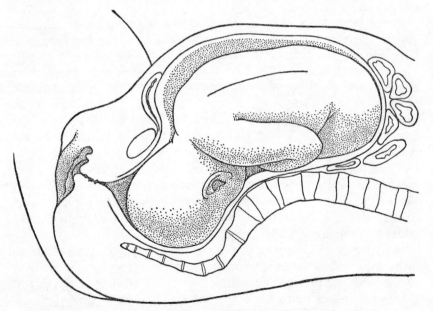

Fig. 22. The uterus after nine months' development of the fetus. The cervix has not yet been dilated and opened.

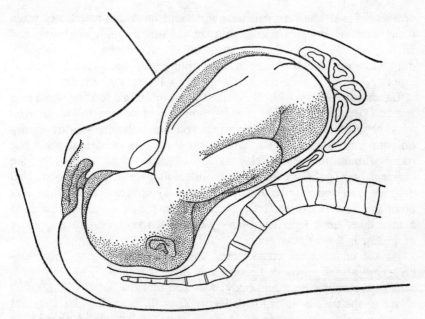

Fig. 23. The onset of labor with the cervix effaced and opening.

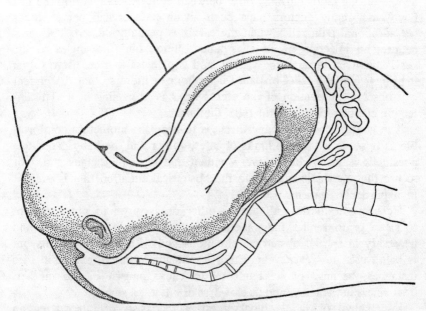

Fig. 24. Childbirth, with the head of the infant passing through the fully dilated cervix.

you to believe. The pregnant woman should not listen to tales of pregnancy and labor which friends tell; these yarns are only confusing and frightening. When you have a question or any uncertainty, discuss it only with your doctor. Keep your ears plugged when friends talk about labor and delivery, since much of what they tell you is unreliable.

Labor may begin with a small amount of blood oozing from the vagina. Usually after this "bloody show," contractions follow shortly.

After notifying your physician that you are in labor, you are finally on your way to the hospital. You will probably be whisked to the labor room without the usual delay at the admitting desk. Generally, the perineal hair is shaved for the sake of cleanliness in examinations and delivery, and you may be given an enema. The average time of the first labor is about twelve to sixteen hours, from the onset of the first mild contractions until delivery. Many women deliver in six to ten hours and a few in three to five hours.

As the contractions come closer together, every three to four minutes, indications are that the cervix is dilating, opening, to allow passage of the baby's head and body; and also that the baby is descending closer to the pelvic outlet for delivery. Your doctor will order Demerol or other pain-relieving drugs to keep you comfortable. You will be awake during labor but may doze between contractions. During the last few years, many doctors have been giving paracervical nerve blocks for additional pain relief when the cervix is partially dilated. This procedure, an injection of an anesthetic solution into the angles of the cervix, is given through the vagina, and is painless to administer. Often it brings complete relief of pain for an hour or more so that the patient can observe contraction of the uterus but has no feeling in it. This injection can be repeated as the relief diminishes.

The goal in obstetrical anesthesia is to keep the mother as comfortable as possible within the limits of safety to her and the baby. No single anesthetic is just right for every patient and most physicians endeavor to use the anesthetic suitable to the obstetrical situation that is present in a particular patient.

General anesthesia with gas or other drugs given to put a patient to sleep or to render the patient insensible to pain is indicated and necessary in special obstetrical situations and with certain patients but is being used less each year. Ether is not administered, except in rare instances, because of its tendency to cause nausea in the mother, drowsiness in the baby, and its slowness of onset.

Low spinal or saddle block anesthesia consists of introducing an anesthetic agent into the spinal canal between the third and fourth lumbar vertebrae. This blocks all sensation of pain in the area, corresponding to that part of the body which rests on a saddle when riding. Caudal anesthesia gives similar pain relief, but this anesthetic is given into the space near the end of the spinal cord and is administered by an injection under the coccyx, the tailbone. Saddle block and caudal anesthesia are usually given only in hospitals with a special obstetrical service staffed by anesthesiologists, physicians who specialize in administering anesthesia.

Pudendal block anesthesia is being used in more hospitals each year. This particular anesthesia usually is given just before delivery by the physician who is delivering the baby, and consists of an injection of Carbocaine, Xylocaine, or Novocaine into the area of the pudendal nerve, through the vagina. The resulting numbness facilitates delivery. Pudendal block anesthesia is often used in conjunction with a small mask containing Trilene or Penthrane which the patient administers to herself at the onset of each contraction. Both media have a pleasant aroma, quickly relieve pain, and yet permit the patient to remain awake between contractions. Penthrane and Trilene are quite safe and when used in conjunction with pudendal block, give excellent results.

The term "natural childbirth" has a variety of meanings to different people. To most physicians this implies that the patient is well informed so she has no fear and is able to relax more during labor. The doctor can, therefore, use a minimum of pain-relieving drugs and have the patient awake and able to co-operate during the baby's birth. In many hospitals now, classes are available where exercises and special breathing and relaxation technics are taught to expectant mothers.

Hypnosis is recognized by the medical profession as a useful adjunct during labor and delivery. This technic requires training and considerable time during pregnancy in order to use it successfully during labor. Not every patient is a suitable candidate for hypnosis and only a few physicians find it practical, timewise, to use it. In selected cases, hypnosis is possible as the sole agent during labor, delivery and even with Cesarean section.

A CHILD IS BORN

An episiotomy, a surgical incision of the external region of the vagina, is commonly done in most primagravida patients, with first baby, so that they will not have lacerations of the vagina. With the aid of an anesthetic to dull the pain, the vaginal opening is cut about two and a

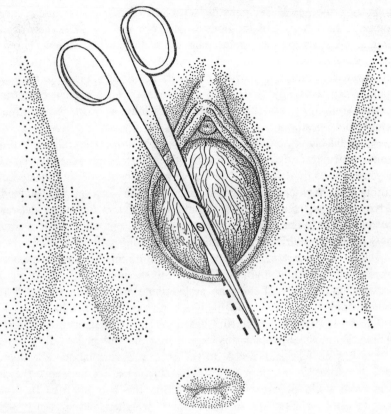

Fig. 25. An episiotomy is a simple cutting of the tissues to prevent tearing during childbirth.

half inches either to the side or in the midline, just before emergence of the baby's head.

Forceps are often used to assist delivery of the head, thus sparing the mother several minutes of pushing. This procedure is also easier on the baby's head. The placenta, afterbirth, is usually expelled from the vagina a few minutes after delivery of the baby and after the episiotomy is closed with absorbable sutures.

A Cesarean section, incision through the abdominal and uterine walls to deliver the baby, is sometimes done before the patient goes into labor if measurements indicate that the pelvis is too small for delivery or if the baby's position makes vaginal delivery impossible. More often, however, abdominal delivery is necessitated when some unexpected situation occurs during labor. Among the more frequent indications for Cesarean section are bleeding from the placenta which develops in the lower uterine segment in the zone of dilatation, or premature detachment of the placenta, prolapse of the baby's umbilical cord, or failure of the cervix to dilate properly. A Cesarean operation can be done at any stage of labor, when indicated, and the mother and baby usually do well.

Twins are less frequent in those having a first child than in those who have borne children previously. The incidence of twins in the first pregnancy is approximately one in eighty. The physician may suspect twins about the seventh month if the patient is unusually large, and an X-ray will then be taken for confirmation. Toxemia and premature labors are more common with twins; therefore, the patient is usually advised to get more rest. Sometimes complete bed rest may be required. Some twins, of course, are undiagnosed until delivery; then both the patient and the physician are taken by surprise.

If the newborn baby is a boy, the parents will be asked if they wish to have him circumcised. Sometimes the circumcision is done at the delivery table with a plastic bell device. In some hospitals, the custom of circumcising the baby five to eight days after delivery may prevail, and in some religions, the circumcision is performed on the eighth day with a special ceremony.

Most hospitals give the patient some choice of room after delivery and usually tentative reservations are made in advance. Some patients prefer the sociability of a two- or four-bed room and others prefer the privacy of a room alone. Many hospitals wisely limit visitors to maternity patients to one or two during visiting hours. New mothers need rest and should encourage their friends to wait until they have been home a few weeks before visiting. Some hospitals are quite cautious and permit visiting only by the husband.

If she has not already done so before the baby is born, the mother must now decide promptly whether or not she wishes to breast-feed her baby or provide the formula. Advantages are on each side and ultimately the type of feeding is a personal choice. If a mother plans to be at home most of the time, breast feeding is probably more convenient. Nursing also transmits to the baby certain antibodies that the mother has developed in her own system which provide immunity against infection. Nevertheless, excellent formulas are available and millions of healthy babies have been raised on them.

Hospital routines vary considerably but most modern ones today have some plan for teaching new mothers how to feed, change, and care for their babies and themselves. Some hospitals are set up for elective "rooming in" so that the baby stays in a bassinet beside the mother's bed and during the day she can feed and change her baby. Usually, however, with this routine, the baby is returned to the central nursery at night so that the mother can have a more restful sleep.

In this discussion on the birth of the first baby, we have followed a patient as she went into labor spontaneously and then to delivery. In certain cases, the physician may advise induction of labor. For this the patient must be in the hospital where labor can be started with medication. Usually to assist the onset of labor, Pitocin, a substance that stimulates uterine contraction, is given either in the form of an intravenous solution in the arm or with tablets which are dissolved in the mouth. Sometimes the membranes are ruptured to facilitate labor. Induction of labor is safe when certain criteria such as softness of the cervix and proper size and position of the baby are met.

Ideally, the patient should stay in the hospital about a week after delivery but because of shortages of hospital beds and because of financial problems, most patients today stay fewer days, some only two or three days. When she goes home, the newly delivered mother should, if possible, have some help for a week or two. She should plan to rest part of each morning and each afternoon for several weeks. Climbing stairs, in moderation, is not harmful and walking in fresh air is advisable.

Mothers who are not breast feeding their babies may find their breasts swollen and painful for seven to ten days after delivery. Usually, applications of ice packs to the breasts, bed rest, and two aspirin taken four times a day will give relief.

Postpartum depression after childbirth, crying without reason, having the "new baby blues" may occur any time after delivery and usually is due to hormonal changes in the body. The patient must not delay in notifying her doctor if emotional upset occurs because it can readily be relieved with medication.

Doctors differ, but not seriously, on the proper time to resume tub bathing after delivery. Many physicians permit tub baths as soon as the episiotomy has healed after one or two weeks. Occasionally, if the episiotomy site continues to be tender, applications of hot wet towels will give great relief. The use of an inflated rubber ring when sitting on a chair is also helpful.

Most physicians examine their patients in the office six weeks after delivery. The customary advice is to abstain from douches and intercourse until after this visit. Menstrual periods frequently are not resumed until nine to twelve weeks after delivery, and later if the mother is breast feeding the baby.

Pregnancies spaced at sufficient intervals so that the mother can regain her strength have been found to be better for both the mother and the children. The patient will find it advisable to consult her physician about family planning at the six-weeks visit. Frank discussion will aid the best planning. Rhythm control, a diaphragm fitted by the physician, an intrauterine contraceptive device inserted by the physician or "birth control" pills may be recommended. No single birth control method is suitable for all patients, and the physician and patient together must work out the solution in each case.

Most physicians see their patients again after six months and at this time repeat the Papanicolaou smear test for cancer of the cervix. At this time the physician usually evaluates the adjustment that the patient is making to her husband now that she is a mother, since her attention to her husband is now shared by the baby. Sometimes mothers must be urged to resume their usual marital relations, and if they are having problems, discussing them with the doctor has been found invaluable.

Having your first baby is one of the most delightful, thrilling, exciting, and interesting experiences that a woman can have. Every week, something new is happening to your body and to your growing baby. This is equally true after delivery. The adventure of taking care of your new baby is thrilling, tiring, and trying, but most satisfying. Children are interesting, ever changing, ever amazing, and the challenge of helping them to enjoy childhood and to mature into useful adults is, in itself, the greatest reward.

Chapter VI

HEALTH OF THE WORKING WOMAN
Ruth R. Rauschkolb, M.D.

INTRODUCTION

Woman has always worked, but her entry in the open-labor market is a product of the twentieth century. Today women, young, middle-aged, and older, single and married are employed full-time or part-time, regularly or intermittently in an infinite variety of jobs in almost all industries. Women workers are not only here to stay but are becoming an ever-increasing component of our total labor force.

During any work week, about 36 per cent of all women work either full-time or part-time; 53 per cent are full-time housewives and the rest are younger and mainly in school.

Many reasons are manifest for the dramatic increase in women working outside the home. This phenomenon is entirely consistent with the rapid growth of the population, yet the female labor force in 1962 was five times as large as that of 1900, whereas the number of women in the nation over the same period did not quite triple. Social and economic factors are even more significant. Most women give financial reasons for going to work. Some have no choice, others feel the extra earnings relieve money worries and help achieve the desire for a higher standard of living. Escape from loneliness, the mental stimulus and satisfaction in work away from home are intimately related to the long-term decline in the size of the family. Furthermore, the shift of the population to urban areas, the availability of modern appliances and labor-saving equipment, changes in traditional attitudes toward women working outside the home, and the increase of white-collar jobs have been overtures to the change. The reasons why women work may, in part, be the key to success or failure on the job.

Few differences between men and women have to be taken into account in the placement and utilization of women employees. The problem of female employment is not a health problem but a general question of labor policy. However, the duty of those concerned with occupational medicine should be to study the special health and socio-medical issues related to the employment of women and to make suitable recommendations that will prevent health hazards and preserve their health.

PHYSIOLOGICAL CONSIDERATIONS

Women, because of their physical strength and size, cannot lift, pull, and strain at the same weights as can men, and their work should be assigned accordingly.

Certain physiological states peculiar to women—menstruation, pregnancy, and menopause—are sometimes disturbed by complications that may require changes or interruption of their work. These will be discussed further.

The belief is widely held that women are tempermentally and emotionally better suited for certain specific tasks and less well apt for others. Their talents are recognized in those jobs that require quick fingers, an eye for color, patience, and in highly repetitive work.

A definite difference in the maximum work capacity exists between men and women. The maximum oxygen consumption of boys and girls is, on the average, the same up to the age of twelve to thirteen years, when a difference gradually develops until the maximum physical capacity of women averages 25 to 30 per cent less than that of men. This difference in maximum work capacity has influenced the legislation of many countries toward lessening hours of female labor.

Similar differences between the sexes in the strength of different groups of muscles may be partly related to woman's smaller muscle mass. A difference can also be noted in the maximal lung ventilation, the vital capacity; the total amount of hemoglobin, the oxygen which carries the pigment of the red blood cell, is measurably less in women.

STATISTICS

The sources of the following statistics are the latest figures on women workers published by the U.S. Department of Labor in April 1962 and the decennial census of 1960. Three and a half million more women than men of working age, fourteen years and older, were listed. In 1900, men outnumbered women by 1½ million. Women have exceeded men in the population since 1942.

These statistics recorded about 24 million women in the labor force, which represented 35 per cent of all women of working age, one in every three persons employed, and exceeded by 3½ million the record of World War II.

One half of the women are forty years of age or older. Seventy-five per cent of the single women between the ages of twenty and sixty-four years are working. An outstanding change in the past two decades has been the sharp increase in the percentage of married women gainfully employed. More than half of the women who work are married. About one in every ten working women has preschool children, and one out of three has children under eighteen years of age. Labor force participation rates are at their peak for single women between the ages of twenty-five and thirty-four years, and for married women between the ages of forty-five and fifty-four years.

Six of the fifty states, New York, California, Pennsylvania, Illinois, Ohio, and Texas have over a million women workers. Women's representation in the labor force varies considerably throughout the country, attaining its highest proportion of 44 per cent in Washington, D.C., 36 per cent in New Hampshire, and lowest, 27 per cent in North Dakota and 24 per cent in Alaska.

Women account for more than two-thirds of the clerical workers. This continues to be the largest group of working women and represents three out of ten employed women. Three-fifths of the female labor force is engaged in clerical work, in services, including 1½ million waitresses and cooks and those in operative pursuits, chiefly in factories. Nearly 3 million American women are vocational or technical workers. Teaching heads the professional occupations for women, accounting for nearly half the group. Nursing is the second most popular career. By 1970, according to projection by the Woman's Bureau of the U.S. Labor Department, a million more women may be engaged in professional work, with greater proportion than ever before in executive positions.

ILLNESS AND INJURY

Information on absenteeism is still fragmentary and generally limited to studies in individual plants or industries. For both men and women, absenteeism bears an inverse relationship to income; the lower the income the higher the absence rate. The findings in a two-year study of 28,000 employees in a leading oil company confirmed the widely held impression that absences due to sickness tend to be concentrated among a relatively small number of employees. This high-absence group was less content and had more emotional and nervous disturbances than workers with better attendance records.

Women have a higher rate of absenteeism and lose more days per year than do men. This difference is apparent largely because women have more days of disability due to acute illness and more non-medical absence. More absences occur among married than single women, for which home and family obligations are probably at least partly responsible.

Differences in the incidence of acute illnesses in men and women are almost entirely attributable to about a dozen conditions. These include the common cold, "grippe," sore throat, acute digestive disturbances, painful menstruation, various rheumatic complaints, minor cuts and bruises, headaches, and skin, eye, and tooth disorder. Minor disturbances of mood, thought, and behavior and brief episodes of tension, anxiety, weakness, and depression also have been found to cause some acute indisposition. The excess of illness reported for women is largely made up of minor ailments. In the United States at the present time, opinion is tacitly accepted that women will be more expressive of their aches and pains and minor emotions. Culturally determined differences in attitude have been ascertained toward what constitutes illness and what is an acceptable reason for disability in men and in women.

Whereas women have more days of disability due to acute illness, men of comparable age have greater incapacity from chronic illness, tuberculosis, asthma, heart conditions, hernia, and peptic ulcer. The cause of chronic disease among women has been found more commonly to be the result of elevated blood pressure, varicose veins, arthritis, rheumatism, anemia, goiter, gall stones, and valvular heart disease.

Whether or not women are more sensitive to toxic substances than men has been the subject of much discussion. Aside from the following possible exceptions, no scientific background for such differences in sensitivity has been proved. The pregnant woman may have a somewhat different status, particularly when exposed to substances potentially damaging to the liver or kidney. Exposure to quartz dust is another exception, and women have been found to show a higher incidence of silicosis than men.

The belief sometimes expressed that women are more susceptible to occupational disease, particularly of the skin, lacks foundation. U.S. Public Health Service authorities estimate that skin problems account for about 60 per cent of all occupational disease in the United States. Industrial health physicians maintain that 90 per cent or more of all occupational dermatoses are preventable. Many of these ailments could be avoided by protective clothing and proper cleansing.

Other hazards, such as toxic chemical and dust residues, can be engineered out by ventilation systems or chemical extraction processes. The actual problem is that 75 per cent of the work force is employed in small industries that either do not know about protective measures or consider them too expensive. The prevention of industrial skin disease and accidents is as essential to industry as to the worker.

Occupational skin diseases are not necessarily the result of a single physical or environmental factor. Such illnesses may result from a combination of different conditions, both physical and psychological. The same anxiety triggered by the skin disease itself can aggravate the condition and even turn it into a psychosomatic disorder, into the itch-scratch cycle.

Paradoxically, although woman has a higher sickness absence rate than man, her life expectancy is longer. Women are more easily incapacitated than men, but hardier. However, in the long run they are more resistant to disability than men, a fact that may be related to a difference in hormones.

ACCIDENTS

As to whether or not women are more prone to accidents than men, opinion and pertinent evidence seem about equally divided. In recent years a notable decrease has been noted in job injury rates, which is a reflection of many factors. High on the list of these should be mentioned improvement in safety legislation and notable co-operation between labor and management in safety programs. An ever-increasing number of labor contracts today contain provisions for committees concerned with plant safety, sanitation, and employee health. In addition to these joint efforts, management is greatly interested in acquiring safety devices and equipment and fostering safety training courses, and is always seeking ways to make work areas less hazardous.

Shorter work days, shorter work weeks, and coffee and rest "breaks" have been found to reduce fatigue and monotony and improve morale. Special controls are directed toward the potential ionizing of radiation hazards.

The influence of automation on the future volume of labor injuries is speculative. Some authorities believe that a reduction in hazards to which machine operators are exposed can be anticipated and that many accident-causing operations will be eliminated, but that automation signals a sharp rise in work related to machine maintenance which could increase hazards. These tasks, however, generally will be performed by men, so that automation may well decrease accidents among women.

The same preventative measures against occupational hazards should be applicable to men and women alike. Included in these recommendations are rules prescribing proper garments, gloves, shoes, and other items of clothing and devices designed to insure safety and protect health.

Laws prohibiting women from working at night or underground were designed to protect family life and exclude women from heavier labor such as work in mines. A medical reason is not valid today for such legislation providing the work environment corresponds to standards set for ventilation, hygiene, lighting, and air pollution.

Health services at places of employment are of special value for working women. Pre-employment and regular health examinations are valuable in aiding to discover disease and signs of maladjustment at an early stage.

PROBLEMS RELATED TO SEX FUNCTION

Women present problems peculiar to their sex. These challenges must be reckoned with in the placement and utilization of women in the labor force and may necessitate changes and interruption in their work. Menstruation, pregnancy, and menopause are normal physiological processes. No reason can be offered to suspect any significant difference in these biological functions between non-working and working women. Nevertheless, variations from normal in any of these conditions may affect the efficiency and attendance of the woman worker and account for a significant percentage of time lost from work.

Normal menstruation does not present a problem; abnormal menstruation may do so. The commonest menstrual abnormality is painful menstruation, or dysmenorrhea. Other complaints concern extended delay or absence of menses, amenorrhea, and excessive and irregular bleeding. Women with these conditions should be advised early to seek appropriate treatment by physicians qualified to advise them.

Painful menstruation may cause temporary reduction of work capacity and absence from work. The incidence of dysmenorrhea may be as high as 30 per cent in workers, but it is estimated that in only 6 per cent is the working capacity influenced. Dysmenorrhea seems to be higher in the younger groups, those fourteen to twenty-nine years of age. Then it tends to decrease gradually and is reduced considerably after the first pregnancy. Extensive studies of this disorder in large groups of women employees have given insight as to the cause of dysmenorrhea and have shown the value of simple exercises and other individual and group measures for its correction. The seriousness of dysmenorrhea has often been exaggerated. Although some women lose considerable time from work because of it, of these many appear to "give in" unnecessarily and take, charged off as sick leave, more "time off" from work than is warranted, apparently because of poor motivation to continue at work. The industrial nurse, who sees patients with repeated episodes of dysmenorrhea, should not content herself with providing symptomatic relief but should refer the woman for examination and treatment.

Pregnancy and the weeks immediately following delivery, the puerperium, account for the most significant physiological changes in women workers. The healthy woman, during a normal pregnancy, can, with proper medical supervision, be employed for at least twenty-eight weeks in a wide variety of positions with minimal limitations imposed for health and safety. Women in exceptionally good health and with only light housework to do may continue until the thirty-second or even thirty-sixth week of pregnancy in certain types of work such as in clerical positions. However, non-medical conditions may be present that require discontinuance or change of work, though the pregnancy itself remains uncomplicated. Non-medical reasons for the absence from work of pregnant employees should be recognized and should not be permitted to count as sickness absences.

It is imperative that the woman make her pregnancy known promptly to the appropriate person at her place of employment, to her immediate supervisor, the nurse or physician if the company has one, or to the person in charge of personnel. The company policy should encourage the reporting of pregnancy. Concealment of pregnancy invites complications, particularly in the first three months when concealment is easy. Having reported her pregnancy, the worker should be encouraged to avail herself of care and guidance, including the initial and periodic visits to her own physician.

As a safeguard, certain restrictions should be placed on the hours and nature of work permitted women during even normal pregnancy. Such precautions should be dictated as much by common sense as by obstetric, gynecologic, or toxicologic considerations. All employees should, of course, be afforded maximal protection against moving machinery at all times.

A healthful work environment should be provided for women as well as for men workers, with concentration in the air of substances harmful to health kept at a practical minimum and certainly within established Threshold Limit Values. However, certain harmful substances, forms of energy, and conditions are known from which, according to available scientific evidence, pregnant women should be spared to an even greater extent than men or healthy, non-pregnant women workers. Among such substances are those containing chlorinated hydrocarbons which may damage the liver and kidneys, those containing benzol and lead which may cause anemia, and those which may cause anoxemia, an abnormal condition due to lack of sufficient oxygen in the blood. Another occupational exposure which may exert a specific effect on pregnancy is ionized radiation, excessive exposure to which may produce definite injury to the fetus or harmful genetic effects.

Blood volume and the cardiac output rise gradually to a maximum approximately at the end of the second month of pregnancy and will later decrease to normal values toward delivery. The venous pressure in the legs rises gradually during pregnancy and the pregnant woman tends to develop swollen ankles more easily than before and may develop varicose veins. Therefore, she must not put stress on her heart by hard physical work and she must avoid continuous standing positions.

Awkwardness in movement and shifting of the body's center of gravity with advancing pregnancy must be taken into account. Particular care should be taken to minimize the amount of lifting a pregnant employee is required or permitted to do. She should be assigned tasks that do not involve undue stretching or reaching, because of the danger of losing her balance. She should not climb a ladder, stand or work on a scaffold, or in other ways incur risk of falling.

The pregnant woman should observe good personal health habits for the sake of her own health and that of her unborn baby. Insofar as practical, she should work days so that she can have the evening and night hours at home to care for her family and get the required amount of sleep with as little interruption as possible. She should not work more than five days or forty hours a week and should have at least a fifteen-minute rest period during the first and second halves of a work shift, and also a midshift break long enough to visit the rest room and have her lunch. Should complications or other health impairment occur, her personal physician and the appropriate person at her place of employment have the joint responsibility of determining whether or not the work assigned should be changed or the woman discontinue work.

The length of time that a woman should be kept off work after delivery should be determined by agreement between her personal physician and the responsible person representing the company. The decision will depend on many factors: the previous general health of the woman, the nature and severity of any complications of pregnancy or delivery, the subsequent course, the nature of the job and the conditions and environment prevailing in the place of employment. No matter how favorable these factors may be, the new mother should ordinarily not return to work for at least six weeks after delivery. If she nurses the baby, it may further delay the return to work. This and other non-medical considerations may influence the decision as to when to return to work.

The menopause is a normal physiological process. Its manifestations are more emotional and functional than physical. If disability does occur, the duration is generally short. The menopause is the most overworked physiological state in the book. Proper health education and counseling at this time, supplementing the care and reassurance of the woman's personal physical being will generally enable her to pass through the menopause easily with minimal distress and incapacity and will aid her to regain stability and comfort.

THE DUAL ROLE

The majority of women continue to be homeworkers whether or not they also have jobs. Most women in the labor force work at two jobs, one at the office or plant and the other at home. Many employed women work harder for shorter periods of time at home than at their places of employment. The chief burden of the double job falls on the woman herself although husbands of today are taking a greater share in domestic duties. Concern for the welfare of her husband and children and her home responsibilities is quite reasonable and understandable. If a conflict arose between responsibility to the job and responsibility to the home, the woman would put the interest of her family and home first, and in most cases this would result in absence from work. Employment will certainly be facilitated if housework is made easier by a high standard of living and with labor-saving devices and help from other members of the family. Organization of part-time work for married women has proved quite useful and also is probably of real value in preventing stress and strain.

Woman herself, however, must see the situation as it is, appreciate the overloading, and set about to tune body and mind carefully and deliberately to keep this much-used instrument on key. She needs the best health care possible and her health habits must be exemplary.

The working woman should begin with attention to her diet. Too often satisfactory meals, including all the basic foodstuffs, are provided for the family but somehow not eaten by the woman herself. Schedules need to be studied, housework streamlined, duties apportioned, and hours of rest so arranged that she can arise early enough to be ready and yet have time for the all-important, universally neglected breakfast. The value of the breakfast will not be decreased one bit by its simplicity, providing one recognizes that it must contribute to the day's full quota of the basic elements of good diet: protein, carbohydrate, fat, minerals, vitamins, fluid, and bulk. Appetite and hunger do not necessarily go hand in hand. Eating between meals, snacking, and piecing in ordinary daily life is a bad habit and has much which can be condemned. Close attention should be paid to the "creeping pounds." The least disadvantage of being overweight is one's inelegant appearance. Far more significant is the overloading on heart, circulation, and body frame.

A definite uninterrupted block of hours, seven at least, should be devoted to rest, undressed, in bed. Sleep cannot be imposed, but lying there quietly can be and is the next best thing to sleep. It makes a difference, too, where in the twenty-four these hours are fitted. Time flies at home with many things to occupy the woman returning from her job, and too often bedtime is postponed and time runs out next morning too when she must start again.

Exercise is of more than ordinary consideration for the working woman. Although it would seem that she has been moving about enough, actually she has overused some muscles and underused others. If exercise can be a part of recreation, so much the better. Conditioning and maintaining the body in health and vigor has come into its own again, and we are all better off because of it. Newspapers and magazines make readily available information and instruction for selecting one's own program.

The woman working at two jobs should always take prompt notice of any sign or symptom of change in her body and its behavior. For her, preventive medicine is the best way of life. Early consultation with a qualified physician will relieve her anxiety and afford her advice and treatment.

Recreation is of greatest import to the working woman. If anyone needs to put back in, after taking so much out, it is she.

A few words about potential harm from unwise sun exposure should be discussed in this connection. All skin ages, eventually, with sun exposure, the fair more quickly than those with more pigmentation. The relationship of ultraviolet light to malignant changes in the skin is indisputable. Proper ways of combating it are known and available.

A bit of advice, too, should be given about clothing, other than protective clothes and uniforms, where they are applicable. A good, properly fitting foundation garment and brassiere give support and comfort increasingly as the hours of being up and about continue. To this undergarment, stockings can be fastened with garters, unless socks suffice. At any rate, constriction on the legs will not occur as with round garters, rolled, twisted stockings, or socks with elasticized tops.

Every moment spent out of the horizontal position imposes maximal stress on the lower limbs, bones, joints, muscles, tendons, ligaments, and vessels. Attention to delay, if not to prevent, decline in these tissues, is of the greatest significance. Obesity should be avoided or remedied. Support may be given to the legs with the increasingly popular support-type hose. The sheer ones will suffice as prophylaxis, but if the circulation begins to falter, proper advice should be sought promptly. The woman should know that when she is standing erect she should move, if only in place, to gain the advantage of muscle contraction and to decrease stasis, stagnation of the circulation. When she sits, the ankles only may be crossed and the feet should be elevated; a little is better than nothing.

The feet should be kept clean and dry and should be properly shod. Shoes for work are usually quite different from dress shoes. Oxfords are best for workers who are much on their feet. With their laces, adjustment can be made as the hours pass, and the thicker soles and medium heel give comfort. Shoes should be fitted every time they are bought. It is a mistake to think that the shoe size attained when growth stops will remain fixed and constant. All too soon, the woman who pays them scant heed will find that she has "legs and feet" for the rest of her life. Corns and calluses should receive professional attention.

FORECAST

Our country's present and future needs for skilled personnel continue to grow. The rising trend in formal education, since the woman worker eighteen years of age now averages twelve years of schooling, will affect occupational choices of women and their opportunities for job advancement.

The complex nature of many jobs will place new emphasis on the quality of the labor force. The demand will be greatest for those with specially needed training and experience. Woman's goal must be to develop individual talents to the fullest extent possible.

The woman with a college education is likely to find a job more quickly, earn more money, and advance faster than her less educated sister. She is also more apt to find greater job security and improved employee benefits.

Should the college worker leave her job to rear a family, her advanced training makes it easier to re-enter the labor market when and if she wishes to do so.

According to the President's Commission on the Status of Women, almost 70 per cent of all women college graduates do return to work eventually, their "second" careers lasting, on the average, about twenty-three years.

From the pamphlet "Womanpower," published by the National Manpower Council, we quote:

"Women constitute not only an essential but a distinctive part of our manpower resources. They are essential because without their presence in the labor force we could neither produce and distribute the goods nor provide the educational, health, and other social services which characterize American society. They constitute a distinctive manpower resource because the structure and substance of the lives of most women are fundamentally determined by their functions as wives, mothers, and homemakers."

Chapter VII

MENTAL HEALTH OF THE HOUSEWIFE
Klara Glottmann Tulsky, M.D.

What is *mental health?* Many definitions are known and some are lengthy; simply it is "a balance of frustrations and gratifications."

Frustrations are unavoidable ingredients of human life. With the best of life situations, perfect plans, superior preparations, financial and professional success, and naturally gifted endowments, a certain amount of frustration cannot be eliminated.

Such frustrations affect our lives in great measure, dependent on each person's emotional make-up. The masochist, a person who enjoys mistreatment, dwells on incidents of frustration and manages to perpetuate them; the sadist enjoys cruelty and punishes others; the pessimist, who sees only the bad side of things, never sees a way out of his difficulty; and the optimist, who sees only good, hopes for improvement but still suffers in greater or lesser fashion.

Seldom, in the midst of our frustrations, do we remember our gratifications. These, too, are inherent in each life. No matter how unsatisfactory the life situation may be—in poverty or failure, in ill health, loneliness, or despair—if the individual can dig deeply enough into herself, she can find some area of gratification which may balance the negative. Unhappily, this is not easy, since our frustrations weigh heavily on us and, like children, we wish mostly for that which we cannot have.

The mental health of the housewife is a complex term. What is a housewife? She is in essence the mistress of the house, whether she is responsible for herself alone in a rented room or for a large family in a big home; whether she is solely responsible for the housekeeping or has a staff to help. She may have no education or may have acquired a Ph.D. in higher mathematics. Her income may be minimal or in the highest brackets and she may be young or old. Regardless of all these facts, she still falls in the category of housewife, and the image of the housewife is thus exceedingly complex.

In her mode of living, the housewife becomes even more diversified. She functions in a full-time capacity, dedicating all her time to her family, home, and personal or civic interests. Her life can be easy or difficult according to her financial circumstances; it can be stimulating or boring, depending on her own view of her position. It can be lonely or sociable, as a result of her surroundings, social capabilities, and interests. These conditions may present themselves simultaneously or alternately, since change and diversity are part of life in its various phases.

The working housewife is a woman who maintains, simultaneously, the responsibility of the homemaker and that of a full-time job outside of the home. Here, too, she does not constitute a homogeneous group, since the reasons and motivations for working lend different aspects to the individual attitude. If she works out of financial need, she may either accept her situation for lack of alternative or resent the burden thrust upon her. In addition, the gratifications, other than monetary, which she derives from her job will modify her life as a housewife. If her work depletes her emotionally and physically, she will have little to give at home and will exhaust herself endeavoring to do her duty. Such a situation can create a vast sense of frustration, conscious or unconscious, and even depression. If, however, her job offers her stimulation, a sense of importance, and emotional nourishment, her physical energy will not falter and she returns home emotionally enriched, ready to give of herself and disposed to enjoy her temporary and different responsibility as a housewife. These general situations depend on individual differences of personality, organizational abilities, and normal variations in good and bad days at work and at home.

When the woman works out of choice, whether motivated by boredom, by a need to express herself in a chosen field, to add some material luxury which she considers significant, or just to be among people —out in the "world"—her attitude will be much different. If she has a young family and necessarily has household help, she will be relieved of housekeeping. Most likely she welcomes this relief but may feel guilty about being away from her children during the day.

The woman who works part-time frequently considers herself in an ideal situation. She is able to fulfill, in her dual roles, her family needs and her desire to be an individual participating in the outside world and proving to herself that she can be independent.

The prelude to becoming mother in a household begins in childhood. Little girls are clad in fancy dresses usually only for special occasions. Mostly, they wear washable pants, slips, and blouses, for laundering convenience.

When we watch their play in nursery school or kindergarten, we see a definite distinction in choice of toys and games between girls and boys. Girls definitely gravitate toward dolls and household equipment toys, while boys will choose more readily mechanical toys or tools for building. Once the child enters grammar school, these tendencies are disregarded by a curriculum that aims toward equal academic achievement. Even in home economics classes, activities are not separated, and the making and wiring of lamps and cooking are activities shared by both sexes. The merit of these programs may be questioned but we must be aware that they express the views of educators in dealing with children as one sex. Yet, inherent intellectual and emotional sex differences have been described in many studies, and the social roles of men and women still follow, generally speaking, the old-fashioned functions of wife and mother for the woman, and wage earner for the man. Education today, however, tends to equalize the social role of the sexes. If such education would prepare children better for life, there would be no objection, but frustrations, for lack of planning, are too evident. Girls are not educated for womanhood; they are encouraged to reach the same goals as men. They compete with men, but are still expected to play feminine roles. Such a paradox creates confusion and may leave a woman's life without pattern.

Competition, so productive and creative in industry, and frequently responsible for progress in physical and intellectual achievement, is not necessarily the healthiest aspect of human life and development. It pervades our lives from infancy when mothers compete about the weight and achievements of their babies, to the grave when even funerals have status.

In such an atmosphere of competition, little time and room are left for learning and for developing the skills and joys of human relationships which nourish and comfort the soul.

Adolescent girls not only compete scholastically with boys, but also compete socially with other girls for "popularity." Youngsters who are unprepared are thrust into a struggle for social and emotional survival. Without the element of competition, this could be an exciting time of discovery of the world, of each other, and of themselves. In a stereotyped mass society, man cannot wait for individual development and readiness. Many women have to overcome the wounds inflicted on them during that period for the rest of their lives. The psychiatrist hears the wails of too much too soon and of too little too late, with incriminations of mother, father, and, worst of all, oneself. Seldom can the health of social forces and values be examined; this factor is too overwhelming and no psychiatric couch is big enough to deal with it.

Many of our problems are culturally induced and are shared by other persons. Recognizing this, we are sometimes able to rise and re-shape our lives with personal wisdom.

The young adult female is usually a housewife of some sort. She is either already married and discovering the joys and responsibilities of marriage, or, as is frequent, she lives away from home, studying or working. In any case, she is involved in some form of housekeeping.

The young married woman steps into a situation to which she brings dreams and unrealistic concepts to deal with the tasks of cleaning, shopping, cooking, interior decorating, being a loving wife and even-tually a devoted and informed mother; and then before long she begins to suffer from the common syndrome of the frustrated housewife. The most frequent symptom the physician hears about from women is fatigue, often physical but more often emotional.

The frustration of the housewife is not due to a single source but to an accumulation of causes and effects during different periods of her life in a fast-changing modern world.

The low status conferred on the housewife in our society is a definite cause of this feeling of inferiority and dissatisfaction. Paradoxically, the mass media of communication—newspapers, magazines, television, and radio—in the process of influencing consumers, create an image of modern women which is not only impossible to fulfill, but which consequently fosters feelings of inadequacy.

In a society in which status is measured by what a person does and how much he earns, not by what he really is, the homemaker receives a silent treatment which depreciates her. As a non-earner she feels unproductive by accepted standards.

In her search for identity, many of the landmarks are lost. In a highly mobile society, the woman is often separated from family and friends, thus losing the opportunity to follow a model.

The specific aspects of her way of life, whether she lives in an urban, suburban, small town, or farm area; in a house or in an apartment; whether her finances are limited, moderate, or unlimited; whether she is socially aggressive or retiring, will greatly influence and even con-trol her conduct of living.

Loneliness can be a destructive factor induced by sheer geographic location. The city dweller who lives among millions of people can often be more lonely and isolated in his house or impersonal apartment building than the farmer's wife with her established relationships. Especially during the early years of motherhood, a young woman may spend long periods of time without any contact with adults during the day. Unrelieved by adult stimulation, the continuous companionship and demands of babies and small children can create depression and doubt in her ability to fulfill her role as wife and mother.

Once her children enter school, a woman's horizon broadens. The PTA and the mothers of her children's classmates can help her find a niche in her small or wide world. Frustrations, however, are still unavoidable. Having conquered loneliness, the woman becomes part of some group and inevitably finds herself comparing herself, her children, and sometimes even her husband with the prevailing standards. She may compare herself with a woman of high achievement, ignoring those factors such as older children, more household help, or constitutionally greater energy and capability which may have made it possible for that woman and infeasible for her.

When our technological progress is examined from a philosophic point of view, its positive and negative qualities become apparent. The automobile has given a fabulous advantage, yet empties the home too often and too easily of parents and adolescents at times when mutual family companionship could be beneficial. Mixes and "ready to serve" edibles, while saving time and energy, can take away from a woman a form of creative expression and gratification that the preparation of food may give.

Husbands and fathers are links in this great and exciting machine of progress, but they are subjected to constant competition and pressures which drain their energies. If they lead very busy lives, come home tired and exhausted, they have little congenial sympathetic reservoir from which to feed the deep emotional needs of women. The emotional differences of the sexes must be recognized. Woman derives her major gratifications from personal responses while man obtains his by accomplishment.

As her children grow older, the housewife finds more time for outside activities and may discover that often these experiences do not correspond with the fantasy of freedom so anticipated during the shut-in years. Charity and community work can have an impersonal and businesslike quality tinged with social competition, yet they will not bring her closer to people nor do they give her direct gratification. At the same time, she may be engaged in unrewarding emotional discussions with inexperienced but independent adolescent children which bruise her ego and create anxieties with which she may not be able to cope. Her dependency requirements may be increased, but knowing that in our society independence is a virtue, she does not dare to confess her need for love, affection, and companionship. The symbol of independence may be carried to such a fetish that the price can become emotional starvation or deprivation.

The menopause period creates panic in some women, chiefly because we live in a youth-worshipping society. Such women feel the loss of sexual desirability and social significance. With proper medical care, self-respect, and a healthful philosophy of life, this phase need not be disturbing.

As the woman grows older, she should be entering a more peaceful way of life. Her children may be married or no longer a responsibility and she can indulge in many of the activities yearned for during the earlier years. These are also the years that a woman may become widowed, or she may be separated geographically or socially from her children, or have to adjust to a new way of life with a retired husband.

We have painted a picture of the frustrations of the housewife. What gratifications can be found to balance them? Gratifications come from usefulness, love, and creativity. The housewife must become more aware of her value to her home, her husband, her children, in a physical and emotional way, and to the subsequent power and satisfaction this entails. Those seemingly long shut-in years are only so because this housewife is needed, and the adolescent tests her because she matters. Her husband may exhaust his energies playing special roles with the outside world and only at home can he be himself and feel accepted. No housekeeper can create this climate. The sense of being irreplaceable should be ingrained in the housewife. Women in glamorous status-symbol professions and occupations are replaceable but there is no substitute for a mother. While child rearing can be confusing, complex, and at times even disheartening, an awareness of the miracle of growth, and development, and the mother's role in this, transcends the artificially formed status ratings, and can be a source of strength, consequence, and fulfillment.

Woman's usefulness, because it does not offer a directly visible product or income, is intangible in its human value and immeasurable in significance and should be a source of self-respect.

Love is a much maligned word, tinged with sex, but still is the moving force of our lives. We all expect to find love, while in reality love must be nurtured, fostered, developed—worked at.

In an overcivilized mass society, not enough time and importance are given to bestowing and teaching the art of loving, to cultivating the enjoyment of warm human relationships and to feeling the satisfaction of giving of oneself to others. The danger of producing alienation and dehumanization is present. If these qualities are not developed in the young, they might disappear in future generations.

The third source of gratification comes from creativity. In an era of automation and cybernetics (which is automation plus computers) the home is still the only place where a person can be most creative and individualistic. Children do not become adults overnight nor can we take a pill to create warm and affectionate relationships. A woman has the opportunity to create a slum or castle out of her microcosmos by influencing the emotional and spiritual climate of her home. When the nest becomes empty, the modern woman can enrich her experience by painting, going back to school, traveling, accepting club work or giving of herself in volunteer work where she can offer unpressured warmth which professionals often cannot afford. When she offers a willing listening ear and pleasant companionship to friends and relatives, her value is immeasurable in human relations. TV and radio programs discriminately selected can keep her informed, stimulated, and entertained.

Woman must work toward the aim of achieving emotional freedom, which would enable her to see all the gratifications. Too much energy is expended in trying to be something other than what one is, which mars the enjoyment of life. The ability to substitute one gratification for the lack of another is imperative. Happiness is many things, some of them often fleeting, and to be accepted for oneself is a significant phase of happiness and of the way to a good life.

Chapter VIII

SPECIALIZED SURGERY FOR WOMEN
Eloise Parsons, M.D.

GYNECOLOGY

Gynecology (jin-e-col'-o-gy or gi-ne-col'-o-gy) is the study of women, their diseases, their physiology, and their hygiene.

Gynecology has become a many-sided specialty. The gynecologist must be an expert surgeon, trained in obstetrics and all its branches. He must have the trained skill to investigate female conditions affecting the kidneys and the bladder and be well informed in pathology. Finally, the gynecologist must be able to recognize and deal successfully with psychological problems which are so intimately related to women's medical problems.

General surgeons, also, perform pelvic surgery. As specialization increases, however, the family doctor usually refers a woman to a gynecologist; or a woman, herself, with a "female complaint" usually consults a specialist in women's diseases.

A woman gynecologist has the skills, knowledge, and training which are demanded by the specialty, but also the unique understanding and sympathy which one woman has for another. No doubt this aids her judgment when making decisions as to treatment. This special attribute may give confidence to the patient, allay her fears, and promote her sense of well-being after successful treatment.

DIAGNOSTIC PROCEDURES

Every person should have a physical checkup at least once a year. You take your car in for a periodic checkup even if it is running well. The human machine, with its complicated mechanism, surely deserves as much attention as you would give your automobile.

For a woman, special attention should be given to the breasts and the pelvic organs.

"PAP" SMEARS

If every physician who performs a pelvic examination of any woman twenty years of age or older would routinely prepare cervical and

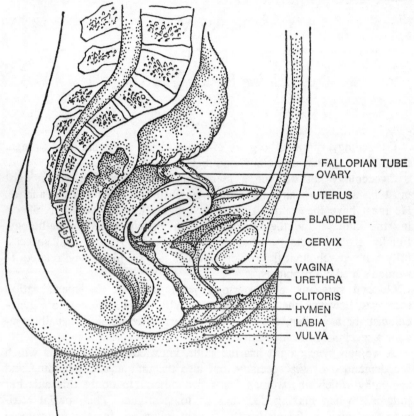

Fig. 26. The female organs.

vaginal cytology slides of the patient and encourage her to have this done annually, invasive cancer of the cervix would become rare and mortality from this disease would fall to almost zero.

More than twenty years have passed since Dr. George N. Papanicolaou demonstrated that cells in the vagina and cervix shed and that the type varied with the stage of the menstrual cycle. Early cancer, he showed, also shed particular cells which could be detected in smears long before there was any obvious sign or symptom of cancer. He perfected the technique of taking the smears and staining them; hence, the test is named for him, with the abbreviation, "Pap." At least seven to nine years prior to the development of evident cancer, most of the eventual victims are already harboring a small focus of cancerous cells of the cervix, detectable by the smear examination.

The smear may be taken in the doctor's office, transferred to a glass slide, put into a fixative solution, and sent to the cytologist for staining and diagnosis. If the smear is positive, that is, if the cells are suspicious of cancer, the patient then must have further diagnostic tests to confirm or eliminate the possibility of the invasion of cancer.

The Pap smear is also useful in conditions other than cancer. In fertility examinations, the vaginal smear gives information about ovulation, and in hormone treatment, the effects can be demonstrated by the cells found in the vagina.

Cells typical of inflammation may be seen in the smears, and at times, also, the organism which causes the inflammation. Yeast cells and trichomonads too can be found stained in the smears.

BIOPSY OF THE CERVIX

The cervix is that portion of the uterus (womb) which protrudes into the vagina and surrounds the os, opening, of the uterus; in the adult woman it is about one inch long. The cervix is covered by a smooth mucous membrane and contains mucous glands. This remarkable structure, capable of stretching enough to permit a baby to pass through it, is, in the non-pregnant state, scarcely larger than a man's thumb.

Erosions of the cervix are areas which appear "raw" to the gynecologist because they are denuded of the covering membrane or mucosa. In a young girl, the erosion may be due to a failure of the mucosa to cover it, and may be the cause of a constant mucous discharge of varying degree. In an older woman, the erosion may be the result of childbirth or inflammation and may also produce an annoying discharge. If the Pap smear is negative, these erosions can be treated by the doctor in the office, usually by superficial cautery.

Any erosion that persists after suitable treatment, especially in older women, even if the smears are negative, deserves a biopsy for microscopic examination. All cases in which the smear is positive or suspicious demand a biopsy to rule out the possibility of cancer.

Some gynecologists perform a biopsy in the office, with a punch instrument that removes a "bite" from the eroded area, which can be examined by the pathologist after fixation and staining.

If the area of erosion is large, or if the smear is positive without any obvious clinical area, the biopsy should be done in the hospital where a sizable portion can be excised. In looking for early cancer, the whole cervix may be coned out and serial sections made so as not to miss any small nest of cancer cells which may be present. In such cases, the cervical canal is also curetted.

Any vaginal discharge, whether it is mucus from a simple erosion or due to inflammation, is not normal. Leucorrhea, or a whitish discharge, should never be permitted to persist without investigation. If the discharge continues after office treatment, the physician will advise a biopsy, since it is impossible to differentiate a benign condition from a cancerous one without a microscopic examination.

Cervical polyps—little growths hanging on stems—are seldom cancerous, but they do produce a vaginal discharge and often bleed at irregular times. They should be removed, preferably in the hospital, because the cervix may need to be dilated to reach the base of the pedicle. Other polyps may be found which do not appear until the cervix is dilated. They should always be examined under the microscope since they may have cancerous cells.

DILATATION AND CURETTAGE, "D & C"

Dilatation of the cervix is performed as a preliminary step to curettage of the uterus. Dilatation of the cervix is also done as a therapeutic measure for acquired or congenital stenosis, narrowing of the cervical opening and canal; for dysmenorrhea, painful menstruation, in women who have never borne children; and also in some cases of sterility to permit the introduction of instruments for insufflation of the tubes.

Curettage of the uterus is the most frequent of gynecologic operations and is generally a simple and harmless procedure, as described below.

The chief purpose of curettage of the uterus is the removal of endometrial tissue (the lining of the cavity of the uterus) and of cervical tissue for microscopic examination in those cases in which there has been abnormal uterine bleeding.

In irregular menstruation, *functional uterine bleeding,* probably due to hormone influences, a knowledge of the type of endometrium is valuable for future treatment.

In *profuse bleeding at the time of menstruation,* a curettage may have therapeutic value. Such irregular bleeding is probably due to endometrial polyps which cause the profuse flow of blood, and are removed with the curettage.

In *cases of sterility* a curettage is done, premenstrually, to obtain information regarding ovulation during the current month.

One of the chief therapeutic uses of the curette is the *removal of placental tissue* following abortion, or the elimination of retained portions of the placenta after full-term delivery.

In cases of "spotting" or bleeding after intercourse, or of any bleeding from the cervix not associated with menstruation, a curettage is a diagnostic procedure which must be done to prove the presence or absence of endometrial cancer.

Technique of curettage: The cervix is dilated with graduated dilators. A curette is then introduced into the uterus and the endometrium lining is scraped off and collected for microscopic examination. This endometrium which lines the uterine cavity is loosely attached and changes during the menstrual cycle, being thickest just before menstruation. During the menstrual bleeding this lining is partially sloughed off in the menstrual blood. After menstruation it forms again as it also does after it has been scraped away with the curette.

Curettage should be done in the hospital where every precaution is taken to prevent infection from being introduced into the uterus. The vulva is shaved because hair cannot be sterilized, the external genitals are scrubbed and then treated with an antiseptic solution. The instruments used are sterilized in a steam sterilizer. The gynecologist scrubs and is gowned as in an operation for major surgery. Because of such precautions, curettage is a safe procedure.

This also explains why curettage done in an office or in the home, sometimes for a criminal abortion, may result in infection, even fatal peritonitis.

Curettage is also done in the hospital because an anesthetic is necessary. Pentothal Sodium, injected intravenously, or a mild gas inhalation anesthetic, is frequently used.

PELVIC SURGERY

The pelvis is the lower section of the abdomen; its bony framework is also called the pelvis.

The urinary bladder, the female organs of reproduction, the rectum, and a portion of the alimentary canal lie in the pelvis and are protected by the pelvic bones. Whenever pelvic surgery is done, all the contents are exposed and must receive consideration as each is in close proximity to the other.

HYSTERECTOMY

Operative removal of the uterus is known as hysterectomy. A hysterectomy is the most common major surgical procedure in gynecology. The operation may be performed alone or in conjunction with additional surgery on the tubes or ovaries, or as part of repair of the anterior or posterior vaginal walls. This operation may be done by either the abdominal or vaginal route.

The uterus is the organ known familiarly as the womb, because its

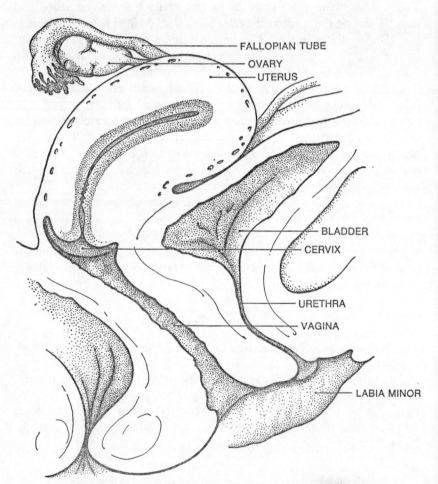

Fig. 27. A cross-section of the uterus and related organs.

function is to nourish and protect the fertilized ovum throughout the forty weeks of gestation, and then to expel the baby by its contractions.

The uterus is a hollow, thick-walled, muscular organ resting in the pelvis between the urinary bladder, in front, and the rectum, behind. This organ is roughly pear-shaped and, in the adult woman, about three inches long. The uterine tubes open on either side of its broad portion, and the small end, the cervix, opens into the vagina. In comparison with the size of the whole uterus, the cavity is a small, triangular-shaped area lined with velvety endometrium. The uterus is balanced in the pelvis by ligaments, which pass from the sides of the uterus to the pelvic wall.

When the uterus is removed, a woman's reproductive life is over. Pregnancy is impossible. The desirability of pregnancy should be of serious consideration. If a choice can be made in the operation to be performed, this decision is based on possible future effects on the patient.

Removal of the uterus inhibits future menstruation. Most women look forward to being relieved of menstruation but others look on the loss of menstruation as the end of youth and the beginning of old age.

Premature menopause ensues if the ovaries are also removed with the uterus. This does not present a problem to the women at or near the climacteric. And for the younger woman, simple harmless hormones, estrogens, can be prescribed to be taken by mouth. These eliminate the hot flashes and nervousness associated with the "change of life."

Interference with the normal sex function is sometimes caused by a hysterectomy, since the vagina may be shortened. This encumbrance seldom follows an abdominal hysterectomy but does frequently occur in a vaginal hysterectomy. Regardless, many women find that their sexual life is more enjoyable with the cessation of menstruation, possibly because the fear of pregnancy is eliminated.

The most common reason for a hysterectomy is the presence of fibroid tumors, leio-myo-fibromata.

Fibroids are quite common in women. Approximately one out of five women has a fibroid and the incidence is higher in the Negro race. Fibroids are clusters of knots of fibrous tissue and usually are no more significant than warts on the skin. Although they seldom become malignant, the possibility does exist. Because fibroids are dependent on estrogens, they seldom continue to grow after the menopause. They are often multiple.

Fibroids are a reason for hysterectomy if they are the cause of pro-

fuse menstruation which incapacitates the woman and keeps her anemic; if they are so large that they produce difficulties because of their
size (fibroids up to 80 pounds have been reported); if they are growing
rapidly; or if they are painful or become twisted on the pedicles.

Myomectomy is an operation in which the fibroid is dissected out
from the uterus, leaving the body of the uterus intact. This procedure
is done in a young woman who is anxious to have children when the
fibroid is either the cause of her sterility or would interfere with the
growth of the fetus. Fibroids may cause spontaneous abortions.

Pregnancy may occur in a uterus that contains fibroids, and it often
does, with the baby going to term and being delivered without difficulty.

Chronic bilateral inflammatory disease of the tubes and ovaries, or of
the ovaries alone, may be a reason for hysterectomy and removal of
the tubes and ovaries, salpingo-oophorectomy. Surgery is not done in
the acute or subacute stages. Moreover, if sufficient and specific antibiotics are given early in the acute stage, surgery may be entirely
avoided. However, if the tubes are so involved, together with the
ovaries, that they should be excised, then the uterus also should be
removed. In the absence of ovarian function, a uterus is a liability if it
remains. If the tubes and ovaries are removed, the uterus has no function and often causes tenderness and discomfort. It may become the
seat of cancer or tumor later so that another operation may be inevitable.

A hysterectomy may comprise a part of any surgical procedure in
which all of the ovarian tissue must be removed.

Endometriosis of the uterus, inflammation of the lining of the uterus
and ovaries, may require a hysterectomy and salpingo-oophorectomy.
However, with the development of oral hormones, which prevent ovulation, this operation now is seldom necessary.

Cancer of the cervix. Hysterectomy may be done in the early stages
of cancer. With the aid of "Pap" smears, more cases of cervical cancer
are being found early enough, before the cancer has spread to the ligaments, so that more hysterectomies are being performed for cancer of
the cervix. Radiation, followed by hysterectomy, may be done in cases
still early, but extending beyond the confines of the cervix. Every case
of cancer of the cervix must be evaluated by the gynecologist or team
as to the kind of cancer, its extent, and its rate of growth before the
decision is made whether to use radiation or surgery for that particular
growth.

Cancer of the endometrium, lining of the uterus, within the body of the uterus, is usually treated by hysterectomy. At the time of the curettage, if the tissue is definitely cancerous, the cavity is sometimes filled with small metal tubes containing radium or cobalt which remain in for a specified time, forty-eight to seventy-two hours; and the hysterectomy is performed four to six weeks later.

Cancer of the ovaries is treated by the removal of both ovaries and tubes, together with complete hysterectomy. The same is true of cancer of either Fallopian tube.

Uterine prolapse, fallen womb, is a reason for vaginal hysterectomy. Vaginal hysterectomy is also done to repair extensive childbirth trauma which is manifest in the form of a large projection of urinary bladder into the wall, prolapse of the bladder, and bulging of the rectum into the vagina. Removal of the uterus disposes of the prolapse but with its excision, a better approximation of uterine and fascial supports can be obtained.

Uterine bleeding, from any cause, which cannot be controlled by other methods of treatment, is an indication for hysterectomy.

Cesarean hysterectomy may be performed at the time of a Cesarean section for various conditions which may be present, related to either childbearing or to situations in the pelvis.

THE OPERATION

In abdominal hysterectomy, the uterus is removed through an incision in the abdominal wall. One of two types of operative procedure may be used, the midline operation extending from the pubic bone up toward the umbilicus, and the curved transverse incision below the hair line, extending up on both sides toward the hipbones. The midline incision is preferable in most cases because it requires less time to perform, permits better exposure, and heals faster. However, the scar of the transverse incision is concealed by the hair, which is the chief advantage of this procedure. The gynecologist decides which operation should be done.

After the organs are exposed, the technique depends upon whether or not the ovaries are to be retained and further, the extent of the tissue to be removed. In a woman past the menopause, the ovaries are usually removed since they are functionless and may be the site of cancer later in life. If the operation is done because of cancer, a wide dissection is made to remove all the tissue in which secondary extension to the glands may be present. The urinary bladder is separated from the uterus, and the ureters, coming from the kidneys to the bladder, are identified so that they will not be injured. The ligaments connected to the uterus are divided and the blood vessels are clamped and tied. The cervix is seldom retained unless some special reason is determined for its retention. The vagina is cut from around the cervix and the uterus. Then, with or without the tubes and ovaries, they are removed together.

An appendectomy, removal of the appendix, is often performed at the same time as a hysterectomy.

The abdomen is closed in layers and the skin may be closed by clips or removable sutures.

An anesthetic is always essential. It may be of an inhalation type or, more usually, a low spinal injection.

Vaginal hysterectomy, which is usually performed for a prolapsed uterus and for repair operations, is popular with some surgeons, who use it routinely except for especially large tumors. The vaginal hysterectomy requires greater skill by the surgeon. This procedure has the disadvantage of not allowing for exploration of the abdominal organs at the time of the operation, and is quite difficult if adhesions are present.

OTHER PELVIC OPERATIONS

Operation for *retrodisplacement of the uterus* is rarely indicated. At one time, the suspension operation performed by shortening the round ligaments was a common procedure. Today this technique is rarely used except in some cases in which sterility is thought to be due to the position of the uterus or when the position of the uterus causes severe pain.

Vulvectomy is an operation by which the labia are removed from both sides of the vagina. This is a mutilating procedure and is done for cancer and precancerous conditions, leucoplakia and kraurosis. When cancer is present, the glands in the groin are also removed.

Excision of Bartholin's glands. Two mucus-secreting glands, which are found on either side of the vagina, often become infected. They may require incision for relief of an acute condition, but for permanent cure, the gland must be removed by dissection.

Operation for imperforate hymen. While rare, there have been cases of a vagina without an opening. In such a case, the menstrual blood would be dammed up in the vagina, and cause pressure symptoms. To correct this abnormality, the hymenal membrane is excised and an opening made. Operations to enlarge the hymen so that coitus is possible is usually a simple plastic procedure.

Episiotomy is an operative procedure which is designed to enlarge the opening of the vagina so that the delivery of the baby will not cause irregular tears in the perineum, which will not stretch sufficiently to allow the expulsion of the baby's head. This operation prevents damage to the bladder, lacerations of the soft tissue, and pressure on the head of the baby.

Surgery of the Breast

Women are always conscious of their breasts, from the time the breasts develop until they shrink at the menopause. The breasts are specialized organs which consist of glands arranged in sectors, usually

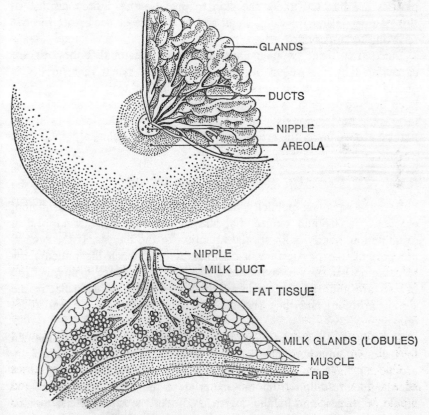

Fig. 28. A cross-section of the breast.

sixteen, each with a duct which opens into the nipple. The gland tissue is surrounded by connective tissue, padded with fat, and covered with skin. The purpose of the breast is to produce milk.

Breasts vary in size from person to person and often the same person has one breast larger than the other. The type of nipple also varies. Usually they are everted, but they may be flat or retracted. Accessory nipples are sometimes noted often below the breast; they are flat, like the breast of a child. Accessory breast tissue may be found in the fold of skin above the breast, near the axilla (under the arm). This also swells after the birth of a baby.

Plastic operations to change the size of the breast. Many women are unhappy about the appearance of their breasts. Those with small breasts want them larger; there are plastic surgeons who have devised operations to do this. Inert material, such as paraffin, sponges, and plastics are inserted under the skin to produce the desired results. In this day of "falsies," a woman can add to the size of her breast without resorting to surgery.

In contrast, some women have such large breasts that they are incapacitated by the weight and bulk to such an extent that surgery is necessary. For such an apparent abnormality, a few techniques have been devised to remove the excess breast tissue. The nipple is left intact, and the incision is planned so that the resulting scar is in the natural groove under the breast and will not be disfiguring.

EXAMINATION OF THE BREAST

Because so much publicity has been given about cancer detection, every woman should realize that she should have a general physical examination, yearly, with special attention to the breasts. If the breasts are normal, the physician will demonstrate and teach the patient how to examine her own breasts, which she should do once a month. The breasts are uniformly soft, when palpated by the hand held flat in the supine position, and they should be without sensations of tenderness or pain.

The skin of the breast is subject to any condition that may happen to the skin anywhere else on the body. Simple pimples, especially around an "ingrown" hair, may appear or a rash from the heat, or an allergic manifestation from the material of the "bra," eczema of the nipple or redness and itching, intertrigo, under the breast if it is pendulous. Psoriasis and ringworm may even occur on the skin of the breast.

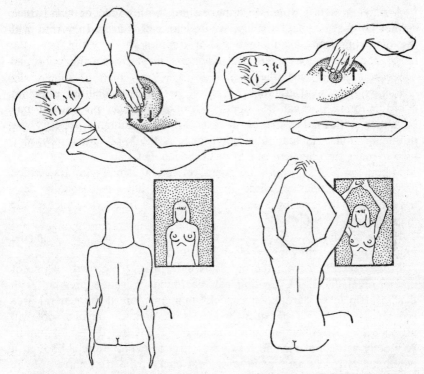

Fig. 29. The technique of self-examination of the breasts for early detection of unusual growths.

Any of these simple conditions should be diagnosed by a physician and not treated by home remedies.

Abscesses may form in the breasts of nursing mothers. These usually produce redness, swelling, and fever and may require incision and drainage.

A physician must be consulted without delay if any of the following conditions are present:

a painless lump in the breast

a lump with pain or tenderness

secretion from the nipple, bloody, opaque, or clear

pain or discomfort in the breast, without any abnormality

any localized puckering in the skin of the breast.

Cancer is suspected by every woman who finds a lump in her breast. The physician's first thought is to establish or rule out the possibility of cancer.

A painless mass, which is firm or hard, with vague borders which cannot be pushed about readily, is suspicious of cancer. In addition, if the overlying skin is adherent and if dimples in the skin, over the mass, can be demonstrated, the diagnosis must be considered to be cancer until it is proved otherwise.

Benign lesions. If the lump is firm, has sharply defined edges, is ovoid or round, and can be "popped" around by finger pressure, it may be either a fibroadenoma or a cyst. Transillumination, done in the physician's office, or mammography, taken in the X-ray laboratory, may help to make the diagnosis of cyst or fibroadenoma.

Mammography may also be useful in finding small nodules, which are not even palpable. These X-ray pictures have occasionally been the means of discovering the earliest cancer in a breast, in which cystic mastitis was present.

In the physician's office, a cyst can be proved by inserting a needle into the lump and drawing off clear cyst fluid.

Bloody secretion from the nipple is indicative of a growth in one of the terminal ducts. Its location can be found by gentle pressure with the fingertip in an "around the clock" manipulation in the general area around the nipple. If the growth does exist, pressure on one spot will produce the secretion, and underneath this point lies the small tumor. A bloody secretion may necessitate a surgical exploration. Although a papilloma is rarely associated with duct cancer, the true nature of the underlying tumor cannot be determined by physical examination alone.

The breast occasionally secretes a clear, yellowish, or milky fluid for which a localized origin cannot be found. This usually occurs after lactation. The diagnosis is probably "non-puerperal secretion" or mastitis with secretion.

Pain without a lump in the breast is not suggestive of cancer. Furthermore, pain is rarely present in an early cancer of the breast. Painful breasts often are noted a week or ten days before the menstrual period and disappear with the onset of menstruation. Such discomfort is apt to occur to women in the late thirties or early forties, and may be so severe that hormones may be necessary for relief. The breasts are also swollen at such a time, and the swelling may be localized in part of one breast or the other, before the menses. Shifting pain and shifting swelling are never indicative of serious disorders. Usually mastitis is the cause of these changes in the breast and does not require more than regular attention and examination to be certain that the diagnosis is correct.

Biopsy of the breast or excision of a breast tumor. A physician cannot determine accurately and positively that a nodule in the breast is or is not malignant without microscopic examination.

A persistent nodule, or "lump" in the breast, must be proved to be benign or malignant, cancerous. In order to perform a microscopic examination, the nodule is excised, if possible, or a portion is removed for biopsy so that the pathologist can examine it.

The physician will explain this to the patient. She will go to the hospital, the mass will be removed, a quick-frozen section will be made by the pathologist, and if cancerous tissue is not found, the incision will be closed and the woman can return home the next day. If cancer should be present, the surgeon will immediately remove the breast. In that case, the woman should be prepared to remain in the hospital for a week or more, depending on the extent of the necessary surgery.

Emotional preparation should be part of the care of the patient. If cancer is ruled out, there is no need for worry. The nodule was removed for examination and found to be benign. If the tumor proved to be cancerous, the patient is also fortunate. It was found early, and was correctly removed; the chances are that it will never recur. The removal of an early cancer saves the pain and agony which often accompany the later stages when metastases develop.

The incision which is necessary for the biopsy is usually only 3 to 4 cm. in length and is made over the nodule, if the tumor is near the surface. If the lump is deeply embedded, the incision may be made under the breast and the breast lifted up to expose the tumor. The tumor is completely excised, together with the surrounding breast tissue. The small blood vessels in the area are clamped and ligated so that little or no blood is lost.

Sometimes a local anesthetic is given. However, if the mass is deep or large, the patient may be put to sleep with an intravenous Pentothal Sodium or a gas anesthetic. A drain may be inserted. Sutures, which can be removed, are used to close the incision. The resulting scar on the breast does not leave any residual pain or discomfort.

MASTECTOMY

Mastectomy is the operation by which the breast is removed.

In a simple mastectomy, only the breast is excised.

In a radical mastectomy, a wide dissection is done so that the breast, the muscles of the chest wall, and the glands in the armpit, axilla, and under the clavicle, collarbone, are also eliminated.

Simple mastectomy. In the operation known as "simple mastectomy" the breast is removed but the surrounding tissue remains. This operation is usually considered inadequate for malignant conditions and too radical for benign lesions. However, often in special cases, a simple mastectomy is advisable. Some of these conditions might be multiple papillomas which involve the ducts in more than one quadrant of the breast, or recurrent nodules, other than cysts in adenosis, or this operation may be recommended in benign conditions. It may also be the procedure of choice in cancer, in its earliest stage, before any metastasis has developed, or in the latest stage of cancer when the growth has already spread and for fear that the original growth in the breast might break down and ulcerate. In such cases, the simple operation is followed by radiation or chemotherapy or both.

To perform the operation, an incision is made enclosing an elliptical area of the skin with the widest portion at the nipple. The incision may be either longitudinal or transverse, depending on the size and shape of the breast, but usually it is transverse so that the resulting scar will be across the chest. However, the incision may be made lengthwise so that the scar will be up and down. The tissue is removed down to the muscles. The small vessels are tied with fine cat gut, a drain is generally left in, and the edges of the skin are brought together with silk, cotton, or nylon sutures, which are usually removed in about a week.

Radical mastectomy. Although radical mastectomy is no longer the sole method by which cancer of the breast is treated, this procedure does account for the greatest percentage of survivals.

The operation attempts to remove, in one mass, all the structures which are liable to immediate invasion by the tumor. This conclusion is based on the assumption that the spread of the disease from its original focus proceeds by continuous permeation in all directions. The plan of operation, for radical removal of the breast, is to excise, in one piece, a safe margin of normal tissues together with the cancer, to include the adjoining pathways, lymph nodes, and lymphatics, along which the cancer spreads, and to guard against the transplantation of malignant cells during the operation by the careful manipulation of the affected tissues.

The palpable tumor is considered as the center of the skin to be encircled and for the removal of the tumor, while the apex of the axilla, the armpit, is taken as the upper limit of the dissection. After cutting through the skin, subcutaneous tissues, and muscular attachments, the dissection is begun in the apex of the axilla to avoid mechanical and traumatic dissemination of cancer along this pathway during the operation. All the fatty tissue in the axilla, with the lymph glands and areolar cells, are removed; the pectoral muscles are freed from the sternum and the chest so that the breast and all the surrounding tissue is removed in one mass.

The skin is sutured and drains are left. Since the serous drainage from such a large area may be profuse, the drains are often attached to a suction apparatus so that dressings need not be changed. Skin grafts may be advisable if the edges of the skin cannot be brought together.

In addition to this dissection, the excision of the internal lymph node chain may be performed. This operation requires rib resection and also opening of the chest, since this chain is located under the ribs parallel to the breastbone, the sternum. Fortunately such radical surgery is rarely necessary.

OTHER BREAST-ASSOCIATED OPERATIONS

Ovarectomy following mastectomy. Since the breasts are influenced by hormones, and the major source of such hormones is in the ovaries, the removal of the ovaries has been advisable following mastectomy. Particularly, this procedure is advisable if metastases have occurred, and it is usually done in premenopausal women. In some clinics, irradiation of the ovaries instead of surgery is the method of treatment, but surgery is ordinarily advised because of occasional ill effects of radiation on the bowels, and the side effects of pelvic radiation.

Adrenalectomy of metastatic breast cancer. The adrenals are another source of the production of estrogen hormones, and their removal has encouraged remissions from metastatic symptoms. In cases of painful metastases, adrenalectomy often brings noticeable relief of the pain and a sense of well-being.

Hypophysectomy for metastatic breast cancer. The development of simple and safe techniques for the removal of the pituitary gland, hypophysectomy, has brought remissions in cases of recurrences of the tumor following cancer of the breast. This operation not only eliminates pituitary hormones, but also suppresses ovarian and adrenal function, comparable to surgical removal of these glands. Hypophysectomy may prove to be the treatment of choice in metastatic cancer of the breast.

RADIATION THERAPY

Most women who have cancer of the breast usually get some type of radiation therapy. Some tumors are treated by radiation before mastectomy, and excellent results are reported in such cases. Radiation, following radical mastectomy, is usually done if the metastases are found in the glands at the time of operation. Radiation is also advised in some instances in which the glands are not involved. X-rays and cobalt therapy, either near or distant, are used to treat such metastases if they occur. Each person is an individual case as far as radiation is concerned, and each woman must be studied and evaluated for the type of radiation to be used.

CHEMOTHERAPY IN CANCER OF THE BREAST

The number of antitumor drugs available for use in the treatment of cancer is increasing as research is progressing and the use of these chemical agents is becoming more widespread. The fact that so many are being used means a perfect one has not yet been developed. Any drug which is powerful enough to kill cancer cells must also have toxic effects on normal cells, so that it must be administered with extreme and cautious care.

The research in progress on viruses in relation to cancers, on antibody and immune reactions to cancer cells, together with antitumor drugs, makes the medical profession hopeful that soon a safe, effective means to combat cancer will be realized.

HORMONES IN CANCER OF THE BREAST

The exact relationship of hormones to cancer of the breast is, as yet, unknown but it is apparent that the pain of metastatic origin is relieved, and often the growth itself does disappear, when treated with hormones.

Chapter IX

THE MENOPAUSE
Beatrice E. Tucker, M.D.

Ever since Eve was driven from the Garden of Eden, women have been emotionally involved and intensely preoccupied with that period in their development known as "the change of life." Even in our enlightened time, the occasion is dramatic. Bizarre and fanciful tales have been invented which, in a frightful manner, correlate with the menopause a variety of physical, emotional, and social difficulties. These tales have been passed down through the ages and created the illusion that the menopause is mysterious and an event to be dreaded.

The stubborn persistence of such senseless tradition speaks for the natural tendency of people to exaggerate and elaborate trouble and to seek a whipping boy to blame for real or imagined ills. Because of these inherited myths and rumors, a natural event has been exaggerated out of all proportion to its real significance. The menopause has become a bugaboo. Fear and anxiety concerning the menopause lurk in the minds of many women, and too often lead to unnecessary physical and psychological suffering.

The explosion of old wives' tales, in itself, does not relieve all fear and anxiety. Few, if any, women completely escape a strong emotional jolt at this time and mixed feelings inevitably occur. For some, menopause brings relief that childbearing is over, and for others it causes regret in regard to the now positive inability to become pregnant. Most women find fulfillment through marriage and motherhood. Nature's forced ending of the childbearing cycle causes varying degrees of insecurity and rebellion. However, if husband and children will assure the woman that she is the same loved person she has always been, self-confidence can be restored and rebellion and hostility lessened. *For the woman who is reasonably secure as a person and as a functioning human being, the physical discomforts of this period, if there are any, will be easily tolerated.*

Life continually demands physical and emotional adjustments. Ideally, the individual passes through each stage of life naturally, with a specific sense of well-being and satisfaction. As stated so beautifully in Ecclesiastes, "To everything there is a season, and a time to every purpose under heaven." Changes occur in both men and women which enable them to meet the demands of living. Biologically, these are primarily concerned with reproduction and the care of the young.

A time comes in the life of every woman when she may no longer suitably have children. The duration of life itself is limited and if reproduction continued into old age, there would be no mother to care for the offspring. This is nature's reason for the menopause. The menopause not only prevents motherless young but guards the woman's health by preventing conception at a time when her body needs rest from childbearing.

A large part of a gynecologist's practice is composed of women who seek help and comfort during the few years which precede and follow the cessation of menstruation. Women may be perturbed because they do not understand what is happening. Many, unfortunately, are physically strangers to themselves. The complaints may be physical or mental, real or imaginary. Some women have serious difficulties; others do not have any specific symptoms but feel that a physical checkup is in order. Occasionally, serious conditions are uncovered, but early knowledge usually guarantees a cure of these perplexities and many are found to be unrelated to the menopause. The doctor must determine whether or not the symptoms are due to the menopause or to some other circumstances which have nothing to do with the change but which occurred at the same time. The menopause is a natural phenomenon and ordinarily is not responsible for ill health. The doctor must have unusual tact, sympathy, understanding, and forbearance to aid him in making the right diagnosis and to plan the best treatment. Probably essential for the best solution is time; time to listen and time to hear. The problems recited by the patient may not seem genuine to the doctor but they are truly vital to the patient. Most women must be reassured in regard to their health and can manage quite well without any drugs. However, a few simple remedies invariably will give great relief. The knowledge that the climacteric, the change of life, is self-limiting and usually lasts only two years or less encourages the woman who is really miserable.

The word menopause implies just that; it is a landmark in life when one phase of existence ceases and another begins. At a time between forty and sixty years, but usually at forty-eight to fifty years of age, menstruation permanently stops and the last menstrual periods are known as the menopause. After this cessation, pregnancy cannot occur and childbearing is at an end. For a few years before and after that last period, changes take place in the body which in most instances are gradual and cause women little or no discomfort. Approximately twenty per cent of women are frankly disturbed and experience some difficulty. The common name for these years before and after the menopause is the "change of life" and the medical term is the climacteric. This period may last one to ten years but the usual duration is two years. The experience is so exceptional that women of all races and social position talk about it. A Sioux Indian, married to an Irish accountant, told me that in her language the change of life is called "the affliction." This would intimate that it was not a happy time. Since Indian women in primitive society did much of the hard work for the entire tribe, they probably had little rest and endured more fatigue at this time of life. Perhaps, however, it was the other way round, that their household duties were limited so they could sit around and talk about their symptoms. Today, however, the menopause need not be an affliction.

This change scarcely ever occurs before the age of forty and if it does, it is referred to as a premature menopause. The removal by surgery of some or all of the organs of reproduction can bring about a premature menopause but this is usually known as a surgical menopause. The organs of reproduction are the ovaries, the tubes, and the uterus, womb. If the patient is properly prepared psychologically before such an operation, she need not have any neurotic effects afterward.

A renowned English philosopher once wrote, "Nature never makes excellent things for mean or no uses." Even a brief glimpse into the reasons and working of the female body will readily attest to the truth of Lessing's immortal line, "Nature meant woman to be her masterpiece."

In order to understand what changes occur in the cycle preceding the menopause, one should know what is considered a normal cycle. A menstrual cycle lasts from the beginning of one menstrual period to the beginning of the next menstrual period and recurs every twenty-four to thirty-two days. Vaginal bleeding, the menstrual period, persists from three to seven days and usually a woman soils from four to six napkins every twenty-four hours. Spotting, that is, bleeding so scant that a pad is unnecessary, may occur at the time of ovulation which is usually midperiod. As a rule, menstrual blood does not clot. This monthly phenomenon, which so many young girls have bemoaned during the hot summer months, may be considered as nature's way of saying that she is a woman and has the ability to bear children.

Scattered throughout the body are a number of glands which may be considered laboratories and which, at different ages of life, secrete specific chemicals in variable amounts. These chemicals are picked up by the bloodstream and carried to distant parts of the body where they affect organs and tissues and the way in which they function. This group of glands is called the endocrine system and the chemicals are termed hormones. All of the glands and hormones are interrelated and operate under a timing system directed insensibly by the brain. Part of the system is concerned with sex and reproduction. Although the entire

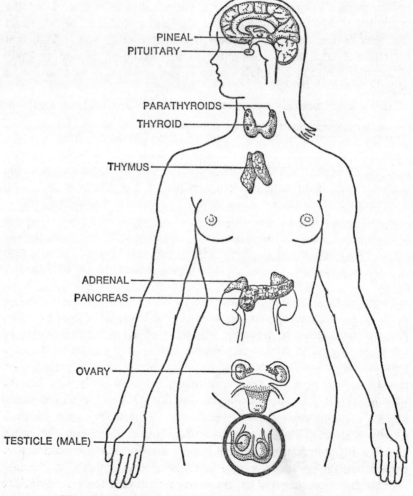

Fig. 30. The glands that control our body mechanisms.

system is quite similar in males and females, the sex glands differ in men and women and secrete different hormones in each.

The sex glands of the female are the ovaries, and nature has provided woman with two, one located on either side of the pelvis. The ovaries develop the female sex cells, called the ova or eggs. They also manufacture two sex hormones, estrogen and progesterone. Estrogen stimulates the development of the breasts and determines body contour, fat distribution, quality of the voice, and the character of the skeleton and the hair. Beginning at puberty and ending at the menopause, these two hormones cause ovulation, the preparation for fertilization of the female sex cell, the ovum. In addition, these hormones aid in the growth and development of the fetus if fertilization and pregnancy occur. If pregnancy does not ensue, the sex hormones are partially withdrawn from the bloodstream and excreted in the urine. Their withdrawal causes death of the lining of the uterus, which is cast off with vaginal bleeding; this is termed the menstrual period.

The majority of women know that ovulation and menstruation are closely related. Ovulation anticipates pregnancy and is usually without symptoms. If conception does not occur, the woman menstruates about two weeks after ovulation. If pregnancy does eventuate, menstruation stops for forty weeks. The reproductive life of the female lasts from thirty to thirty-three years.

In the premenopausal years, many changes occur in the endocrine system and the aging ovary works irregularly. These changes account for many cycles without ovulation and for variations in the menstrual cycle. These variations occurring after forty years of age are suggestive that the menopause will take place in two to three years.

An exception to these changes is the woman who menstruates regularly without shift of pattern, until the periods suddenly stop. As a rule, cycles become longer and the periods shorter and more scant. The time between the periods may lengthen from three to six months and vary decidedly. Cycles may, however, become shorter and heavier. Flooding is not unusual and, occasionally, an alarming amount of blood is lost, liquefied or in clots. Another variation is spotting before and after a menstrual period. If a year passes without a period, one may safely assume that the menopause has occurred. Any bleeding after the ordinary menstrual cycles have ceased is cause for alarm. Spotting, other than just before and after a period, is also reason for concern. A cycle of less than twenty-one days is abnormal.

How is a woman going to know whether or not these irregularities are normal? Unfortunately, in medicine as well as in life, hard and fast rules that apply to every individual or situation do not exist. Women today in this and in most European countries are more enlightened than at any other time in history. They have a healthy respect and regard for their bodies and usually possess a goodly amount of common sense about taking care of their health. A woman need not be unduly apprehensive during the change of life. Certain variations will occur and she should be prepared for them beforehand. However, to play safe and allay any unnecessary anxiety, the woman must report any irregularity of the menstrual cycle or any intermenstrual bleeding to her physician.

Fear of cancer during the climacteric is common since it has been fairly well established that cancer of the female genitalia, reproductive organs, and breast occurs more frequently at this time of life than at any other. As just stated, a frequent symptom of cancer of the womb is intermittent vaginal bleeding. For this reason, patient and physician should be concerned about any irregularity or changes in the menstrual cycle. While most of these are not due to serious conditions, a few are related to cancer. Because *time* is such a significant factor in treating this disease, a thorough investigation of all irregularities is recommended in order that anything pertaining to this condition will not be overlooked.

Fortunately many women, alerted to the great advances made in preventive medicine, have periodic pelvic examinations every six months of adult life. This examination includes cytocervical smears, the Papanicolaou or Pap smear. The Pap smear is a routine office procedure which takes less than five minutes to perform and is painless. A vaginal speculum is placed in the vagina and the cervix is exposed. A tongue depressor or swab is then passed lightly over the mouth of the womb, that part which is in the vagina, and the material gathered is then placed on a glass slide. The slide is then sent to a pathologist who specializes in cytology, the study of cells. He will examine the material to see if any abnormal cells are present. Conditions other than cancer, most frequently infection, can cause abnormal cells. The patient need not become panicky because of any abnormal smear. The infection should be treated promptly and a repeat smear made at a later date. If this smear is abnormal, pieces of tissue are removed from the cervix for microscopic study or the entire lining of the cervix is removed for examination. Removal of the entire cervical lining is known as conization, and many physicians prefer it to spot biopsy. The operation requires a hospital stay of a few days. The Pap smear enables discovery of cancer of the mouth of the womb five years in advance of invasion, when it really becomes dangerous. Early diagnosis and treatment leads to cure in most cases.

Although cancer of the mouth of the womb can be diagnosed by the Pap smear, cancer of the body of the womb usually cannot be distinguished by this method. In order to secure material for study from the body of the uterus, the part of the abdomen, dilatation and curettage are necessary. This is a minor operation usually requiring two days of hospitalization. Under anesthesia, the mouth of the uterus is opened with dilators and the lining of the uterus is scraped off with a sharp, spoon-shaped instrument. The tissue is then sent to the pathologist for study.

Profuse vaginal bleeding which may occur in the premenopausal years usually is not caused by cancer. Endocrine disorders, submucous fibroids, non-malignant tumors beneath the lining of the uterus, and polyps are the most frequent culprits. The bleeding may be controlled by curettage. If the ailment is due to lack of hormones, hormones may be given safely once cancer has been ruled out. Hormones will not control bleeding from fibroids. A hysterectomy, surgical removal of the uterus, may be necessary in either case to control serious loss of blood.

If the patient has an excessive flow of blood or if the periods are too close together, anemia occurs. The amount of blood lost is considered abnormal if twelve sanitary pads are saturated in twenty-four hours, or if pads as well as tampons are needed. The blood count is the best index as to the amount of blood lost. Signs of anemia are excess fatigue, dizziness, faintness, headache, and a sense of chill.

Cancer of the breast is most likely to occur in the years just preceding the menopause. The incidence is more than the sum of cancer of the womb and of the ovary together. Cancer forms a palpable mass in the breast. In 90 per cent of the cases when the breast is involved, the lumps are found by the patient herself and not by the physician. The size of the lump is immaterial, nor is the degree of pain of consequence; many early cancers are painless while non-cancerous lesions may be distressing. If any lump is discovered in a breast or beneath the arm, a physician should be consulted immediately and the mass promptly removed and studies for cancer made under the microscope. To repeat once again, early diagnosis determines the rate of cure. To insure early diagnosis and treatment of cancer of the breast and ovary, a physician must see the patient at least every three months.

The astonishing fine feature of the endocrine system and of the other vital systems of the body is that they are self-regulatory. Imagine how complex life would be if we had to order our lungs to breathe, our heart to beat, the ovaries to make eggs, and the glands to secrete hormones. Although the endocrine system functions without conscious control, fear and anxiety can upset the applecart, as the saying goes. If a woman is emotionally disturbed, the entire system can get out of kilter, disarranged, and many annoying symptoms can develop. During the menopause women are prone to display more anxiety than perhaps at any other time in their lives. Many myths and jokes have prevailed for years about the menopause. The woman is rare who remains serenely undisturbed and accepts this process as just another natural and normal phase of her development—which it is.

The menopause does not affect the entire body physically or psychologically. The ovary does not completely stop the manufacture of the female sex hormone, and the adrenal gland acts as an auxiliary laboratory that secretes estrogen for many years after the last menstrual period has occurred. This insures the health and well-being of the woman.

Changes due to age, which may occur at the same time as the menopause, are not to be confused with those due to loss of ovarian function. No amount of sex hormone will restore the color of hair, prevent distribution of fat about the middle, sagging breasts, loss of hair, dry, coarse, wrinkled skin, or the growth of hair on the face, arms, and legs. Beauty parlors, plastic surgery, and electrolysis have their legitimate uses.

Only a few symptoms which are caused by a lack of the female sex hormone can legitimately be charged up to the menopause and these are by no means of universal occurrence. They are (1) the notorious "hot flash," (2) changes in the tissue of the genital tract which may be troublesome, and (3) inadequate bone metabolism which is conducive to arthritic pains and backache. However, a warning is in order here. Any of these conditions may be due to other causes, and, if so, estrogens will not help in the treatment.

The hot flash is usually due to a lack of the female sex hormone estrogen. Not all women have hot flashes: 10 per cent have never experienced a flash and 80 per cent have them only occasionally and never suffer any real inconvenience. The remaining 10 per cent are distressed by this phenomenon. The term hot flash is itself fairly descriptive of what occurs. Usually a flush, which is actually a nervous vascular phenomenon, starts on the breasts and spreads upwards to the neck, face, and scalp. The blood vessels of the skin are dilated, the skin becomes red and remains so for three to four minutes. The woman has a hot, burning sensation and the sweat glands grow overly active, causing beads of sweat to stand out on the forehead and slip down the neck. Then, after three or four minutes, the vessels contract and the skin blanches and becomes quite pale. The perspiration evaporates; the woman experiences a cold, clammy feeling. These flashes occasionally recur every ten minutes during the day and night. In milder cases they occur less frequently but often enough to disturb sleep. Needless to say, night after night of sleeplessness can change even the most well-adjusted woman into a nervous wreck!

The woman who is experiencing continuing flashes certainly has no legitimate reason to endure them. Some women are under the impression that the administration of female sex hormone leads to cancer. This is not true. The proper administration of the female sex hormone estrogen is harmless. Estrogen is not prescribed until after the menopause has occurred, except in special cases, and it is not given if a cancer is known to be present. Estrogens can usually completely relieve hot flashes and sleeplessness and the nervousness caused by the flashes; thus the hormone contributes greatly to the patient's health and feeling of well-being. Estrogen may be administered by mouth or hypodermically, as the patient wishes. The drug may come from natural sources, that is, from animals, or it may be synthetic, chemically produced. Most physicians have their own preferences. However, a simple preparation costing about two cents a pill gives as much relief as a "shot" which costs five dollars or more. Shots, however, are necessary in approximately 5 per cent of cases because the oral preparations are not tolerated well by these patients.

The tendency of many women to run for "shots" and to appear obviously disappointed if these are neither given nor prescribed, reminds me of my father and a dog that he purchased on Maxwell Street in Chicago. Maxwell Street used to be a large, open-air market on the west side of the city, and its entrepreneurs were without peer in the art and science of salesmanship. The dog with which my father arrived home was supposed to be a fox terrier, but he had a tail where no tail should be and his ears drooped instead of rising jauntily in the manner of most "legitimate" terriers.

"How much did you pay for that dog?" I asked my father innocently.

"Ten dollars," he replied.

My mouth dropped open. "You could have gotten him for one dollar," I said.

My father regarded me sternly and replied, "I wouldn't own a dog that cost less than ten dollars."

Some people feel the same way about drugs. They are convinced that the more they cost, the better they are. Such an argument is, of course, patently ridiculous and the patient who deludes herself with such a notion is only increasing the cost, not the efficiency, of her medical care.

Excessive fatigue is a common complaint of the climacteric. The patient may tell the physician that regardless of how much sleep and rest she gets, she still feels that she can hardly get about. Upon questioning, many times the doctor finds that for years the woman has not been getting enough sleep, due to overwork or nervousness or lack of planning for some definite rest or relaxation. Insufficient rest for a prolonged time has finally caught up with her. This extreme fatigue has no doubt caused a break in her physical stamina which has resulted in depression and exhaustion, which she incorrectly blames upon the menopause. A poorly working thyroid gland may also aggravate the case. A complete physical examination which includes blood counts, basal metabolic rates, and other laboratory tests should be made. The disorders unrelated to the change of life which may occur at the same time include thyroid irregularities, high blood pressure, diabetes, heart trouble, obesity, and other ailments. Proof that fatigue is due to lack of ovarian function has not been indicated. The administration of estrogen will only give a sense of well-being if feeling of lassitude is due to insomnia. Prolonged, too frequent, and too heavy menstrual periods may lead to anemia and great weariness. To recover energy and health, each specific problem must be corrected. After rest has been attained, rest and more rest is essential. Furthermore, we must remember that many women are not really tired at all, but simply terribly bored with the monotony of domestic life. Many have not had a vacation for years. A variety of new and interesting experiences can bring about an amazing cure of the doldrums.

As the witty and wise Washington Irving so aptly wrote, "There is a certain relief in change, even though it be from bad to worse; as I have found in traveling in a stagecoach, that it is often a comfort to shift one's position and be bruised in a new place."

With ovarian failure, certain changes occur in the reproductive tract which may cause a woman some distress. One difficulty is painful intercourse due to atrophy of the mucous membranes of the vulva, labia minora and to changes in the covering of the vagina with a lack of secretion, which normally is lubricating. These changes may be offset by the use of estrogen suppositories or by the administration of estrogen by mouth or hypodermically. The use of a hormone not only increases secretion but causes changes in the lining of the vagina which makes it more resistant to injury and infection. Unfortunately, unless the drugs are properly administered, they may cause bleeding from the uterus and it is difficult to determine whether this is due to the drug or is a new growth.

Many women complain of indefinite joint and bone discomfort and backache. Recently, much research has been done on the relationship to bone metabolism of both male and female sex hormones. The administration of these hormones may alleviate these symptoms and may prevent the development of osteoporosis, fragile bones which break easily. One group of physicians believes that women should take these hormones throughout life, after the menopause.

Again, we must emphasize that not all changes that occur in mid-life are due to lack of female sex hormones. Some that are attributed to this deficiency are not correctable by hormones. Body contour does change and fat distribution may be different. The flat-chested woman may develop larger breasts. This is one of the reasons why the middle-aged figure is considered more attractive by many men. The increased deposit of fat on the abdomen and thighs is not unattractive if obesity is avoided. Actually, these deposits of fat help to offset changes in the skin which otherwise lead to sagging. The thyroid gland, located in the neck, determines the rate at which food is converted into fat. If a weight problem develops, tests of the functioning condition of this gland are made. If the examination indicates a lack of thyroid hormone, the hormone will be given by mouth to the point of proper function. Restoring the thyroid gland to its proper working order will not correct the problem entirely; it may improve the feeling of well-being, but loss of weight will not ensue without decreasing the intake of food.

The gain of weight after the menopause is most likely the result of a change in the pattern of living. Excessive fatigue, which many women experience, limits physical activity and this leads to a more sedentary and less active life. The body needs rest and should not be driven. The less active the body, the less food it needs, so that cure for obesity, as always, is the intake of less food, unless some medical difficulty is at fault.

Another factor in weight gain is the tendency of some women toward nervousness, irritability, and boredom. Consciously or unconsciously comfort is sought by way of the stomach. Constant nibbling on snacks can turn those snacks into fat. If the fat were to be distributed favorably over the body, it wouldn't be too bad, but inevitably the fat leads to the pear-shaped figure, which turns few heads.

However, it is better to be fat than to be a hellion. Few, if any, households can tolerate a woman on a crash diet. Nothing is more boring than a calorie-counting wife who is constantly snapping and insists that her family pay for her frustrations. If a rapid major weight loss is in order, treatment should only be undertaken with isolation of the woman in a hospital or sanitarium, under the strict supervision of a physician.

Every human being needs a well-balanced diet and almost every sane person enjoys eating and drinking in moderation. Some drugs, designed to reduce appetite, increase nervous irritability so that sedatives are often taken to offset this difficulty. As a consequence, the nervous system is insulted two ways; it is flagged upward and then sedated. After a time, the system is completely worn out and excessive fatigue is added to an already jaded mechanism. A haggard shrew with possible hypertension may be the result.

Amphetamines are drugs that decrease appetite, increase energy, and act as an anti-depressant. However, this drug is only a crutch to bolster will power, and is to be avoided if possible, or used sparingly under a physician's supervision.

Many sensible people maintain that the good life includes good liquor and good food served with imagination and shared with interesting company. Calorie intake should be planned to allow for this type of relaxation and enjoyment, even if one is 10 per cent overweight. This does not mean that a person should be either an alcoholic or a glutton.

During the change of life, some women do experience restlessness, sleeplessness, forgetfulness, and feelings of inadequacy and depression. These symptoms rarely, if ever, reach a serious state and usually can be controlled by reassurance from her family and from her physician and by the temporary use of sedatives. Ordinarily a woman will have a major psychological problem only if she has previously experienced serious emotional instability. This problem is not due to the menopause, but rather to the accumulation of years of emotional stress, which now give way to severe emotional disorders. Fears of insanity or of erratic behavior due to the cessation of ovarian function are absolutely unwarranted; they are unrelated.

Probably the nervous symptoms manifested during the menopause are not due to the physical, but rather to the emotional, turmoil stirring within the woman. An indifferent or hostile family increases a woman's emotional difficulties, for she finds herself afraid or unable to communicate her feelings to them. If the woman is unstable and has had a previous nervous breakdown, the anxiety and fear of her home situation may aggravate an earlier existing problem. If emotionally unstable, unoccupied and unfulfilled, the woman may seize upon the advent of the menopause as the perfect target upon which to vent her anger and frustration; unfortunately, it is those around her who suffer her wrath, while she herself contributes to her own destruction as a loving and lovable human being.

The administration of estrogens will not prevent nervous breakdown. It will enable the patient to sleep and be less nervous, if her symptoms are caused by the hot flash.

The menopause brings on anxieties both valid and imaginary. The fear of pregnancy is almost universal at this time of life. Although some women voice regret that the childbearing period is over, pregnancy is not really wanted. A woman who wishes to avoid an unwanted pregnancy must exercise great care and continue to utilize contraceptives for one year following what is assumed to be a last period. We delivered a baby to a fifty-four-year-old woman; the oldest recorded case of pregnancy was in a woman seventy-two years of age who miscarried. Contraceptive precaution for a period of one year following the last menstrual period is an absolute necessity for the woman who does not wish to become pregnant, because ovulation can take place many months after a seemingly last period. If menstruation should occur during the apparently "last" one-year interval, then this period is to be considered the last one and contraceptives again are to be used for another full year.

The fear of loss of sexuality disturbs most women at the menopause. Sexuality implies sex drive, desire, and gratification. Sexuality is independent of ovarian function and of sex hormones. Women who have had their ovaries removed surgically do not experience any change in sexuality after the operation nor is there any difference in the sex pattern of a woman after the menopause unless she develops a fixed idea in this regard. Sexuality is primarily a psychological, emotional, and sensory reaction, ideally inspired by love. After the menopause, the desire for sexual activity is often greater than before, and the pleasure induced by gratification is frequently more intense. This phase may be prompted by the assurance that pregnancy no longer can occur. No longer must the woman depend on contraception and there can be more freedom in the act of intercourse. Furthermore, there is also an added factor of time; lovemaking is not confined to schedules nor is there the disturbing and inhibiting factor of small children in the home.

The pleasure of intercourse is dependent physically on the sensory stimulation by touch of various parts of the body. This includes preliminary play with mouth, breasts, neck, and other areas and stimulation of the clitoris and the vagina during the sex act. Every healthy, well-adjusted, emotionally stable female has the ability to finish coitus with a climactic orgasm most of the time. The primary excitement of sexual urge is optimally based on love, or at least affection. If indifference is present, intercourse is not only a waste of time, it is a travesty on the nature of both man and woman. Rather than fixing the menopause as the reason for a seemingly diminished sexuality, women should look into their hearts and their heads. The ovaries, or lack of them, are completely blameless.

Problems of frigidity will be neither caused nor cured by the menopause. In general, frigidity is evoked by a multiplicity of complex factors, among which are painful intercourse, fatigue, poor health, guilt, fear of pregnancy, dissatisfaction with the partner, lack of self-confidence, poor sex education, and boredom. Any one or combination of these will rob the act of intercourse of its delight.

The fear of loss of attraction for the male bedevils many women and at the menopause can become almost an obsession. Many such women strive to emulate themselves as they were at "sweet sixteen." They wear clothes that ill-befit them, make-up that too obviously screams its purpose, and demeanor that robs them of their natural stature and dignity. Much of this frenzied pursuit of the so-called "joys of youth" has been generated by the extravagances of advertising which find a gullible market. The full-blown rose is almost always preferable to the bud; and the mature woman carries an aura that the girl must take years to attain. Certainly, as one grows older, the difficulty of maintaining the illusion of vibrant sex appeal increases. Ability at maturity to maintain the mate's interest is dependent on character of sexuality, which is a complex quality made up only in part of physical appearance. The capacity for sympathy, understanding, respect, love, tenderness, and unselfishness is the basis of mature sexuality.

For the woman in her mid-years, all too often the sex act is considered more of an obligation and duty than a joyous participation in something that can be fun and sheer, unadulterated delight. To be sexy, a basic approach not related to duty or obligation, but to pleasure and desire, is essential. Women who confuse sexuality with appearances should read the ancient proverb, "To marry a woman for her beauty is like buying a house for its paint."

The woman who feels herself diminished because she is no longer the beauty she once may have been, is far less a woman, in the truest sense of the word, than she may wish to realize. The buildup and maintenance of self-confidence is essential to every human being; without it, one is lost. Rather than neurotically dwelling on the mirror's unvarnished message, women should realize that their men stare into that same mirror each morning and endure the same pangs of self-doubt and fear. For men, there is no "menopause" to blame or on which to hang their eccentric behavior. To be able to confide his fears and doubts and longings to the woman of his choice, unashamedly, is to a man the profoundest idea of marriage. The woman who understands this and infuses her husband with a continuing sense of his desirability to her is the woman who will never be driven to count her wrinkles or to fear that her attraction for her mate has lapsed with the passage of years.

Although divorce may occur at the time of the climacteric, the menopause is not responsible. The seeds of marital disaster must have been planted many years before. Neurotic dependency is not a substitute for love in holding a mate. The middle years become crucial for many reasons. Perhaps for the first time, the man may be financially able to make a move, or he may be struck by the passage of time and determine to change his life while he is still vigorous enough to enjoy it. For too many women, self-complacency has often led to a lack of interest and vigor; and a selfish person cannot permanently retain sex attraction for the same mate. Sexual interest and drive are a significant part of life between forty and sixty years of age, and the wise woman knows this. The ball game is not over; it has just begun.

The healthy middle-aged woman can be beautiful. Every age has its own special appeal. The adolescent appears half-baked compared with the middle-aged, mature, fulfilled woman. Character is reflected in her face. If a pervading spirit isn't already there, it is time for it to be nurtured. Not since girlhood has a woman been able to enjoy the relative freedom from childbearing that the menopause brings. The cessation of menstruation is only that; it is not the end of life. The unmarried, busy woman usually has less trouble at this time than the married one, chiefly because she has sought and achieved fulfillment through work rather than through marriage and motherhood. If unmarried, inactive, and with life unfilled, and by fulfillment I mean emotional satisfaction, she will have problems.

The wife, after the menopause, is much like the professional man or woman who is forced to retire after a certain age. Now she has more freedom and time and doesn't know what to do with them. For thirty years, more or less, the household and family have required most of her attention. No doubt she is still needed, but in a less demanding way. Naturally, at first she feels lost and depressed. Many women find satisfaction in the care of their grandchildren. However, this is a good time to take stock of one's physical and emotional capacity. Many wives have helped with the financial support of the family. In a way, these women are quite fortunate because their horizons have been broadened and they have interesting things to do outside of the family. The wife and mother from a sheltered home cannot be expected to become a breadwinner, unless her interests and demands lie in that direction. Many women anticipate and plan for their well-earned freedom before it takes place. This is wise. The unprepared need not lose hope, because most of us have talents and desires which have never been developed or satisfied. This is a good time to seek them out and add a new zest to living.

Chapter X

THE YEARS AFTER SIXTY-FIVE
Janet R. Kinney, M.D.

The years after sixty-five are said to be the "age of serenity." If this were true, you would not be reading this chapter and I would not be writing it. Many persons who reach these years face some of the most difficult situations of their lives; they will probably face them alone, and will encounter problems not only new to them but new to all our society.

In 1900, life expectancy for a baby girl was forty-nine, in 1960 it was seventy, and in 1965 it reached seventy-five. Married women outlive their husbands by an average of eight years. This prolongation of life brings problems for womankind and for society. How can we make the added years happy, creative, and productive? Is it better for older people to live together or to be with all age groups? What kind of retirement policies are best? How can we use all the experience and knowledge that age brings to the greatest benefit of the community? How is medical care most efficiently provided? These are problems to which each member of society should give thought, but those persons directly involved should be particularly concerned. It is the supreme challenge that can make these years rewarding, and to face this quest we must muster all forces—physical, economic, intellectual, and emotional.

Physical problems are signally obvious and the most easily faced. It should be noted, too, if a person has reached the age of sixty-five, he must have started with a fairly good, healthy constitution and maintained it. Now this status must be preserved if possible. Another person particularly concerned with this problem is the doctor. He must know his patient and the strengths and weaknesses of his background. Great emphasis is placed on babies receiving continued pediatric care, and the importance to the physician of the baby's medical history is well known. How much more important it is then that the physician know the seven hundred and eighty months of the aging person's history. One should not wait until an emergency arises. The physician should be carefully chosen. He should be one with whom the patient can establish a relationship of mutual trust and faith. One does not like or trust every physician. Not every physician is prepared to care for older people nor will the patient always be completely satisfied with the first physician he visits. It is significant that the patient know his doctor and that the doctor know his patient. The patient must never try to be his own doctor or endeavor to make his own diagnosis. Even physicians' diagnoses need confirmation, and self-diagnosis is prone to err.

The story of Ellen W. is apropos. A nurse of sixty, she came to the office looking like a depressed skeleton. Ten years before she had been referred to a surgeon for a radical operation for a small cancer of the breast. In the past year she had lost forty pounds of weight. At the insistence of her family she had come for consultation although she was convinced that she would soon die. Upon examination, to the amazement of the physician who had the same idea, there was no evidence of cancer. A urine specimen was checked and was found to be loaded with sugar; a blood specimen was drawn and was similarly filled with sugar. And as Ellen watched, she knew she had diabetes, not cancer. Suddenly she looked like a rainbow after a storm. She accepted her diet, her insulin, and her tests as the tools of a new life. She went back to her nursing profession with a new spirit and a will to live, not only to do her duty but a bit more. She always gave a little extra—a hand if the procedure was difficult, a little encouragement to the new intern, an extra back rub to an uncomfortable patient. She often cheered patients who were alarmed and depressed by the diagnosis of diabetes. She died peacefully at seventy-four of a heart attack. Those fourteen unanticipated years she had used as a precious gift for herself and others.

Just as important as it is to abstain from self-diagnosis, so it is to attend to all chronic health problems. Although a person may have lived years with arthritis, high blood pressure, or heart disease, during this period it is essential to avoid the complications of these conditions. This is best done by regular supervision and checkups.

Certain problems are common sources of worry. Surgery is one of these. Many older people fear that they cannot survive an operation. The great advances in anesthesia, transfusions, fluids, and early ambulation have made older people amazingly good candidates for the great modern surgery. A prominent vascular surgeon said, "We no longer ask people how old they are, we go about finding how young they are." This remark was made on the successful conclusion of surgical removal of an abdominal aneurysm from a spry eighty-year-oldster.

Another fear is that of heart attack, which is caused by a stoppage of the blood supply to the heart muscle. Such attacks are rare in women unless they are diabetic, hypertensive, hypothyroid, or have other metabolic problems. Today the majority of people survive first heart attacks to resume reasonably normal lives.

Stroke (impairment of the blood supply to the brain) is a great source of fear. Today, although more definitive approaches to blood vessels are known in only a small proportion of cases, for the great majority, care and courage can result in some degree of rehabilitation. The single most important factor in the success of rehabilitation is the desire to be rehabilitated.

Cancer is a word which still causes fear that hinders treatment. Checkups and early diagnosis help strikingly, but even more significant is the reporting of symptoms. After diagnosis comes treatment. If the physician suggests surgery, X-ray, or medical treatment, follow his suggestions, for chances of recovery are often better in the old than in the young.

Modern treatment of fracture of the hip has revolutionized the outlook for the older patient.

A cause of concern more than worry to most of us today, but particularly to the aging group, is the skin and hair. Lincoln said, "After the age of forty, we are all responsible for our faces." The character that a face reflects is of far more consequence than a youthful appearance. However, if you hate your gray hair, you should dye it. If wrinkles bother you, have plastic surgery. One may "wash away the gray" but not disappointment and frustration, and wrinkles can be removed but not worries, hates, and fear.

At this time, senior citizens—as older persons are often referred to—may notice some loss of acuity of the senses of sight, hearing, taste, and touch. Because contact with our environment is maintained through these senses, they should be preserved. One of the interesting sidelights of the medical studies relating to manned space flight has been the import of stimuli in keeping people alert and in contact with others. Healthy young people, deprived of external stimuli for long periods, sometimes become emotionally unstable and hallucinate. Is it any wonder then that an older person who is blind or deaf may easily become confused? Therefore, every effort must be made to keep these faculties. If the physician suggests cataract surgery, it should be accepted; if he advises a hearing aid, it should be sought and if he recommends lip reading, this should be tried; and if he advises eye drops, they should be used. More important than these, however, is the retention of a sense of humor.

The other change that may be noted is loss of elasticity. This may be noted in the face and feet, or in the joints. When these conditions arise, a good rule to follow is to slow down—to do less at one time and do it oftener. Let's consider this in regard to eating. If the routine has been a cup of coffee for breakfast, a sandwich for lunch, and a "Henry VIII" menu for dinner, these meals can be divided more evenly—a good breakfast, a real lunch, and a light supper. Three lighter meals with mid-meal feedings and an evening snack might be relished. Now, how much and what to eat? Weight should be checked first. If the oldster and his doctor agree that it is normal, fine. If not, he can suggest ways to modify it. If a woman is five feet four and weighs 180 pounds, she is not going to become a Marlene Dietrich but she could reduce her weight to 175. And if she is a skinny 100, she could get up to 105. Then a proper caloric intake should be translated into meals, and this means preparation and cooking, not tea and toast. Selection of the proper diet at this time of life is as essential as when a child is growing. Change is going on inside the body and the body must be given the building blocks for repair. These building blocks are protein, meat, fish, fowl, eggs, milk, and cheese, and fruit and vegetables are needed for vitamins. Next let's consider sleep. Here a woman may find that her sleeping needs work better with an afternoon nap in addition to the night's rest. Most older people require more, not less, rest; therefore, they should adjust to shorter but more frequent intervals of sleep. The same general principles apply to work and to exercise. If the washing has always been done on Monday morning, remember that it is not a sin to do half of it on Thursday. Don't make yourself play eighteen holes of golf if nine holes two days a week is more fun.

Economic challenges center around retirement. The problems of when, where, and how are multiple and individual. The woman who had been truly happy in her work or home will be happy in retirement. A woman who has put her whole life into work (and this is not a happy adjustment) will have problems in her old age. If she continues in her work, she is apt to resent new ideas and new people, and if she retires, she will resent retirement. These people are rarely so constituted that they can accept a position of less responsibility in the same work. In the professions, consultative work where experience is appreciated but responsibility is lessened can be a most happy solution. Community or charity service may give a woman the feeling of usefulness that is necessary. Sometimes starting a new job or business will be the best solution. For the woman who has gone to work in "quiet desperation," retirement may be wonderful release. One of the happiest patients I have known is a seventy-five-year-old former grade-school teacher who worked part-time in an adult education program for immigrants. She taught the subject she loved but in a different environment and to a different group.

The woman who works has her problems in retirement, but so does the housewife whose husband retires. As one woman said, "my marriage vows included in sickness and in health but not for lunch." This can be a second honeymoon but it still calls for the same adjustments, compromises, love, and understanding as the first one.

Several years have passed since Ethel K. called on her physician, fearing that she was losing her mind. Her husband, a mild, slightly deaf accountant, had retired six months previously. He had no outside interests and spent all his time at home. He kept the television on loudly all day, and daily his wife grew more nervous and irritable. Ethel was advised to look for a part-time job, while other solutions were suggested for her husband. Now she works happily in a bakery three mornings a week, and her husband, with a hearing aid, helps the minister with his accounts two afternoons a week. The rest of the time they enjoy each other's company.

Intellectually, the years after sixty-five can bring great rewards. There will be leisure to follow personal interests, but this must be combined with the discipline to learn, and the courtesy and will to adjust to new situations. There are few finer pleasures than at last to have the time to follow an interest that has intrigued one for years, and few more sad and hollow moments than finally to have leisure and discover that you have lost or never cultivated any interests or hobbies. The pleasure of leisure requires practice just as much as does work. If you want to travel, you should take some trips or start to learn a language before retirement. If you have a desire to paint, you should start lessons now, and if you dream of building a house, you should begin at once to collect information on it.

Although muscles and joints must lose elasticity, the brain need not. Psychological studies have shown that the slight decline in learning abilities is made up by added retentiveness. The blocks to learning are lack of practice and lack of emotional drive and confidence. Fifty years ago a person might have finished school and practiced a trade or profession without further study. Today, whether one is a construction worker, housewife, or doctor, he is forced to learn new techniques ranging from preformed concrete to frozen foods to radioactive isotopes. Perhaps this has been as important a factor in prolongation of life as medical advances.

Finally the courtesy of adjusting must be considered and evaluated. Adjusting to the times, particularly to new moods of the present, is really a necessity, for unless this is done, the woman can be as truly isolated as if she were deaf and blind. Preference for Bach may be perfectly natural, but you had better know something of the Beatles. It is fine to like Shakespeare, but one might also enjoy John Osborne. You may prefer the paintings of Raphael but also like those of Andrew Wyeth.

EMOTIONAL PROBLEMS

Emotional problems are most difficult. Fear and loneliness haunt many. Most of the older people whom we have seen have lost their fear of death. Dr. William Osler, professor of medicine, observed the deaths of 500 patients at Johns Hopkins Hospital and noted that "about nine of the 500 suffered bodily pain, eleven showed mental apprehension, two were terrified, one expressed exaltation, and one suffered remorse, but the great majority (476) gave no sign one way or the other; like their birth, their death was a sleep and a forgetting." Nevertheless, fear of incapacitation and dependency remain. These should be dispelled. Let us consider ways to allay such anxieties. First, talk about these fears with some trusted person—your doctor, minister, or a friend. One patient we saw had a slight stroke from which she made an excellent physical and mental recovery, but she remained depressed and constantly expressed a wish to die. Her mother had had a series of strokes, and she kept reiterating that this would happen to her. Further discussion revealed that her mother had been a most domineering woman whom she hated and resented. When her mother became incapacitated, she had come to live with our patient, who had taken care of her and suppressed her resentments. The patient was informed that, in the first place, she had made a good recovery, that she was financially independent, and finally, that she and her own daughter had a fine, mature, and understanding relationship. She began to realize that much of her fearful emotion about illness and death was complicated by guilt feelings about her mother and fear of her relationship with her daughter. It was explained and emphasized to the patient that however she may have felt, she did her best for her mother. The daughter was encouraged to express her love for her mother. The depression lifted and the patient was able to face her physical problems with equanimity and courage, and to enjoy the many years, twenty in fact, before she died in her sleep at eighty-eight of a massive stroke.

Another way to handle fear is to replace it by concentrating on the maintenance of health rather than worrying about disability.

Loneliness is a most difficult problem. For a woman who has had a happy married life, to face widowhood is desolating. When I need courage I often think of Jane L. She and David were devoted. They were both reserved and outside their marriage did not have much social life. When Jane was sixty-seven she had surgery for cancer of the breast; three years later her husband developed cancer of the bowel and two years later had a recurrence. His terminal illness was difficult and one day Jane said to me, "I pray to God every night that I will live to see him through this illness," and I prayed so too. Two weeks after his death she came to the office and cried, "What will I do now?" I said, "Your prayer was answered, wasn't it?" She looked startled for a minute, said, "Yes," straightened up, dried her tears, and left. A month later she came in to ask about being a volunteer at the hospital and as she left she said, "I am living up to a bargain."

To withstand the death of a child when one would be more than willing to go oneself takes even more courage. Loss of friends must be met with a willingness to make young friends and new friends. True, there may be "no shield against fate," but it is heartening to see the number of women who have the inner resources to meet it. These women grow by their courage and they help others by providing an example of fortitude and faith.

As I consider the adjustments that must be made to be happy and contented, I think how much easier it would be to write a prescription for unhappiness. First, be a martyr. Constantly emphasize that you have sacrificed your life to your husband, children, or employer. This will drive a husband to a club, hobbies, or drink; children to foreign climates; and an employer to urge early retirement. Second, complain constantly about your health. Don't follow your doctor's suggestions. After all, he is too young to know anything, and even his father, although more mature, was prone to error. Obviously, he misfits your glasses and hearing aid because he is in such a hurry; not, of course, to quite the extent that the dentist has misfit your dentures. Tell everyone about your sleepless nights. Even if you look well nourished, explain that you are unable to take a bite without repercussions. Let people know that you feel that government, religion, and education have deteriorated, and that modern literature, art, and drama are for delinquents and degenerates. Merely following one or two of these directives can bring a modicum of unhappiness. To be sorry for oneself brings great unhappiness and despair. These should be shunned, avoided, and discarded, even if the effort needed seems too great.

For the fortunate ones, the senior years can be the harvest years and the years of fulfillment. As John Donne wrote, "No spring, nor summer beauty hath such grace/As I have seen in one autumnal face."

PART TWO

A Concise Medical Encyclopedia
for Women

abasia. Inability to walk or stand, due to lack of co-ordination. May be caused by disease or, sometimes, by hysteria.

abdominal enlargement. When confronted with this condition, the doctor looks for excess fat, fluid in the abdomen, an ovarian cyst, gas in the digestive tract, a loaded colon, fibroids (fibrous or muscular tumors), a normal or false pregnancy. Excessive enlargement may signify multiple pregnancy.

abdominal pain. Because the abdomen contains so many important organs, pain in that region can arise from various causes. Diagnosis in this area is one of a doctor's most difficult and delicate tasks. A "stomach ache" may be caused simply by overeating or by highly spiced foods, too much smoking or drinking, nervous tension or anxiety, emotional strain, fear, or by gas in the stomach or intestines.

Abdominal pain that continues, even if it is not severe, or that comes on suddenly and severely, may mean a more serious condition. Laxatives must not be taken to relieve such pains.

Inflammation of the appendix is a frequent cause of abdominal pain. It is usually a dull pain that gradually localizes in the lower right sector and hurts when pressed. In adults the gall bladder may be the cause of the pain. The gall ducts may be blocked by a stone or the gall bladder may be swollen or infected. The body's attempt to pass a stone from the kidney or gall bladder may cause serious pain.

Worms and other parasites may also cause acute pain.

Deficiency conditions, such as pernicious anemia or sprue, also can cause considerable distress. In children particularly, communicable diseases such as pneumonia and infectious mononucleosis can also bring on abdominal pain.

Young children can also develop an intestinal obstruction with severe cramps and spasms known as intussusception. This occurs when part of the bowel is telescoped into itself. It requires immediate medical attention.

A sudden, agonizing pain in this part of the body may be the result of a perforated ulcer of the stomach or duodenum and such an attack demands a doctor without delay.

Women may have abdominal pain related to the uterus which develops cramps. A twisted ovary may cause abdominal pain on the side involved. Interference with the flow of urine may also produce pain. Especially serious is pregnancy in the tube which passes from the ovary to the uterus. This is known as ectopic pregnancy.

abdomen. The cavity of the body below the chest and above the pelvis. The principal organs in it are the stomach, the intestines, the gall bladder, liver, spleen, pancreas, lymph glands, kidneys, and bladder. In women it also contains the ovaries, uterus, and Fallopian tubes. The skin over the abdomen shows special gray streaks after pregnancy.

aberrant. Wandering from the normal place, as an aberrant kidney or spleen; in cancer, aberrant cells.

ablatio placentae. In pregnancy, premature displacement of the placenta. The symptoms are bleeding, pain, and contraction of the uterus. Treatment is for shock and the replacement of the lost blood.

abortion. The expulsion of the fetus from the uterus during the first three months of pregnancy. Abortion may be spontaneous (due to some abnormality in the growing fetus) or induced. Induced abortion may either be therapeutic or criminal. The Roman Catholic Church forbids induced abortion. Therapeutic abortion is considered necessary for the sake of the mother in toxemia of pregnancy, in heart disease when failure is probable, when there is the possibility of starting again a once inactive tuberculosis, in malignant and other diseases of the uterus, in insanity, or when the mother has had rubella (German measles) in the first three months of pregnancy.

Spontaneous abortion can be caused by extreme exertion or an accident such as a bad fall. Infectious diseases or poisons may also cause abortion. A first symptom of spontaneous abortion may be vaginal bleeding, especially if there is also a pain in the lower abdomen or back. Any such bleeding should be reported to the doctor immediately and the pregnant woman should go to bed at once.

The word "miscarriage" is used when the abortion occurs after the fourth month but before the seventh month of pregnancy. Babies are called "premature" when delivered after the beginning of the seventh month but before full term.

Almost half the women in the United States have had a miscarriage or spontaneous abortion before they are thirty years old. About one-third of the abortions are spontaneous, the other two-thirds are induced.

abscess. A cavity full of pus and surrounded by an inflamed area. It is usually caused by streptococcic or staphylococcic bacteria. White blood cells gather at the point of infection to contain it and destroy the invading bacteria. The painful red area around the abscess is due to the concentration of blood and the pressure of the pus on the nerves. In women, abscesses often occur in the glands of the outer sex organs.

When the abscess comes to a head, it will burst but there is danger then that the infection may spread. A physician makes an incision and drains the abscess before it bursts. Sulfa drugs and antibiotics are frequently effective in controlling such conditions. Abscesses that occur in the lungs or the abdomen are extremely serious and urgently require professional attention.

absorption. The action of the skin, mucous membrane, and other organs in taking in the substances necessary to function.

abulia. Inability to exercise "will power." Hesitation, indecision, sometimes seen in the mental state called schizophrenia.

acarpia. Barrenness or sterility.

accommodation. The action of the lens of the eye in changing its shape when focused on objects at varying distances. After the age of forty, when the lens tends to harden, the ability of the eye to accommodate diminishes and glasses often become necessary.

Normal vision is acquired only gradually during growth and thus close work such as sewing or reading small print is difficult for young children.

accouchement. Childbirth (French).

acetone. A colorless liquid found in the blood and urine. Increases of acetone in the blood of diabetics is a dangerous sign, so tests are made regularly to determine its quantity.

acetylsalicylic acid. Aspirin. Used for the relief of the milder forms of pain and to reduce fever.

achlorhydria. Absence of hydrochloric acid in the gastric juices. These juices in the stomach aid in digesting food. Reduction of hydrochloric acid may occur normally, especially among older people. Small doses of the acid may be taken in water, before meals.

achondroplasia. Also called dwarfism. Abnormal development of the bones of the embryo causes the head to be unusually large, the arms and legs curved and dwarfed, but the torso normal. Most such infants are stillborn. Those who live to adulthood have unusually strong muscles. Sexual and mental development are not affected nor is longevity.

Achromycin. The trade name for a yellow-colored antibiotic similar to Aureomycin or chlortetracycline. Chemically known as tetracycline.

acidosis. *See* DIABETES.

acne. A chronic inflammatory disorder of the sebaceous (oil) glands of the skin, usually resulting in surface eruptions. These eruptions, caused by the overactivity and blocking of the tiny glands and hair follicles just below the skin surface, include whiteheads, blackheads, and pimples.

Acne usually occurs between the ages of twelve and twenty, beginning just before puberty and ending with adulthood.

acne rosacea. A skin disease similar to common acne. The face is flushed, usually about the nose, though redness may spread to the forehead and neck. Small dilated blood vessels then appear and later the flushed areas develop tiny pimples which are more superficial than in acne and do not leave scars.

acrodynia. A disease that occurs in children, usually between four months and three years of age. Painful red swollen hands and feet, muscular pains that make movement difficult, loss of energy, and general mental and physical sluggishness are the chief symptoms. Acrodynia is also called "pink disease" because of a rash which colors the skin. A dietary deficiency is believed to be responsible.

acromegaly. A chronic condition in which the extremities and some soft parts of the body continue to grow after normal growth has stopped. The jaws and mouth, the nose, and the hands and feet are most often affected. The condition results from excessive action of the anterior part of the pituitary gland, which secretes the special substance, or hormone, which ordinarily brings about normal growth during childhood and youth. A related condition is giantism, in which overgrowth affects all parts of the body.

The first symptom of acromegaly is enlargement of the soft tissues, which may include the lips, tongue, ears, and nose. This is closely followed by excessive growth in associated bones, such as the lower jaw and the hands and feet. Gradually the face assumes a gross appearance, the hands become pawlike, and enlargement of the vocal cords deepens the voice. The entire body begins to show hair growth. The function of the sex glands is disturbed and, contrary to popular myth, the sexual power of the acromegalic is impaired rather than heightened. Women who have the disease rarely bear children.

ACTH. An abbreviation of adrenocorticotrophic hormone. The adrenocorticotrophic hormone of the pituitary acts upon the adrenal gland to produce cortisone. ACTH is not manufactured synthetically, as is cortisone, but is secured from the pituitary glands of cattle and hogs, and has been widely used in the relief of rheumatoid arthritis and of pain provoked by a variety of other diseases. The hormone is also used in a number of other conditions. *See also* CORTISONE.

acute illness, acute pain. In describing an illness, the term "acute" indicates a relatively abrupt onset with evident symptoms and limited duration. Acute illness is distinguished from chronic illness, in which pain or discomfort is present at a less intense level for an indefinite period of time.

addiction. Known to medical science

also as pharmacopsychosis, is the habitual use of alcohol, drugs, and similar substances. *See also* DRUG ADDICTION.

Addison's disease. When the two adrenal glands, each of which lies above a kidney, become infected or damaged in any way, the resulting condition is Addison's disease, named after a British physician who identified the disorder. Although the severity varies, the disease is always serious. The adrenal glands are so vital that death comes quickly if they are completely destroyed or removed.

adenitis. An inflammation of the lymph glands which occurs in the neck, armpit, groin, and other parts of the body. The area is generally swollen and tender. Among women particularly a rather frequent complaint is infection of a gland called Bartholin's gland, which is part of the structure of the external genitals. This gland may become involved in an infection and thus become inflamed. When inflammation occurs, it becomes red, swollen, and painful, and squeezing may cause a flow of infectious material exactly as with a pimple. Since even moderate movements may cause pain, doctors recommend rest in bed, the giving of a suitable antibiotic drug, and sometimes Sitz baths. Occasional application of an ice bag relieves pain and a hot-water bag will also give relief from pain through decreasing inflammation. Should the infection become worse, the physician can usually do minor surgery exactly as he would for a boil or furuncle.

adenoidectomy. The surgical removal of the adenoids.

adenoids. Enlargements of the band of lymphoid tissue situated in the back of the nose where the nasal opening joins the throat. When adenoids become inflamed or infected they enlarge, and because of their location obstruct the passage of air from the nose into the throat. This condition is one of the most common causes of ear infection and sinusitus in children.

Infected adenoids, if untreated, usually remain enlarged and cause other disturbances. Breathing is done through the mouth, and the air inspired is not filtered and warmed as in nasal breathing. Colds and other infections are common, appetite decreases, and listlessness develops. Characteristic structural changes of the face may take place. The mouth hangs open and the upper teeth become prominent and give the face a rabbitlike, dull expression.

A child with troublesome adenoids is apt to suffer from disturbed sleep and bed wetting, and will often awaken irritable and peevish. Hearing is often impaired.

In addition, infected adenoids are usually associated with infected tonsils. The child becomes inattentive and seems dull. Therefore, adenoids which are repeatedly inflamed must receive medical attention.

Early, mild cases can be controlled with antibiotics which usually will prevent more serious complications, such as deafness, kidney disease, rheumatic fever. However, the removal of diseased and enlarged adenoids and tonsils is ordinarily recommended by the doctor. The operation, though simple and short, is most effective. *See also* CHILD CARE.

adenoma. A form of tumor which occurs in the cellular tissue of a gland.

adenosis. Any disorder of the glands, particularly one that involves the lymph nodes.

adhesiectomy. Scientific term for surgical removal of adhesions.

adhesions. Generally the cohesion of adjacent organs or surfaces which are normally separate. When tissues heal, for example, fibrous scars are formed which cause the segments to adhere to each other. Following operations within the abdomen, adhesions sometimes cause pain when pulled or stretched because fibrous tissue is not elastic.

adiposis. Corpulence or obesity; an excessive accumulation, either general or local, of fat in the body.

adnexa. The adjunct parts of any organ. Adnexa uteri, for example, are the ovaries and Fallopian tubes, and adnexa oculi are the lids of the eyes.

adolescence. The period in human growth between the ending of childhood and the attainment of full physical development. During this period anatomic development and glandular changes culminate in puberty, at about the age of twelve for girls and fourteen for boys. In girls, menstruation begins at this time, although it may occur a year or two earlier or later. The breasts develop, the pelvis broadens, and the body becomes more rounded, acquiring distinctive female characteristics. In boys, hair grows on the face, sexual organs mature, and the larynx enlarges, causing the voice to "break."

In both sexes the physical changes are associated with emotional and mental development. The rapid growth at this time is likely to make heavy demands on the adolescent and adjustment to the glandular changes as well as the whole growth process is often difficult. Reactions to situations are apt to be keener and more immediate; feelings, whether of joy or depression, become more intense than previously. The boy may become concerned that he is not growing as fast as his friends, or that his voice cracks, or by the appearance of hair on his face and body. The girl may regard with embarrassment the beginning of menstruation and its recurrence every month.

Parents, during this period, may be alarmed at what appears to be erratic growth and rapidly shifting moods in their children, who want love and attention one minute and "to be left alone" the next. However, if the proper foundation of love and security has been laid during infancy and childhood, the adolescent years can be productive and rewarding for both parents and children. By gradually preparing the child for the physical changes that will take place, including giving her the necessary information about sex and reproduction, the shock of the onset of awakening maturity can be softened.

Even with understanding and sympathy, the adolescent will often still be subject to tensions, rebellion, and conflicting emotions. The pe-

riod of adolescence may demand a large measure of patience and tolerance from the parents. Faced with hostile parental attitudes, the growing child may develop feelings of insecurity that find understandable but often undesirable outlets. While the adolescent may rebel against authority in the home, acceptance and approval by her group is of paramount importance to her. Few influences will shake her from conformity to teenage standards and values. The change from dependence upon parents and home to identification with her peer group is a natural step in the process of maturing.

Hero worship, romantic attachments that may ripen and wilt in rapid succession, called crushes, and an intense desire for privacy are normal behavior manifestations of the adolescent. Unless the phase becomes too intense or prolonged, authorities on child development consider that parents should not intervene since ordinarily time and growing maturity will limit or terminate it.

The proper attitudes on the part of the parents can be of immeasurable help in assuring that the period of adolescence is a significant and meaningful step toward maturity. *See also* Chapter II.

adrenal glands. The adrenals are a significant part of the system of endocrine glands which control and co-ordinate, by means of specialized secretions, many of the body's most essential functions.

So essential to life are the adrenals, particularly the cortex, that when they are removed experimentally from an animal, it dies within a few days. Similarly, destruction of the adrenals by infection or injury causes death.

The adrenal cortex secretes many hormones, including cortisone, dihydrocortisone, and aldosterone. The cortical hormones are significant in the basic defenses of the body against various infections, poisons, and other invasions or threats. They are also concerned with the regulation of the supply of salt and water and the maintenance of correct blood pressure.

Adrenalin. The trade name for epinephrine, is a hormone produced by the adrenal glands.

This drug stimulates heart action, elevates blood pressure, constricts blood vessels, and tends to stop bleeding in wounds. Adrenalin is used to relax the muscles in the bronchial tubes, thus making it an invaluable aid in the treatment of severe asthmatic attacks. This drug is also used extensively to counteract hypersensitivity and allergic reactions.

aerobic. Refers to the need of free oxygen or air required for life. The term is used in connection with bacteria that demand oxygen to survive. Anaerobic bacteria live only without oxygen.

aero-otitis media. A painful condition of the ear caused by inflammation of the middle ear. This disorder affects some people during changes of altitude—for example, when descending in airplanes from high altitudes. Swallowing helps to relieve the condition. Symptoms like congestion and painful inflammation may be followed by temporary or permanent impairment of hearing. Relief usually follows quickly. However, if the pain continues and is not relieved by simple ordinary medication, a physician should be consulted.

aerophagia. A condition caused by swallowing an excessive amount of air either consciously or unconsciously. It is apt to cause belching and stomach discomfort and is most common in children and hysterical persons.

afferent nerves. Sensory nerves that transmit impulses from the outside to the central nervous system.

afterbirth. Or placenta. A tissue which carries nutrition and oxygen to the child while it is in the mother's womb. Together with the umbilical cord and membranes it is expelled from the uterus after the child has been born; hence "afterbirth."

afterpains. Spasmodic cramps in the lower abdomen which resemble labor pains, though are not as severe, and may occur for two or three days after childbirth. These pains develop from the efforts of the uterus to contract to normal size again, and are stronger in women who have previously borne children.

agalactia. The condition following childbirth when the secretion of breast milk is absent in the mother.

agnosia. Lack of power of perception or recognition in one or more of the senses.

agoraphobia. Morbid fear of open, unenclosed places; as opposed to claustrophobia.

agranulocytosis. An acute, fever-producing disease characterized by high fever, ulcerative lesions of the mucous membrane in the mouth, throat, and other areas, and a great reduction in the granular white blood cells. The disease is rare, especially in children, and occurs more often in females than males.

Excess number of white blood cells, called leukemia, is extremely serious. Even more serious may be a sudden decrease in the number of white blood cells or their disappearance from the blood. The white blood cells are the chief defense against infection, and their sudden decrease or disappearance from the blood can lead to an overwhelming attack by dangerous germs which can cause death in a day or occasionally in a few hours.

In agranulocytosis, or granulocytopenia, the number of red blood cells is normal in amount, but the white blood cells may drop from 7500 per cubic millimeter to 1000 or even much less. Since, as a result, the white blood cells are so many fewer in number than the red blood cells, examination of one specimen after another may fail to indicate the presence of even a few white blood cells.

The severity of agranulocytosis is such that about 75 per cent of those affected die. Treatment of the disease includes—most essential—immediate rest in bed, cleaning of the infected areas, drinking fluids, and antibiotics like penicillin or Terramycin to control infection which develops easily in the absence of white blood cells. Any remedies must be prescribed by the doctor, in conjunction with regular examination of the blood to indicate the

progress or remission of the disease.

ague. The former name of malaria. It also describes chills associated with intermittent fever and various other conditions.

akinetic. Refers to loss or impairment of muscular action and power of movement from any cause.

albino. A person in whom melanin, the dark pigment which gives color to skin, hair, and part of the eye, is absent. The hair of the albino is platinum blond, and the skin is pink, since the blood circulating in the skin capillaries shows through the skin. The eyes have a distinctive pinkish hue because pigment is absent from the iris and the blood vessels are reflected through the pupil. Sometimes this lack of pigmentation of the eye may cause defective vision and create extreme sensitivity to light, and therefore direct exposure to the sun should be avoided by albinos. Ordinarily an albino has less energy and is more delicate than other persons. While the condition is abnormal in these respects, albinism is not considered a disease. If both parents carry the albino gene their offspring are certain to be albinos. The condition, however, tends to be recessive and about one person in 10,000 is affected. When albinism is present in a family, a physician can usually estimate the chance of its recurrence in future generations.

albumin. A clear, thick substance soluble in water and coagulated by heat, is one of a group of protein substances, the chief element of most animal and vegetable tissues, and the most significant part of blood serum or plasma. The largest component of egg white is albumen. If there is albumen in the urine, it coagulates when heated.

albuminuria. The presence of albumin in the urine which can be easily detected by examination. It is an early sign that the kidneys are not functioning properly. Sometimes, however, albuminuria may occur temporarily as a consequence of a high protein diet or following strenuous exercise. *See also* KIDNEYS.

alcohol. Ordinarily alcohol refers to ethyl alcohol, a clear, colorless fluid which is fit for human consumption when diluted. Alcohol is inflammable and has a characteristic taste and odor. It is obtained by distilling fermented solutions of sugar, grain, or starchy substances, or it may be prepared artificially. Whiskey, gin, rum, beer, ale, stout, wine, and brandy are some of the alcoholic beverages in common use.

Small doses of alcohol are stimulating and produce a temporary sense of warmth and well-being. Alcohol dilates the blood vessels of the skin and brings an increased flow of warm blood to the skin surfaces. However, the blood in the body is cooled off by this action and body temperature drops. Alcohol also depresses the central nervous system, and acts as an anesthetic upon the cerebral cortex, which controls behavior. When a person brightens up after a drink or speaks and acts more freely than usual, she does so because the restraining influences which she usually exercises have been diminished. Moderate drinking, even as a daily

habit, is practiced by many people without harmful effects. However, excessive amounts of alcohol may act as a poison and seriously damage the body.

Alcohol is quickly burned in the body and has little food value. The body does not have a way of storing alcohol, and excessive amounts irritate the stomach and cause chronic gastritis. Constant excessive drinking may also damage the liver, the kidneys, and other body organs. The central nervous system becomes depressed, and with continued indulgence the entire system is damaged. Co-ordination of muscles and nerves is diminished, speech becomes thicker, gait and sense of balance are impaired, judgment suffers, mental changes are apparent. Constant excessive use of alcohol often leads to stupor, delirium tremens, or other manifestations of serious damage.

alcoholism. Poisoning by alcohol, or the severe results of prolonged and excessive consumption of alcohol. The alcoholic has a compulsive need for alcohol and can abstain only with great difficulty or not at all. Usually she is totally unable to help herself out of her situation. The causes of alcoholism are deeply rooted in the varying needs and insecurities of the person affected. There is no such thing as an "alcoholic type." An alcoholic may drink steadily day after day or she may have short periods of abstinence followed by a drinking bout.

The effects of alcoholism are serious, both mentally and physically. The compulsive drinker gradually loses her desire for food and may develop dangerous malnutrition with all its varying symptoms. The liver may become enlarged, the heart damaged, and other organs affected. The central nervous system is depressed, and a steady and progressive disintegration of personality takes place.

If alcoholism continues, the person will eventually develop delirium tremens, in which she loses all sense of time, space, and surroundings and is racked by terrifying visual hallucinations. During this time, many alcoholics have seriously injured themselves in their efforts to escape from their hallucinations. The condition lasts for from three to seven days and requires emergency treatment. Afterward the alcoholic will usually revert to her usual state. Death may result from an attack of delirium tremens if hospitalization and competent medical care are not secured.

Hospitalization is desirable in treating the compulsive drinker who wishes to be cured. Physical factors are a significant part of alcoholism, and treatment includes both medical as well as psychological care. The influence of the endocrine glands, hormones, metabolism, and diet on alcoholism is being investigated. New tranquilizing drugs, such as chlorpromazine and Miltown, when used with discretion, have been helpful, and a drug called Antabuse is sometimes used to condition the alcoholic against drinking. After the first stages of recovery have been reached, the alcoholic may respond to psychiatric treatment. Group therapy, in which victims of a common affliction meet and talk, has proved helpful.

Among the many organizations dedicated to helping the alcoholic, the best known is Alcoholics Anonymous, a group of men and women who have overcome alcoholism, and who actively help others to do so. Their sympathetic understanding of the problems of the compulsive drinker, based upon their own experiences, and their philosophy of mutual help have proved to be one of the most effective adjuncts in treating alcoholism. Alcoholics Anonymous has branches in almost every city in the United States and in many countries throughout the world.

The combined efforts of medicine, psychiatry, and organizations like Alcoholics Anonymous have brought about an increasing rate of recovery in what was once considered a hopeless problem. *See also* ANTABUSE; DELIRIUM TREMENS.

alexia. Sometimes called word blindness, a form of aphasia in which the victim is unable to recognize or understand printed words. The difficulty may result from damage to the brain by disease or injury.

alimentary canal. The digestive tract of the body is a long muscular tube which begins at the mouth and ends at the anus. The stomach and intestines hold, digest, and prepare food for absorption into the bloodstream, and eliminate the indigestible residue. By this route the body rids itself of any excess accumulations of mineral substances. *See also* DIGESTION; STOMACH.

allergy. A reaction to a particular substance by a person sensitive to that substance. The condition was originally called hypersensitivity, but allergy is now the term most frequently used.

Allergy is among the most common of all human disorders. It can be associated with an innumerable variety of substances, including pollens, foods, dust, animal dander, drugs, cosmetics, toilet articles, dyes, chemicals, and fabrics. Asthma, hay fever, and other major allergic disturbances affect a tenth of the population; and a much greater number of persons are subject to more limited allergies such as poison ivy, which is so common that it is rarely recognized as an allergy. Allergic symptoms may result from substances inhaled (dust, pollen, and animal dander), eaten or drunk (foods), touched (soap, wool, and cosmetics), and injected (insect bites). Sunlight and heat or cold may aggravate allergic response, as may bacteria, microorganisms, or other large parasites in the intestines.

When the substance called an allergen enters the body, the body reacts just as it does when attacked by virus or bacteria. It protects itself by setting up antibodies to neutralize any further attacks. These antibodies which the body has produced attach to tissue surfaces, and when the allergen, or allergy-producing agent, again enters the body it is believed that the antibodies separate from the tissue and attack the invading substance. A slight tissue damage results which apparently causes the release of histamines, chemical substances, which are carried by the circulation to skin and mucous membranes, with subsequent allergy symptoms.

As can be seen, two conditions are necessary to produce an allergic response. (1) The person must be first sensitized to a particular substance; she may not even notice the sensitivity. (2) A second exposure to the substance must occur, which then provokes the allergic symptoms. The reaction may be localized, if only a small area of skin is exposed to the substance, or it may be generalized, if the substance has entered the system. One part of the body may have a greater reaction than another because tissues in that part are more sensitive. The reason why a sensitivity to a particular substance exists in one person and not in another is extremely complex. Probably an individual structural or functional change is involved, a theory supported by the fact that, in some cases, allergies may be inherited. The adrenal glands probably contribute to allergic responses, and emotional attitudes also seem to be associated.

A wide variety of symptoms are caused by allergies. Since many of these symptoms are also characteristic of other disorders, it is necessary in treating the condition that the diagnosis definitely establish the cause to be an allergen. Hay fever affects the mucous membranes of the upper respiratory tract, the nose, and the eyes. Asthma primarily involves the lower part of the respiratory system. Some allergies produce digestive upsets, severe headaches, dizziness, and nausea. Sometimes a skin change, as in hives, eczema, and erythema, is the only symptom.

Food allergies are relatively rare and are almost always caused by the protein in the food. Foods which most frequently produce allergic reactions are milk, eggs, shellfish, peas, and beans, and hives is the usual symptom. In infants, milk, egg white, corn, oats, wheat, and barley are most often responsible and the allergic reaction is commonly severe eczema. Many chemical substances can act as allergens. Although skin change is the usual symptom, cramps, ringing in the ears, nausea, sore throat, leg and arm pain, and fever may be present. Many women are allergic to face powder, lipstick, or other cosmetics. The number of substances to which persons can be sensitive is vast and isolation of the allergen is often difficult.

To treat an allergy, the doctor compiles a detailed case history of the patient, including the first occurrence of the allergy, when it customarily appears, the patient's occupation, diet, cosmetics, clothing, habits, and many other small details. To establish what substance or substances are producing the sensitivity, the doctor may give the patient a patch test or a scratch test. In the patch test, small squares of absorbent gauze or cotton are dipped in various solutions containing suspected allergens and taped against the patient's skin, usually the forearm. In the scratch test, a minute quantity of possible allergens is placed in small scratches made on the arm. In both tests, the doctor watches for skin reaction to the different patches or scratches such as redness, blistering, or itching, which may indicate that the allergen has been isolated. Expert medical attention is indispensable in diagnosis and treatment, and the services of a dermatologist, or specialist in skin conditions, may be necessary. Basically treatment consists of locating the allergen and then avoiding the allergen as much as possible. When other methods are unsuccessful, injections of minute amounts of the allergen may be given to the patient to increase her tolerance for the allergen, a process called desensitization. However, desensitization may have only a small or temporary effect.

Drugs such as the antihistamines, Adrenalin, and ephedrine are often effective in relieving allergic symptoms, but do not cure the condition. In severe cases, the hormonal substances ACTH and cortisone may be used.

Allergies often appear to involve emotional factors as well as organic, and conversely the allergy may induce tensions which did not originally exist. The doctor must determine the place of these emotional factors in the patient's condition; sometimes all treatment for the condition fails until the psychological problems are uncovered and dealt with. *See also* ASTHMA; ECZEMA; FOOD ALLERGY; HAY FEVER; HIVES.

aloes. Aloes is used in chronic constipation for its stimulating effect on the large intestine. Large doses taken too frequently may irritate the kidneys.

alopecia. Loss of hair that may follow a number of different illnesses. The loss of hair may be partial or total, premature or senile. If hair falls in patches, the condition is known as alopecia areata. Alopecia cachectica is baldness as a result of general malnutrition.

alveoli. The small air cells of the lung.

amaurosis. Loss of vision due to nervous disorders and not to any structural defect of the eye.

ambivalence. The coexistence within a person of opposite or conflicting feelings, such as love and hate. It refers to impulses, conscious or unconscious, that contradict each other and may be symptomatic of schizophrenia. *See also* SCHIZO-PHRENIA.

amebiasis. An infection caused by an organism called endameba histolytica. Amebic dysentery usually develops and occasionally the condition spreads to the liver, in which case amebic hepatitis follows.

amebic dysentery. Inflammation of the colon, caused by invasion of a single-celled parasite, endameba histolytica. It has been estimated that from 1.5 to 10 per cent of the population of the United States is infested with this parasite, which enters the body in contaminated food and drink. Amebic dysentery is more prevalent in economically poor areas and in hot climates. The number of persons infested in any area usually remains constant, but occasionally an epidemic occurs.

Symptoms of amebic dysentery may be mild, with only fatigue and depression, or may include constipation, nausea, slight appetite, gas, and abdominal cramps. When the organisms spread throughout the wall of the bowel, there is severe diarrhea with excretion of blood, pronounced weakness, prostration, vomiting, and pain on the right side of the abdomen. Usually fever is not present or only slight.

Recovery is slow and the condition may become chronic, with anemia and occasional occurrences of more severe diarrhea. When the dysentery is not cured, the organisms enter the liver and lungs and form abscesses.

Amebic dysentery is often difficult to control and repeating the treatment may be necessary. If the liver and lungs have been invaded, special drugs are given.

The organisms causing amebic dysentery are hard to destroy, and can be carried on fruit, vegetables, flies, cockroaches, and water. Careful personal and public cleanliness is the best means of avoiding the illness.

amenorrhea. Absence of menstrual periods. False amenorrhea is most commonly caused by a congenital obstruction. A girl may show all the other signs of puberty but no menstrual flow. This may be accompanied by a general feeling of malaise. The symptoms become severe if untreated. The correction is usually minor surgery.

True amenorrhea may be caused by pregnancy, hormone misfunction, thyroid disease, Addison's disease, ovarian tumor, disturbances of the hypothalamus, alcoholism, morphinism, or chronic lead poisoning. Unusual emotional strain, such as major changes in living conditions which require great adjustment, can also cause amenorrhea. In adolescent girls the condition may occur during a severe emotional disturbance, such as an unhappy love affair.

amentia. Subnormal mental development. It is mental deficiency, such as idiocy which begins in infancy, adolescence, or is congenital. Amentia is contrasted with dementia.

amino acids. Organic compounds often called the building blocks of protein. They are absorbed into the blood from the digestive tract and distributed throughout the body to the tissues, which use them to build new proteins. Protein is essential to the living cells. The body uses amino acids to replace the parts of the body proteins which are constantly being destroyed or lost.

Amino acids are supplied primarily by meat, fish, poultry, cheese, milk, and eggs.

ammonia. A strong and rapidly acting stimulant used in smelling salts for relief in cases of fainting or exhaustion. The solution and vapors are extremely irritating to the mucous membranes, and concentrated solutions will burn the tissues, as do all corrosive poisons. The antidote for ammonia poisoning is olive oil taken by mouth with large quantities of water, or weak vinegar or lemon juice in water.

amnesia. Loss of memory, especially inability to recognize ideas represented by words.

The symptoms of amnesia are varied. Anterograde amnesia is loss of memory directly following severe shock or trauma. Auditory amnesia is an inability to recognize the spoken word. In retrograde amnesia, memory of all previous events is obliterated, and sometimes those incidents occurring after an accident are also effaced (posttraumatic amnesia). The latter is of variable duration and is a yardstick of the severity of the shock or injury.

Amnesia may be partial—as, for instance, losing one's memory for sounds, names, or colors—or it may be general with a loss of the greater part of memory. It frequently involves a sudden emotional conflict, and memory will begin to return when the conflict is resolved. Doctors often find it difficult to decide in these cases whether the inability to remember is actual or simulated. If someone simply refuses to remember, the diagnosis is difficult.

Occasionally one reads of a person who cannot recall her name or address. Psychiatrists believe that such persons suffer from amnesia because they have been unable to cope with certain situations which apparently were so painful that the only solution was to deny their identity.

Even in total amnesia certain habits are remembered, such as writing, walking, and reading.

amnion. The inner fetal membrane of the sac or bag which encloses and protects the embryo. It contains the amniotic fluid which surrounds the fetus until the sac is ruptured at birth.

amputation. The removal of a limb or an organ of the body, in whole or in part.

amyotrophic diseases. Those disorders that cause degeneration of muscle.

anaclitic choice. An early expression of psychosexual development, the opposite of narcissism. The object of love is influenced by the dependence upon the mother, inhibiting other expressions of the sex instinct.

anal erotic. Anal refers to the outer rectal opening. An anal character is one who has persisted in sexual emotion related to the anus. Psychiatrists characterize such people by orderliness in all habits, obstinacy, sometimes by miserliness, spite and a spirit of revenge.

analgesia. Insensibility to pain. May be produced by drugs known as analgesics, by anesthetics, or by nerve block. Analgesic drugs relieve pain without producing loss of consciousness. Among the milder analgesics are acetylsalicylic acid, commonly known as aspirin, and acetophenetidin, or phenacetin, both of which may be obtained without a prescription. However, recent investigations indicate that these drugs should be used with caution, and should be kept inaccessible to children.

Among the stronger analgesics, used for the relief of severe pain, are morphine, opium, and codeine, all habit-forming drugs which should be used only under the supervision of a physician.

analysis. In psychology, the diagnosis and treatment of emotional disturbances.

anaphia. A defective or absent sense of touch, or an abnormal sensitivity to touch.

anaphylaxis. The opposite of immunity. It denotes abnormal sensitiv-

ity and susceptibility to infection.

androgen. A male hormone that produces and controls the secondary male sex characteristics, such as the beard, muscles, deep voice. The male sex hormone itself, testosterone, is the primary androgen. The secretions produced by the testes include the androgens.

Women of childbearing age also produce androgens. Synthetic androgens are sometimes used, after menopause, to treat breast cancer and other sex-related conditions.

androgyny. Or pseudo-hermaphroditism, is the state of having congenitally malformed external genitalia resembling those of one sex while the gonads are those of the opposite sex.

androsterone. One of the male sex hormones.

anemia. In a healthy body, a balance is maintained between productive and destructive blood processes. Anemia, which occurs when the concentration of hemoglobin in the blood falls below a normal level, can result from any of a number of causes. Hemoglobin is the red coloring matter whose main function in the blood is to transport oxygen through the arteries to the body's cells. It is formed in the bone marrow and is normally found in the blood in a ratio of about 16 per cent. Anemia can be caused simply by loss of blood or it may result from a destruction of cells or from inadequate formation of cells. To treat an anemic condition, the doctor must first determine just what type of anemia it is and when this is established, correct the basic fault causing the anemia.

Anemia in a pregnant woman is caused by an attempt by her system to care more adequately for the growing baby. Since the blood of the woman must carry food, oxygen, and waste products for two beings, demands on the circulatory system are increased, which can lead to a dilution of blood, with fewer red blood cells per cubic centimeter of blood. Inadequate diet or vomiting tend to increase the possibility of iron deficiency and the doctor may prescribe iron and protein supplements to the mother's diet. Normally, a baby is born with enough iron in his tissues to last several months but if the iron supply of the mother is low, the baby will have a low reserve and develop anemia unless diet supplements of iron are given. Milk is a poor source of iron.

Anemias can follow a sudden blood loss from an injury or from internal hemorrhaging. In this case, the cells themselves are normal but reduced in number. Following a hemorrhage, the body compensates by adding fluids to the blood to restore it to its original volume. The blood is diluted by these fluids and the ratio of hemoglobin to total blood volume is lowered, causing anemia. It often takes time for the body to manufacture sufficient red blood cells and other substances for the blood to become normal. Symptoms of blood-loss anemia which result from the inability of the blood to carry enough oxygen include headache, general weakness, faintness, and dizziness. In more severe cases of blood loss, vomiting, intense thirst, a fast heart rate, and

weak, shallow breathing as well as the other symptoms of shock are readily seen.

Treatment of this condition includes, of course, stopping the blood loss where such loss is evident—as in the case of wounds. Blood transfusions are sometimes given to prevent excessive dilution of the blood. In less serious hemorrhages, rest and proper diet, including iron and protein for building cells, will be sufficient to enable the body to restore the lost blood.

In anemia caused by abnormal breakdown or destruction of red blood cells, called hemolytic anemia, hemoglobin is released at a much greater rate than it can be replaced. This is converted by the liver into other pigments excreted in the bile. When the manufacture of bile pigments is excessive, some appear in body tissue and give the skin and whites of the eyes a yellowish cast, the symptom commonly known as jaundice. In hemolytic jaundice, the cells are so fragile that they are broken down more rapidly than usual by the spleen. Without the spleen, the cells can function properly, and the spleen may have to be removed in such cases to prevent the overly rapid cell disintegration.

This condition is either congenital, as in sickle cell anemia, or may accompany various types of systemic diseases.

An excessive breakdown of red blood cells can also be caused by allergies, poisoning, malaria, severe burns, and other conditions. The treatment in each case depends on the basic underlying cause.

Nutritional anemias, which are caused by deficiencies, are characterized by defective blood formation. Most common and least severe is the type in which the amount of iron essential for hemoglobin manufacture is inadequate. Eighty-five per cent of the iron necessary is released from the breakdown of old cells, but some iron must be supplied in the diet. Symptoms of iron-deficiency anemia commonly include pallor, weakness and fatigue, faintness, and difficulty in breathing. It is easily diagnosed by laboratory tests and responds rapidly to proper diet and rest.

Bone marrow deficiency disease is another anemia caused by defective blood formation from decreased bone marrow formation. The red blood cell formation in bone marrow is highly complex and involves many functions of the body. In the marrow, the prospective red cells are larger than they will be when released and lack hemoglobin. Before the new cells are released into the bloodstream, they shrink in size and gain hemoglobin. When something prevents normal development, or the cells are released prematurely, the result is oversized red cells. To mature properly, the cells must have a substance from the liver called the growth or maturation factor. This maturation factor is identical or closely related with vitamin B_{12}. To absorb vitamin B_{12}, the body uses a substance called the intrinsic factor, which is found in normal gastric juice. Some anemias are caused by absence of the intrinsic factor and others by a poor supply of the maturation factor.

Pernicious anemia is characterized by the disappearance of this intrinsic factor and, along with it, hydrochloric acid in the gastric juice. Therefore, vitamin B_{12} or the maturation factor cannot be absorbed and the red cells cannot mature properly. As pernicious anemia progresses, changes occur in the spinal column, with weakness and numbness of the limbs and eventually a complete loss of their control. As well as the other anemia symptoms of pallor, weakness, and difficult breathing, there may be diarrhea, nausea, sore tongue, and yellow pigmentation of skin.

A specific treatment to restore the intrinsic factor and hydrochloric acid to the gastric juice is not known. However, in 1926, it was discovered that regular amounts of liver in the diet would control pernicious anemia. Today intramuscular injections of highly concentrated liver extract, sometimes in conjunction with vitamin B_{12}, are given instead of liver. However, this is not a cure and must be continued through the lifetime of the person.

Many other conditions exist in which absorption of material from the intestine is impaired as a result of diarrhea, excess fat in the intestine, or impairment of intestinal walls. Other anemias include sprue, pellagra, infestation with fish tapeworm, liver disease, myxedema, and rare ones whose causes are unknown. Most of these conditions respond favorably to liver injections alone or vitamin B_{12}.

Probably the most serious of the

anemias are those caused by destruction of bone marrow. Cells of all types rapidly disappear from the bloodstream until only a small percentage of the normal amount is left. It may be attributable to overdose of radium, X-ray, or severe infection, but usually the cause of the destruction is not known. Sometimes an improvement or cure is effected by repeated blood transfusions.

anesthesia. The absence of pain sensation, with or without loss of consciousness. Three forms of insensibility to pain are recognized: (1) general anesthesia, loss of consciousness; (2) regional or spinal anesthesia, lack of pain in a limited area; and (3) topical anesthesia, lack of pain on a surface area by direct application of an anesthetic agent. The concept of anesthesia is ancient and alcohol and opium were used for many centuries to relieve pain.

An outgrowth of anesthesia was the development of caudal anesthesia, in which the anesthetic is injected into the sacral canal. In "painless childbirth," the anesthetic is injected in small amounts, a continuous "drip injection," into the region of the coccyx and acts on nerves leading to the womb.

Improvements in the methods of administering anesthetics have accompanied the discovery of safer drugs. One of the most significant steps has been the development of the "closed system" of administration. In the past, ether was given by dropping it into an open cone held over the patient's face. In the new system of administering ether,

or supplementary gases, the gas is conducted through a series of closed tubes leading into a mask fitted tightly over the patient's face. This apparatus can absorb the carbon dioxide in the air exhaled by the patient, add oxygen when it is needed to the air inhaled, and add the anesthetic gases in the necessary concentrations. Anesthesia can thus be carried on for a much longer time and with much greater safety.

New and better anesthetics have continued to be developed. Ethylene and cyclopropane are in common use in many hospitals, although they have the one disadvantage, not yet completely overcome, of being highly explosive. *See* TWILIGHT SLEEP.

aneurysm. Dilatation of an artery or vein caused when a weak spot occurs in the wall. The layers of elastic tissue that form the wall enable the vessels to dilate and contract. When they are stretched at any point, because of innate weakness, the enfeebled section pouches out and causes distention, just as in the weakened wall of a rubber tire.

This thinning out, which destroys a section of the elastic tissue, may be the result of an infection such as pneumonia, or of a streptococcal or staphylococcal infection. Often, physical injury to an arterial wall leaves it so weakened that an aneurysm may eventually occur. If the blood-filled sac ruptures, a serious, often fatal hemorrhage may ensue.

Aneurysms are of various types. When one of the layers of tissue of the wall of the blood vessel also becomes the wall of the sac, a true aneurysm results. False aneurysms occur when the layers of the artery are all ruptured, leaving the surrounding tissues to retain the blood. Also the blood may force its way between layers of the arterial wall and separate them.

All arteries are subject to aneurysms, and a most commonly affected artery is the aorta, the large artery leading from the heart. The disorder may develop in a blood vessel as the result of an injury, and even though such aneurysms are smaller they are no less dangerous, and may prove fatal when they occur in the heart, brain, or other vital organ.

angina pectoris. Pain in the chest, a symptom which accompanies any interference with blood supply or oxygenation of the heart muscle. Men are affected five times as often as women, and the symptom is seen most frequently in the sixth and seventh decades of life, though younger people are also affected. High-strung, sensitive, active people are most commonly subject to it, and in 90 per cent of cases, arteriosclerosis, or hardening of the arteries, is noted. Persons with diabetes, high blood pressure, rheumatic heart disease, and anemia are more susceptible than others to angina pectoris.

The pain of angina pectoris is typically brief, seldom lasting more than three or four minutes. When longer, the cause may be something else. The pain is just under the breastbone and often radiates to the neck and down the left arm. Occasionally it may move from the chest to the right arm, the stomach, or back.

Any strong emotion may precipitate an attack of angina, especially grief, anger, or worry. It may occur in persons of any occupation, though less commonly to laborers because of their better muscular development. Angina pectoris is more prevalent in cities and cold climates, probably because of the faster paced life associated with northern cities.

Moderation is of the utmost importance in controlling angina pectoris.

The woman who suffers from angina pectoris should not despair of her situation. It is not a disease, but a warning of danger from the heart. One may live a fairly normal existence if she takes proper care of herself and always heeds the warning signal of pain.

ankle. Sprained ankle. Sudden twisting of the foot may stretch one of the many ligaments which connect various bones in the ankle area, and produce local bleeding, swelling, and extreme tenderness. Immediate application of cold compresses is helpful to reduce swelling, bleeding, and pain during the first twenty-four hours. Strapping the ankle with elastic bandages or adhesive tape relieves tension and mobility of the joint and hastens healing. Daily submersion in hot water and rest are also beneficial and soothing. The latest treatment includes injection of novocaine solutions for relief of pain, as well as hyaluronidase to decrease swelling, to permit earlier use of the foot.

Swollen ankle may occur in many

conditions, especially in pregnancy, kidney disease, heart disease, and in overweight persons because of impaired circulation. Women especially develop swollen ankles in hot weather.

ankylosis. Abnormal rigidity of a joint.

anodyne. Any agent that will relieve pain.

anorexia. The scientific term for loss of appetite.

anorexia nervosa. A condition most frequently found in young neurotic women, is characterized by amenorrhea and by a pronounced aversion to food, due to a hysterical condition. The patient may show an unwillingness to be treated. In extreme cases, the loss of weight may be so great that death may ensue if the malady is not corrected in time. Both psychological and medical treatment are necessary.

anosmia. Complete loss of the sense of smell. Loss of the sense of smell may be the result of a mental state, as in hysteria. In some instances of hallucination, the person imagines that he smells certain odors not actually present. Treatment of anosmia due to mental causes is difficult.

Defects of the sense of smell may be caused by dryness of the mucous membranes of the nose, by infection, injury, obstruction, deterioration of the nasal tissue, or by action of drugs. Certain diseases of the brain, brain injury, or brain tumor may also produce anosmia.

anoxemia. A lack of the normal amount of oxygen in the blood, due to high altitudes, low partial pressure of oxygen in anesthesia, cardiac failure, or strangling.

Antabuse. A recently developed drug used in the treatment of alcoholics to produce a distaste for alcohol. When Antabuse is administered to an alcoholic, extreme discomfort, severe nausea, vomiting, and flushing develop, with intolerance to alcohol.

Antabuse should never be given to a person who is intoxicated, nor should it be given without the full knowledge and consent of the person. The drug is best used in conjunction with psychotherapy. *See also* ALCOHOLISM.

antacid. A substance that relieves acidity and neutralizes acids.

antenatal. Denotes the time from conception to delivery.

antepartum. Refers to any occurrence or condition that takes place before the baby is born.

anthrax. A carbuncle, a serious infectious disease which not only attacks animals such as cattle and sheep but is also transmitted by them to human beings.

antibiotics. Substances produced during the growth of molds or bacteria which inhibit or kill other bacteria that cause disease.

The search for effective and nontoxic antibiotics is unceasing. Molds and bacteria are grown and examined for antibiotic substances by bacteriologists and mycologists. Chemists then purify these substances and prepare them as concentrates which in turn are tested in animal experiments by pathologists to determine their potency and toxicity before they can be employed for human use.

Among the significant ones are bacitracin and tyrothricin, and "broad spectrum" antibiotics, so-called because they are effective against many different types of infectious diseases. These antibiotics include penicillin, Aureomycin, Terramycin, streptomycin, Chloromycetin or chloramphenicol, Erythrocin, Erythromycin, Kanamycin, and the tetracyclines. These are used in the treatment of many bacterial, viral, and fungus diseases.

Antibiotics have been employed with dramatic success in rheumatic fever, bacterial endocarditis, syphilis, tuberculosis, pneumonia, and many staphylococcic infections. However, in some instances they have produced undesirable reactions, such as diarrhea, nausea, vomiting, and abdominal cramps, and may also cause serious damage to the kidneys or other organs. When used indiscriminately, antibiotics may lead to growth within the body of new strains of previously harmless bacteria which become drug-resistant and thus expose the patient to residual infections. Most doctors believe that antibiotics should not be used in conditions such as minor colds and sore throats which are readily controlled by simple remedies. The patient's response to antibiotics should not be endangered or his immunity to disease decreased by the use of antibiotics for minor infections. *See also* BACTERIAL ENDOCARDITIS; MEDICINE CHEST; PNEUMONIA; RHEUMATIC FEVER; STREPTOCOCCUS; SYPHILIS; TUBERCULOSIS.

antibody. A substance, natural or artificial, introduced to serve as a protection against infections or foreign proteins in the body fluids. Antagonistic to factors which are injurious to the animal organisms, an antibody can destroy bacteria adequately and counteract poisons that cause infections. Diphtheria and other antitoxins are typical antibodies. *See also* ANTITOXIN; BLOOD TYPES; GAMMA GLOBULIN.

anticoagulant. A substance or condition which opposes or prevents coagulation or clotting. *See also* COAGULATION.

antidote. Any agent used to prevent or to counteract the effect of a poison. There are specific antidotes for different poisons.

antigen. An immunizing agent which, when injected, produces antibodies.

antihistaminic drugs. Synthetic substances used to alleviate allergic conditions by diminishing the action of histamine.

Antihistaminic drugs are often ingredients of advertised cold remedies. The claim that colds can be avoided by taking such remedies shortly after the appearance of the first symptoms of a cold has not as yet been scientifically established. However, in combination with aspirin or phenacetin, or sprayed into the nose with camphor, antihistaminic preparations are useful in treating colds which begin with a running nose due to allergy. They also may relieve stuffiness, irritated eyes, and similar symptoms.

Antihistaminic drugs are not a cure; they may obscure the real symptoms and are occasionally harmful. *See also* ALLERGY.

antiseptics. Substances that hinder the growth and activity of microorganisms, or germs. Antiseptic agents differ from those which act as disinfectants, germicides, or deodorants. A disinfectant or germicide kills bacteria which cause infectious diseases; a deodorant destroys or covers disagreeable odors. Substances like chloride of lime can be used for either purpose.

In surgery, the use of antiseptics is essential, especially in disinfecting instruments and other materials used in operations. In first aid for accidental wounds and in the care of contaminated or suppurating wounds, antiseptics prevent infection from spreading in the body. *See also* BORIC ACID; MEDICINE CHEST; POISONING; WOUNDS.

antitoxin. A substance that counteracts the effect of toxins or poisons in the body produced by harmful organisms, such as bacteria that cause disease. Antitoxins may be developed by the body itself or by the blood of an animal which has been injected with a toxin. Some of the blood is then withdrawn and the serum containing the antitoxin separated from it. This serum or antitoxin may then be injected into a person suffering from the particular infection. *See also* IMMUNITY; IMMUNIZATION.

antrum. A cavity or hollow space, usually within a bone. Most frequently it refers to the maxillary sinus, one of a pair of sinuses, in the upper jaw. Among others are the mastoid antrum, the pyloric and the dental antrums. *See also* SINUSES.

anuria. An acute kidney failure, caused by an obstruction in the urinary tract or a lack of renal function.

anus. The extremity of the rectum and the outlet of the bowel.

anxiety neurosis. A functional disease in which fear, or the physical evidence of fear, is shown without any obvious, rational reason. An example is the fear that frequently occurs with delirium tremens.

aorta. The largest blood vessel coming from the heart. It distributes blood to every part of the body through its system of arteries.

aphasia. An organic condition caused by lesions in the cortex of the brain which produces loss or impairment of the capacity to use words as symbols of ideas.

aphonia. Loss of voice because of hysteria or peripheral lesion.

aphrodisiac. Any preparation or agent which stimulates sexual desire. Actually desire is mostly mental so that drugs which release inhibitions may act as aphrodisiacs. Certain substances which have an irritating effect when excreted may stimulate congestion of the sex organs. *See also* CANTHARIDES.

apoplexy. In apoplexy, or "stroke" or cerebral hemorrhage, an artery in the brain either ruptures and bleeds or is blocked. The victim is apt to lose consciousness and some part of the body is paralyzed, at least temporarily. Apoplexy occurs most frequently in persons whose arteries have deteriorated with age or who have high blood pressure. Age tends to bring rising blood pressure and degenerative change in the arteries. As the proportion of elderly people in the United States increases, the proportion of people susceptible to apoplexy also increases and therefore apoplexy has become a leading cause of death. When younger persons have apoplexy it is frequently the result of a blood clot from elsewhere in the body obstructing a blood vessel which serves the brain. *See also* CHOREA; EMBOLISM; PARALYSIS; THROMBOSIS.

appendicitis. Inflammation of the appendix, more properly known as the vermiform appendix, a finger-shaped sac three to six inches long which projects from the large bowel, in the lower right quarter of the abdomen.

Infection and inflammation of the appendix are potentially serious because the infection may spread to the peritoneum, the membranous tissue which lines the abdomen. Acute peritonitis is a grave development and may be fatal unless treated promptly.

Peritonitis may result from appendicitis in at least two ways. The peritoneum is shaped to fit over the appendix, just as a glove covers a finger, and is thus in close contact with it. Accordingly, infection of the appendix may spread to the peritoneum simply by contact. Moreover, if an inflamed appendix is left untreated, it may rupture or develop gangrene. In either case, masses of infected matter will be discharged into the peritoneal cavity.

These possibilities demand that the condition be accorded immediate attention by a physician. Delay often unnecessarily permits the development of complications, renders treatment more difficult, and may possibly endanger life. Attempts to diagnose and treat the symptoms of appendicitis without a physician, by ascribing the symptoms to a gastrointestinal disturbance and administering a cathartic or laxative, may have serious consequences. Abdominal pain should never be treated with a cathartic or laxative without the cause of the pain being first established.

Appendicitis usually begins with a sick feeling, accompanied by nausea, lack of appetite, and at first a rather diffuse abdominal soreness. Vomiting may occur, and a rise in temperature is likely. Gradually the pain tends to concentrate on the right side of the abdomen below the navel and the muscles in that region tighten when pressed in examination.

appetite. The recurring and usually natural desire for food. A distinction must be made between appetite and hunger. Hunger pangs result from contractions of an empty stomach and are rarely felt by anyone who regularly eats adequate amounts of food. Appetite arises with the customary intervals of eating and may be influenced by numerous external and internal phenomena. Eating is one of the most firmly fixed of all habits, and appetite is usually a longing for something one wants to eat at a time when one habitually has or expects food. Ordinarily, a good appetite is considered a sign of health.

Appetite, however, can become excessive or subject to distorted impulses. Occasionally, people suffering from specific disorders, such as diabetes, gastric ulcers, or chronic gastritis, develop appetites out of proportion to their needs. In pregnancy or hysteria, unusual and specialized cravings may develop for particular kinds of foods, or even for injurious substances.

A close connection may exist between appetite and individual psychological experience. Children, for example, are apt to develop cravings without realizing the cause. Overeating may be a form of compensation for a major loss or disappointment, or a means of securing attention from adults who otherwise might not notice the child. Some children develop unaccustomed appetite from significant new events taking place about them, such as the birth of a new baby.

A person who has duodenal ulcer seems to have a special form of appetite. Her pain is apt to rise and fall with the stomach's desire for food. In such cases, eating tends to relieve the pain, at least temporarily.

Diminution or loss of appetite accompanies many disordered conditions, and is usually one of the symptoms of tuberculosis and anemia. Loss of appetite and refusal to eat anything is known medically as anorexia nervosa. Ordinarily, this disease is related to some form of emotional instability and is observed more often in women than in men.

Appetite can be artificially decreased by taking such drugs as Benzedrine, Dexedrine, or Pre-sate. These drugs are sometimes prescribed for weight reduction, but should be taken only on the advice of a doctor.

Investigation indicates that small amounts of cocktails and other alcoholic drinks arouse or increase appetite, although they hinder the stomach contractions associated with hunger.

arachnodactyly. Derived from the Greek words for spider and finger, a condition in which the fingers and sometimes the toes are abnormally long and thin. This abnormality has a hereditary tendency.

arches, fallen. A breakdown of the natural arch of the foot which is an elastic spring that supports the weight of the entire body. This arch, made up of numerous bones held in place by a series of ligaments and muscles, is a curved structure resembling an arc. Flat feet, a common complaint, may be caused by the natural weakness of the arch, but usually result from certain occupations which require long standing, or from injury or obesity. The condition may be corrected or benefited by wearing proper shoes or arch supports, or by exercises to strengthen the muscles.

areola. A deeper pigmentation of the area around the nipple appearing about the twelfth week of pregnancy. A lighter secondary areola may be seen, especially in brunettes, in the sixteenth week.

arteriosclerosis. Hardening of the arteries, a disease fairly common among older people. The walls of the blood vessels are clogged by deposits of minerals and fatty material and degenerate, losing their original resilience, and become thicker, tough, and more rigid. Arteriosclerosis represents from 25 to almost 50 per cent of all chronic circulatory disease, and is responsible for many deaths among persons living past middle age.

A healthy blood vessel can be compared to a hose made of elastic material. When the volume of liquid flowing through the hose is increased, the hose stretches to accommodate it, and when the volume of liquid decreases, the hose shrinks. This is exactly what a healthy blood vessel does, stretching and shrinking to accommodate the increasing or decreasing volume of blood flowing through it. But when the walls of a blood vessel become rigid and inflexible, as in arteriosclerosis, this accommodation does not take place and thus when increased quantities of blood flow through a hardened or sclerotic artery, the pressure within the blood vessel rises temporarily, sometimes to the bursting point. Actually the symptoms of hardened arteries develop largely from the effects of this condition on the blood pressure and the circulation of local areas of the body. Generalized high blood pressure throughout the body is not caused by hardening of the arteries, although the two conditions tend to be closely related.

The commonest symptoms of hardened arteries are drowsiness, periods of giddiness, headaches, and other manifestations of high blood pressure. Interference with circulation may cause cramps in the legs, which give them a bluish tinge. The most serious form of arteriosclerosis occurs when the blood vessels of the brain and heart are involved.

The specific causes of the hardening process within the arteries is not as yet fully understood and is the subject of much medical research. One theory, partly borne out by experimental work with animals, places responsibility on excessive consumption of fats. Another suggests that overindulgence of tobacco and alcohol somehow stimulate the condition, although this has never been proved scientifically.

Treatment for arteriosclerosis is generally limited to establishing the patient's comfort and peace of mind as much as possible, and encouraging her to take good care of herself. The patient is urged to relax and eliminate as much as possible the stresses and strains of daily living, since excitement or intense emotion may stimulate a greater flow of blood than the hardened arteries can accommodate, with the possibility of severe consequences from rupture and bleeding. A low-fat diet is often recommended, and heat treatment, either baths or exposure to hot air, has been found useful. Several new drugs are available which often prove beneficial when prescribed.

arthritis. Inflammation of the joints. At least seven million people in the United States are afflicted by various forms of arthritis, causing more days lost from work than any other disability except nervous and mental diseases.

Innumerable forms of inflamed joints affect people, and only a doctor can differentiate them. Arthritis may be caused by infection, by degeneration of joint tissues coincident with overweight or old age, or by deposits of uric acid crystals within the joint space, as in gout.

Arthritis may follow injury or be associated with allergy to medicine or to food. Occasionally joint pain may indicate tumor growth or inflammation of the nerves surrounding a joint.

Arthritis in women may be related to the function of the sex glands or ovaries. In postmenopausal arthritis, which occurs after ovarian activity has ceased within the body, relief is often obtained with small doses of sex hormones.

Arthritis due to infection of a joint resulting from tuberculosis, syphilis, typhoid fever, or gonorrhea is not as common now as in former years, because treatment of these diseases is now more effective. Joint pains due to allergy to penicillin or other drugs can be relieved by simple medications with antihistamines such as Pyribenzamine, Benadryl, or Neohetramine. Inflammation due to gout is treated by drugs such as colchicine, Benemid, Butazolidin, or Anturan. When the condition is caused by old injuries, surgery may occasionally be helpful in mollifying the scar tissue responsible for the pain. Neuritis and neuralgia, mimicking true arthritis, are sometimes relieved by large doses of the B vitamins.

Rheumatoid arthritis is somewhat more complex as well as more frequent than the types mentioned. While the exact cause is not known, certain factors have been established that definitely relate to the development of rheumatoid arthritis. Overfatigue, shock, injury, prolonged exposure to dampness or cold have all been thought to be associated with the development of this type of inflammation. Allergy has been postulated as a cause, as well as hormone defects. Rheumatoid arthritis often begins with pain and stiffness in a single joint months before other joints become affected. It strikes the fingers, hands, wrists, and knees primarily, but may also affect the bones of the back and the hips. The fingers develop a typical "sausagelike" appearance in which the middle joint of the fingers becomes swollen and tender. The toes are seldom involved, as opposed to gouty arthritis in which the great toe is commonly affected. Nodules may occur under the skin in about 10 per cent of cases, usually located around the elbows, wrists, fingers, and occasionally the ankles. They vary in size from a small pea to a large walnut, appearing and disappearing without apparent cause.

Although true rheumatoid arthritis tends to be chronic, sudden complete relief of pain and stiffness may occur for months or years at a time. In mild cases the disability may be scarcely noticed, but in others the victim may become bedridden.

In older people, and in younger ones who are extremely overweight, osteoarthritis or degenerative arthritis may occur. The average age of onset of this type is between fifty and seventy, whereas rheumatoid arthritis usually strikes before forty and may affect children. In osteoarthritis the signs of inflammation are few. The symptoms of pain and disability are due to degeneration or wearing away of cartilage within the joint and, unlike rheumatoid arthritis which may affect almost any joint, the knees, back, and neck are most commonly involved. Swelling may occur in the last joint of each finger, but nodes are not found under the skin. Whereas rheumatoid inflammation tends to produce permanent deformity of the joints, osteoarthritis does not usually have that effect.

Many effective drugs and treatments are now available for persons afflicted with arthritis, depending on the particular type. For those suffering from rheumatoid arthritis, the discovery of cortisone has been most encouraging. With the help of this drug, former cripples are able to lead active lives. Use of this hormone, isolated from the adrenal gland, followed the observation that pregnant women often are completely relieved of arthritis during pregnancy. ACTH, isolated from the pituitary, is another dramatically effective substance.

Unfortunately, cortisone and ACTH do not *cure* arthritis. They do *relieve* disabling symptoms. These drugs must be taken indefinitely, always under the supervision of the attending physician. Although the drugs were originally quite expensive, newer techniques of producing cortisone may soon make arthritis treatment relatively inexpensive.

Rest is essential for the patient with arthritis. While he can continue to work, he should rest for an hour or two each day, preferably lying down after lunch. In severe cases, hospitalization may be necessary.

Diet may be significant. Patients are advised to eat a well-balanced, high-vitamin, high-protein diet, rich in vegetables and fruits.

Reliance is especially placed on treating arthritis with dry heat, diathermy, massage, and exercises, in order to increase circulation to the joints, which may help retard the arthritic process and keep the surrounding muscles from becoming distorted or weakened. Many arthritis sufferers get considerable relief with hot, wet compresses. Aspirin, salicylic acid, and mild sedatives are also beneficial in relieving arthritic pain, especially in milder cases that do not require cortisone. People with rheumatic ailments feel better in warm, dry climates, such as those of Arizona and New Mexico. Wet, damp environments may aggravate the condition.

Orthopedic surgeons can do much to improve the control of deformed bones and muscles in arthritis resulting from any cause. This, plus the amazing advances made in the medical care and treatment of arthritis, should brighten the hopes of everyone who suffers from this disease. *See also* GOUT.

Aschheim-Zondek test. A test for pregnancy. A specimen of the woman's urine is injected into an immature mouse. If, after ten days, the animal shows signs of bleeding and maturing, the woman is 98 per cent certain of being pregnant.

ascites. Fluid in the abdomen. This is a condition rather than a disease. It may be caused by a cardiac or kidney condition or by a tumor.

ascorbic acid. An organic compound found in citrus fruits and juices, fresh green leafy vegetables like kale and broccoli, potatoes, cantaloupe, tomatoes, and straw-berries. Ascorbic acid is essential to the proper development of teeth and bones and the walls of capillary blood vessels. It is an aid in resist-ing infection and its absence leads to the once dreaded scurvy. Vita-min C is significant in infant diet, and is usually added two weeks after birth. Children may need a supplementary form of this vitamin, but only on recommendation of a doctor. An adult woman requires 75 mg. daily. *See also* VITAMINS.

asepsis. The absence of disease-producing bacteria. A wound is aseptic if it is cleansed and in a germ-free condition.

aspermia. Lack of, or failure to ejac-ulate, semen containing sperm.

asphyxia. Suffocation, coma, or un-consciousness caused by depriva-tion of oxygen which results in ac-cumulation of carbon dioxide and fixed acids. When breathing stops, no matter what the cause, oxygen must be supplied artificially or un-consciousness will take place, fol-lowed shortly by death.

The causes of asphyxia or suffoca-tion are many, the most frequent being electric shock, gas poisoning, heart attacks, brain injuries, smoke, and drowning. Babies occasionally suffocate in their cribs.

aspiration. The act of breathing; may also indicate the removal of fluids or gases from a cavity by suction.

astasia. Inability to stand in a nor-mal manner because of lack of co-ordination. Astasia-abasia is a symp-tom of neurosis in which the affected person is apparently unable to walk or stand and seems to col-lapse when she tries to walk or stand.

asthenia. Lack of vitality and loss of strength which creates a general weakness. *See also* EXHAUSTION; FATIGUE.

asthenopia. Weakness of the eye muscles and of visual power due to overuse or to errors of refraction.

asthma. A disorder of the upper res-piratory tract involving the lungs and the bronchi, characterized by wheezing, coughing, choking, and shortness of breath. Asthma is a symptom and not a disease; there-fore, remedial measures involve lo-cating, isolating, and eliminating the cause rather than treatment of the condition itself. Recently, asthma in children has come to be considered largely a psychosomatic disease.

About half the incidence of asthma is due to allergy-irritation of the bronchi by specific allergens breathed into the respiratory sys-tem. The balance of the asthma cases are brought on by specific in-fections in the bronchi. The aller-gens causing allergic asthma are the same as those which are re-sponsible for hay fever, and include pollens, organic dust, house dust, feathers, and so forth. Allergic asthma begins most often between the ages of twenty and forty, while asthma caused by infection tends to occur in older people, although it can occur at any age. The disorder is generally equally divided between men and women. In both types of asthma the mucous membrane of the bronchial tubes swells and the air passages are partially closed.

A sudden asthma attack is apt to

be more frightening than it is dangerous. The affected person finds herself suddenly unable to fill her lungs, and then when she has struggled to gasp in a partial breath is unable to expel it. The person in an asthma attack may bend over slightly to aid her breathing efforts. In prolonged or especially severe attacks, there may be evidence of cyanosis—the blueness of the skin that indicates that the blood had been unable to pick up sufficient oxygen from the lungs. Attacks rarely last for more than a few hours and are often of much shorter duration, although often the condition will persist for a much longer time in milder form with a slight wheezing noise evident in the sufferer's breathing.

Often, people who suffer from allergic asthmatic attacks will outgrow the tendency—however, this is by no means always the case. The asthmatic must learn to avoid the cause of her condition and to control it when it appears. *See also* ALLERGY; BRONCHITIS; HAY FEVER.

astigmatism. Faulty vision which results from irregularity in the curvature of one or more refractive surfaces of the eye. When the eye is at rest, and parallel rays are focused exactly on the retina—the seeing tissue at the back of the eye, vision is said to be normal. The human eye is nearsighted when the object seen is focused in front of the retina, or farsighted when the rays of light focus behind the retina. When parallel rays of light coming into the eye are focused at different meridians, or angles, the eye has astigmatism.

atabrine. A substitute for quinine, used in the treatment of malaria.

ataxia. Disorganization of muscular co-ordination so that movement can be controlled only partially. It is a symptom rather than a malady.

One of the best known ataxias is St. Vitus' dance, in which an abnormal nervous system, perhaps as a result of streptococcus infection, causes constant sharp twitching of various parts of the body. Another ataxia is multiple sclerosis, in which sections of the nervous system degenerate and form scar tissue, which causes partial paralysis, among other symptoms.

Parkinson's disease, also known as shaking palsy and paralysis agitans, manifests itself in trembling and loss of power in the muscles. Locomotor ataxia, characterized especially by muscular disorganization and disordered sensation, is the result of infection of the spinal cord by syphilis. Several other special ataxias are known, including that which affects children suffering from cerebral palsy.

Some particular ataxias are hereditary and make repeated appearances in the same family. Such ataxias, the result of a localized developmental failure in some part of the nervous system, may affect not only muscular movement but also the sense of sight, touch, hearing, taste, and smell.

In cases of cerebral palsy, lack of co-ordination, most commonly associated with generalized muscle weakness, is notable. Treatment consists of muscle-strengthening and co-ordination exercises. *See also* CEREBRAL PALSY; MULTIPLE SCLEROSIS; PARALYSIS AGITANS.

atelectasis. Incomplete expansion or partial collapse of the lung. It may be present at birth or result from diseases of the lungs or bronchi. It is a condition in which the air is lost from the small alveoli, or air chambers, in the lungs, giving the lung a contracted, solid appearance when viewed with the X-ray.

athlete's foot. A ringworm infection or dermatophytosis of the feet, is a superficial fungus disorder. It is not restricted to athletes, but is found in all age groups and in both sexes, although it occurs more frequently in men.

atresia. A pathological closure of a normal anatomical opening or the absence at birth of the opening. Atresia is the cause of crypto-menorrhea, or concealed menstruation.

atrophy. The normal or abnormal shrinking of an organ or cell which has previously reached normal size.

Aureomycin. The trade name for chlortetracycline, one of the newer antibiotics.

auricle. Either of the two upper chambers of the heart which receive blood from the veins. The left auricle admits blood from the lungs and the right auricle from general circulation.

auscultation. The detection and study of sounds produced by the lungs, heart, and other organs to help determine their physical condition. During pregnancy it is used to detect fetal life.

bacillary dysentery. An acute infection of the large bowel caused by bacteria which enter the body in contaminated food and water. The symptoms are diarrhea and cramps, it normally runs its course in about ten days and is rarely fatal. Sulfonamide drugs are usually effective against the bacteria. *See also* AMEBIC DYSENTERY; DIARRHEA.

bacilli. One of the main types of bacteria, so called because rod-shaped. Bacilli of one type or another are responsible for tuberculosis, diphtheria, typhoid fever, leprosy, plague, tetanus or lockjaw, and other diseases. Bacilli are also involved in the decomposition of dead organic substances, in acid fermentation, and in various processes of wine making.

backache. Like headache, a symptom rather than a disorder and, similarly, may originate from a multiplicity of causes. (Lumbago and low-back pain are words meaning no more than that the back aches.) The complex structure of the human backbone makes it subject to a great variety of disorders. Its vertical position, which enables man to walk upright and perform tasks impossible for animals, throws a burden on the spine which most creatures are spared.

Back pain and back ailments may be closely related to occupations in which the spinal structure is required to absorb more stress than it can tolerate. Continued heavy lifting or prolonged standing on the feet impose unusual strains and have a perceptible effect on the body, even during a single day, and may be responsible for back pain. In women, backache tends to become worse just before menstruation and after coitus.

Backache may also result from infection, overstrain, disruption of some part, injury, or failure to function properly in any part of the complicated spinal system. The structure of tissues of the back may have been defective from birth. Perhaps one or more of the many parts of the back have been injured or strained. Occasionally a slight difference between the length of the legs will put the whole body off balance and require abnormal effort on the part of the back to maintain correct position. Infection may attack any part of the back and is particularly troublesome when it affects the joints or the largest muscles involved. Tumorous growths may appear. Disturbances in the glandular systems and in the organs may indirectly be the source of serious back disorders. Malfunctioning of the parathyroid glands, for instance, may cause a general softening of the bones and thus be responsible for a fracture of the backbone. Diseases of the nervous system, meningitis, sciatica, encephalitis, and others also produce backache.

Backache may originate with conditions which primarily affect some other part of the body, or as a by-product of surgery. Conditions as varied as stomach ulcers, gout, and disease of the gall bladder can cause back discomfort. In women, stress and strain on the tissues joining the womb to surrounding tissues, either as a consequence of pregnancy or otherwise, often produce backache. Occasionally abdominal surgery heals in such a way that scar tissue develops in a place that becomes troublesome to the back. Finally, some cases seem primarily to have a psychological basis.

In treating backache, the doctor first endeavors to establish the specific condition involved and its sources. Sometimes this is simple to do, but frequently it includes extensive tests, X-ray studies, and collection of the fullest possible medical history of the patient as well as complete information of the conditions of his work and daily activities.

Excess weight, flat feet, and other structural conditions can and should be controlled. Frequently, braces which support and rest a long irritated tissue will bring relief from backache. Warmth and gradually increasing degrees of massage and exercise are also often helpful. For acute or chronic backache due to strain in the lumbo-sacral region (low-back pain), rest on a flat, rather hard surface is beneficial. Boards can be inserted between the mattress and springs to insure a non-sagging sleeping surface. As long as it does not have too much "give," the bed need not be too hard. Those who suffer from postural backache will obtain definite relief from sleeping on a flat surface and by improving their posture.

Some of the many products sold to alleviate the pain of backache do afford a temporary relief. Persistent back pains, however, are a sign of a deeper disorder and the doctor should be consulted.

backbone. The column of small bones called vertebrae which extends from the head to the seat, also called the spinal column or spine.

bacteremia. Blood poisoning, the presence of bacteria in the blood. When the body's natural defenses around the site of an infection have been temporarily disorganized, bacteria may enter the bloodstream. Such an invasion is called bacteremia. Symptoms are chills, heavy sweating, or general collapse.

Bacteremia is especially severe when caused by the entrance of staphylococci into the bloodstream from abscesses in the skin or bone. The migrating bacteria may set up new abscesses at distant points in the body, in the deeper tissues or in the lungs. Infections of this type can usually be controlled with antibiotics. *See also* PYEMIA.

bacteria. One-celled organisms, scientifically classified as members of the plant world. Bacteria constitute one of the basic and largest classes of micro-organisms. The term bacteria is preferable to the more popular name, germ, which indefinitely indicates almost any invisible, disease-causing organism. Although innumerable kinds of bacteria are known, only a few can live within the human body, and many of these are not harmful. However, other bacteria, known as pathogens, can produce such diseases as tuberculosis, diphtheria, tetanus, typhoid fever, and pneumonia.

Bacteria are extremely sensitive to the conditions under which they live. This renders them relatively susceptible to complete control. For instance, they do not survive a high degree of heat or a lower heat sustained over a longer period, especially when moisture is associated with it. Consequently surgical instruments can be cleansed thoroughly of bacteria by fifteen or twenty minutes of boiling. Complete dryness renders it impossible for bacteria to live, which is the reason that wound dressings are kept as dry as possible. Sunlight retards some bacteria and destroys others. Again, some germs, called aerobic, must have air to live; without it they die. Others known as anaerobic, can live only in the absence of air.

Disease-causing, or pathogenic, bacteria harm the human body by the poisons or toxins which they produce. Some of these are excreted while others are held within the bacterial cell until it is destroyed. One of the protective measures of the body against infectious disease is the production of antitoxins which counteract these bacterial products. In addition the body produces other substances which prepare the bacteria for easier attack by the protective white cells of the blood, which also leads to the disintegration of the bacteria.

Bacteria usually abound wherever any moisture is present within the human environment, and protection against dangerous bacteria is a matter of selective measures rather than an attempt to avoid them entirely, which would be impossible. Eating and cooking equipment must be kept thoroughly clean for the elimination of bacteria. The hands should be washed before eating, especially after prolonged soiling or contact with anything in which dangerous bacteria are likely to live, such as human or animal wastes. Likewise, bathing should be frequent.

Medicine has developed a formidable array of specific weapons against bacteria in addition to cleanliness, clean water supplies, and adequate sewage systems. Antiseptics, like iodine and alcohol, are available to clean wounds and instruments, and immunization procedures ward off many of the worst infectious diseases, such as diphtheria, lockjaw or tetanus. In addition the antibiotic drugs, like penicillin and the sulfas, are effective against a wide range of bacterial infections. The best protection is prevention, which means maintenance of clean conditions in and about the body. *See also* BACILLI; INFECTIONS; IMMUNIZATION.

bacterial endocarditis. An infection of the membranes of the heart cavities, which often attacks people who have had a previous heart disease. This condition also accounts for about 2 per cent of all organic heart disease, usually affecting young adults, although persons of every age group may have it.

Two forms of bacterial endocarditis are the acute and subacute. The acute form strikes suddenly and may cause death within a few days unless treated immediately. The subacute type comes on slowly and may also cause death within a year or so unless medical treatment is begun promptly. About 30 per cent of the cases end fatally, from various causes such as cerebral embo-

lism and cardiac failure, in spite of treatment with the new antibiotics.

A characteristic sign is fever, especially with the acute form, although intermittent fever is usual in the chronic type. Anemia is also a symptom, as is embolism, which may disrupt circulation in acute cases, and in some instances cause nodes to appear in the skin of the fingers and toes. Fingers may also take on a clubbed appearance. Other complications include involvement of the lungs and kidney. Effective treatment of almost all cases of bacterial endocarditis consists of the use of one or more of the various antibiotics, such as penicillin or Erythromycin, over varying periods of time.

For people who have heart defects and who may be susceptible to bacterial endocarditis, special care should be taken in dental or surgical treatment to prevent the possibility of its development. Such persons should be given large doses of penicillin or other antibiotics before any operation. *See also* ANEURYSM.

bactericide. Any substance able to destroy bacteria.

bacteriophage. The name applied to a virus which attacks bacteria.

bacteriostatic. Denotes the power of stopping the growth of bacteria.

balanitis. Inflammation of the foreskin and the tip of the penis.

balantidiasis. Or balantidial colitis, an infection by a species of protozoa, unicellular bacillus, called Balantidium. It is characterized by diarrhea and dysentery.

baldness. Or alopecia, loss or absence of hair. Baldness and spontaneous regrowth often follow infectious diseases accompanied by fever, including pneumonia, typhoid, and influenza. Serious hair loss sometimes follows childbirth and surgery. In all these conditions, normal hair growth returns without help.

The only explanation scientists give for the fact that many men do not suffer from baldness while so many others do is that baldness is largely hereditary. Most popular beliefs about baldness are untrue and exploited by quacks. Dry, brittle hair, dandruff scales, thinning of hair in the crown and temples, tight and itching scalp actually do not cause baldness. Nor is it encouraged by wearing hats, tight or otherwise. Baldness, formerly much more common among men, in recent years seems to be occurring frequently among women. *See also* ALOPECIA.

barbiturates. Derivatives of barbituric acid used in medicine as hypnotic and sedative drugs. Sedatives, or hypnotic drugs, are a valuable requisite to medicine. They can help break the cycle of insomnia in some cases, and restore the sleep pattern in others. Often they help to induce sleep when nervous and physical exhaustion has set up such a pattern of irritability that the person needs to relax for a long time. The inability to sleep can surely increase tension, making sleep exceedingly difficult. Sedation may be essential as the initial step to restful slumber.

Barbiturates differ in absorption and elimination, onset and duration of action. In the United States, the most commonly known barbiturates are pentobarbital (Nembutal), secobarbital (Seconal), amobarbital (Amytal), and phenobarbital (Luminal) which is the most slowly absorbed and longest acting.

Small doses of these barbiturates evoke drowsiness by depressing the functions of those parts of the brain related to mental activities. Therefore, physicians often prescribe these drugs to help patients with ulcers to relax and thus overcome contributing causes such as worry and anxiety.

Barbiturates are often subject to abuse. The physician with a patient who is psychologically disturbed endeavors to direct his treatment toward the eradication of the fundamental cause of the disturbance in preference to treating the symptoms by a long-term prescription of barbiturates. Barbiturates should serve only as a temporary bridge.

According to both state and federal laws, barbiturates are not to be sold without a doctor's prescription and there cannot be any legal refilling of a prescription without specific orders from a doctor.

Barbiturate poisoning may be mild, moderate, or severe. It causes about 1500 deaths yearly in the United States by the acute form, which is the most common. Women are more subject to poisonous doses of barbiturates than men. Some time ago, the U.S. Public Health Service investigated 547 non-fatal cases; 407 of them were women, and 140 men. Of these cases, 254 were accidental and 293 were attempts at suicide. In addition, poisoning may result from a pronounced sensitivity to the drugs. Drowsiness induced by a small dose may pass into a coma with an overdose.

The symptoms of acute barbiturate poisoning resemble, to some degree, those of alcoholic intoxication. Among the numerous mental symptoms are moral deterioration, aggressive outbursts, slurring of speech, and impairment of mental activity. A reeling gait, because of uncontrolled muscular action, rapid beating of the heart, disturbed digestion and vision, and, in severe cases, exceedingly slow and shallow respiration are other signs.

Mortality, which is at present about 8 per cent in all cases of barbiturate abuse, is highest in older people and in those with a weakened physical condition. Care should be exercised not to give barbiturates to people with liver and kidney disorders, since the liver is actively involved in destroying toxins and the kidney in excreting them.

barium sulfate. A compound formed by barium and sulfuric acid, used in taking roentgenograms of the stomach and intestines, because, when taken by mouth, it renders those organs opaque to X-rays, and subsequently the drug passes unchanged through the gastrointestinal tract.

Bartholin's glands. Small glands in the vulva that pour out a clear, thin, mucous secretion to lubricate the vulva during intercourse.

bartholinitis. Inflammation of Bartholin's glands, frequently caused by gonorrhea.

basal ganglia. Groups of nerve cells, situated internally in the brain substance. They control basic emotions

and deter muscles from certain movements which would occur if this area of the brain were injured.

basal metabolism. Metabolism is the conversion of food into energy in a living body. Basal metabolism is a measure of the chemical changes involved in the body at rest. The basal metabolic rate measures the speed at which basic, constant processes within the body are taking place and, in particular, how much oxygen a person uses in a given time. The basal metabolism indicates whether or not heat is produced at a greater or smaller rate than is normal for most people in developing energy from food and oxygen.

The basal metabolism of a pregnant woman remains at its usual level until the last two or three months before birth. Then the rate in this period will represent the combined metabolism of both mother and child.

When a basal metabolism test is made, the person rests after arising in the morning, without having had any breakfast, and breathes from a tank containing a measured amount of air. The rate at which the oxygen in that air is consumed indicates the level of the basal metabolism. A range of 7 plus to 7 minus, relative to the average, is considered normal. Some persons, however, have rates as low as 25 minus without ill-effect on their health. Children who are active and growing have a noticeably higher rate than the average. Various factors cause the basal metabolic rate to be greater than normal. Intense emotions, such as fright or rage, speed up the metabolism, as do certain diseases, such as hyperthyroidism.

The metabolism may also be measured by a chemical test of protein-bound iodine in the blood.

Lowered basal metabolism is noted in such bodily states as sleep or undernourishment. It is also found in persons who are anemic, have certain nervous disorders or thyroid deficiency. Inadequacy of either the pituitary or the adrenal gland may have the same effect, while excessive action by either can raise the basal metabolism.

Basedow's disease. *See* EXOPHTHALMIC GOITER; GOITER.

BCG vaccine. A vaccine used to increase resistance to tuberculosis, which is spread chiefly through direct contact.

bedbug. A common domestic insect pest; small, wingless, and light brown in color. Although it feeds on the blood of human beings, it is not, strictly speaking, a human parasite. It comes to the human skin only for its food and may, in the absence of human beings, feed on other warm-blooded animals. The bedbug lives in the crevices of bedsteads, floors, walls, wallpaper, and furniture. Usually it is carried from house to house on clothing and bedding, but it may also travel from one dwelling to another in search of nourishment.

Usually a 5 per cent spray of DDT, or one of the other exterminating preparations on the market, will be efficient.

bed sores. A bed sore is a degeneration of skin at a particular spot, which exposes underlying tissues and invites infection. At first glance, it may seem rather insignificant but actually, in a bedridden paralytic or aged person, bed sores are potentially so serious that nurses and doctors must continually guard against them. They are much easier to prevent than to treat.

Those persons most susceptible to bed sores are the chronically sick and the people affected by specific disorders of the nervous system. Protracted pressure on a particular area of skin, especially such as occurs from lying in one position too long, is the immediate factor.

Once established, degeneration of tissues in the area involved occurs, and ultimately leads to ulceration. Expert medical care for such condition is imperative to prevent extensive damage in the area of the ulcer.

bed wetting. Urination during sleep after the age of three, by which time normal bladder control is ordinarily expected to be established.

Bed wetting is an early childhood habit that is not easy to control. In the adult, urination is regulated by two nerve centers; one, involuntary, in the spinal cord and the other, which in turn controls that in the spinal cord, in the brain. The newborn infant releases urine automatically and the act is regulated from the spinal center in accordance with the need to empty the bladder. As the child grows and is gradually trained, the brain becomes involved in the conscious control of urination and eventually regulates it during sleep. Some children acquire this control earlier than others, but the average time is two years. If, however, this habit has not been well established by the end of the third year, medical attention is warranted.

The causes of bed wetting vary greatly. Physical reasons alone are often responsible, such as infection, inflammation, or faulty nutrition. A doctor will always examine a child thoroughly at the outset to determine whether or not such a factor is involved. Bed wetting may also be of nervous or emotional origin, and a large proportion of cases are of this kind. In such instances, attempts to control the problem directly are unavailing. Improved psychological adjustment is indicated and is the principal hope of curing bed wetting. Punishment is likelier to work in reverse, to reinforce the habit rather than break it.

Some young children urinate in their clothes during the waking hours, largely because they are too interested in what they are doing to bother to go to the toilet. The preferred solution to this problem is to explain the situation to the child, help him to remember, and praise him for adequate continence. Here again, punishment accomplishes little or nothing.

The following methods will facilitate bladder training:

1. Give the child plenty of water during the day, but no water or other fluid after 5 P.M.

2. A bit of fruit may be given if the child complains of thirst at bedtime.

3. Get the child out of bed to go to the toilet at 10 P.M. Awaken him sufficiently to permit him to urinate thoroughly and consciously.

4. When he awakens in the morning, get the child to the toilet without delay. Bed wetting often occurs a few minutes after the child's sleep has ended, if he does not get to the toilet promptly.

5. When diapers are finally omitted during the day, omit them also at night, but protect the bed adequately.

6. In "dry" suppers, omit milk, water, or cocoa for drinking, and do not serve milk with cereal or with dessert. Cook foods with milk when possible. Whole-grain cereal and bread are preferable.

If it is necessary to take the child to the toilet a second time at night, note the time when the bed wetting occurs, and then plan to awaken him a few minutes before that time. The interval between the first picking up and the second can be regulated to aid the child's progress. *See also* CHILD CARE.

bee stings. The injection of bee poison by a bee into the skin. A blister and a surrounding area of redness appear immediately, but usually all symptoms disappear within twenty-four hours or less. But some people have such a sensitivity to the venom that the symptoms are exceedingly dangerous and have been known to be fatal.

The poison injected by the bee is composed of acid and alkaline materials and a substance much like histamine, a chemical released into the bloodstream by allergies. Ultrasensitive people can be desensitized by being injected with small amounts of bee poison over a period of time, thus building up a resistance to it.

The bee stings by inserting a

sharp, fine, horny needle with two barbs into its victim. The needle with its barbs remains anchored in the skin. The bee, in its efforts to get away, presses on the sac containing the bee venom and the pressure empties it into the skin of the victim. Research has proved that this bee venom is a virulent poison, that it affects the heart and destroys the red blood cells, lowers blood pressure and contracts the muscles of the heart and intestines.

A person who has had multiple bee stings or is known to be sensitive should immediately rest, and the action of the heart and kidneys must be carefully watched. If the blood pressure falls too rapidly, and such symptoms as swelling of the body or collapse appear, a physician should be called. He must also be consulted promptly if the sting is on the tongue or in any other sensitive place. Relief is obtained by injecting or applying locally such antihistamines as Benadryl, Pyribenzamine, or Neohetramine.

Generally, and especially in the case of children, the stinger should be removed with tweezers, if possible. For relief of itching, a paste of baking soda, well-diluted ammonia, or soothing lotions may be applied. Vinegar is beneficial in stings of wasps, hornets, and yellow jackets. The wounds of insect bites should never be scratched.

belching. The eructation of sour substances, including acid of the stomach, air, or gas. People who eat too fast swallow air and then belch it back.

Belching has become a recognized part of baby care and has brought a new word into our language, burping. In nursing, especially with the bottle, the baby swallows quantities of air. As the small capacity of her stomach does not allow for air bubbles, these cause pressure and pain. The process of assisting the baby to bring up the bubbles is called "burping the baby."

Bell's palsy. Paralysis of the muscles of one or both sides of the face.

Benadryl. An antihistaminic drug used in allergic conditions like hay fever, asthma, urticaria, contact dermatitis, erythema, rhinitis, drug sensitization, serum reactions, and irradiation sickness. It has also been used to relieve motion sickness.

benign. When used to describe tumors, it means "not cancerous."

Benzedrine. The trade name for amphetamine, a potent stimulant usually taken orally in tablet form, and rarely injected. This drug has a powerful action on the brain, in addition to its ability to cause physiological changes similar to those produced by action of the sympathetic nervous system. This drug is prescribed by physicians as a stimulant and to cut down appetite in obesity.

The abuse of Benzedrine has become common among alcoholics, barbiturate addicts, and thrill seekers who turn to the amphetamines for the delusive sense of well-being and confidence that they cannot find for themselves. Among the symptoms of overdose and of chronic poisoning are nervousness, apprehension, tremors, insomnia, hypertension, and dilatation of the pupils of the eyes. Hallucinations and delusions of a paranoid type may be a psychotic consequence.

beriberi. A deficiency disease resulting from an inadequacy of vitamin B_1, or thiamine, in the diet.

Beriberi attacks the gastrointestinal tract and causes changes in the nervous system. Manifestations of this disease are multiple neuritis, paralysis, progressive edema, inflammation of the nerves, collection of fluids in the legs, changes in the adrenal glands, mental deterioration, and heart failure. In addition, there is a tingling and numbness in the portions of the body reached by the nerves affected, tenderness of the muscles, wasting of the tissues through secondary infections, fever, and general weakness and disability.

Occasionally invalids on greatly restricted diets suffer from a deficiency of thiamine. After surgical operations on the bowel, in cases of chronic diarrhea, ulcers of the stomach, chronic alcoholism, or after long infectious diseases, signs of thiamine deficiency may appear. Food faddists, living on incomplete diets, may show a moderate form of beriberi, and chronic alcoholics, who stop eating during their periods of drinking, often manifest the same symptoms.

biceps. The large muscle on the front of the upper arm.

bicuspid. A tooth with two cusps, or points. An adult with a full set of teeth has two bicuspids between each canine and first molar, eight in all. The bicuspid is often called premolar. *See also* TEETH.

bifocal. A system of lenses with double focus. Those who need different glasses for near and distant vision can have the proper lenses combined in a single pair of glasses. The smaller lens, for near vision, is placed below the center of the larger lens, which is for distant vision. These are called bifocal lenses and are said to have been invented by Benjamin Franklin.

bile. A bitter, bright golden-red fluid, manufactured in the liver and excreted into the intestines. Its function is the digestion of fat and its absorption from the intestines. Bile stimulates movements of the intestines, prevents fermentation of the contents, and serves as a disinfectant. It is essential for the absorption of vitamins A, D, E, and K, and is also known to have a mild laxative effect in its salt form.

Bile consists of water, bile salts, a little fat, which in part is lecithin, and pigments. Cholesterin is another ingredient, which appears to be a fatty substance but is actually an alcohol. Together with other elements found in bile, cholesterin is the basis of formation of gallstones in the gall bladder or the biliary ducts. Passage of these stones through the ducts is connected with painful spasms known as biliary colic.

Any obstruction of the flow of bile into the intestines results in the absorption of the secretion into the blood, and jaundice occurs when it accumulates there. *See also* DIGESTION; JAUNDICE; LIVER.

biliousness. In popular usage, a condition of digestive disturbance accompanied by headache, nausea, constipation, thick tongue, and other similar complaints. The word is scientifically a misnomer and rarely encountered in medical literature. It goes back to the time, centuries ago, when illness was interpreted in terms of "humors," of which bile was considered the worst.

The amount of bile in the body actually has little or nothing to do with whether or not a person is "bilious." Symptoms that accompany "biliousness" are due to one or more of many different specific causes. If the disorder is serious and demands treatment, the doctor must determine the cause in order to prescribe correctly. The term "bilious" does not convey any pertinent information except to suggest the presence of certain symptoms. Excessively rich food, migraine, eye strain, glaucoma, brain tumor, or other conditions may provoke the symptoms. Liver infections, by ameba or organisms of malaria, may be the source of the trouble. Hardening of the liver from various causes is another possibility. Severe infections induce destruction of liver cells. The liver has a safety factor of unusual size—in fact, seven times as large as necessary for minimum requirements—but even this margin can be endangered by persistent abuse through overeating and excessive drinking. The person who suffers from "biliousness" usually has discomfort and loss of well-being without particularly severe pain. He is easily tired and disinclined to work. The symptoms often disappear at midday when the person develops an increased appetite.

Sufferers of "biliousness" will feel more comfortable if they avoid rich foods such as pastry, chocolate, candy, and eat more protein-rich food. Alcohol should be omitted. Glucose, taken either by mouth or injected, will provide relief.

biopsy. The removal and examination for diagnosis, usually under a microscope, of material from the living body. This material may be removed by means of a needle, punch, sponge, or other instrument. Surface biopsy involves the microscopic study of cells which have been scraped from the surface of suspected areas. This technique is frequently employed when examining for cancer of the uterus or bowel. Scrapings are also studied, including those from the stomach, intestines, or other tissues.

birth, multiple. The birth of more than one offspring at the same or approximately same time, with all having been conceived at the same time.

Twins occur about once in every 90 births, triplets once in 10,000, quadruplets once in 750,000, and quintuplets once in many million births. Eighteen quintuplet births have been reported in the United States in the past hundred years, and approximately 75 authenticated quintuplet births have been reported throughout the world. As is most often the case, few of the infants survived. Sextuplet births have been reported on five occasions, without survivals. Twins are most common among Negroes and least common in Orientals. Frequency of twins seems to be related to hereditary factors in both parents and is more often seen in women past thirty who have had large families. If a woman has had one set of twins, she is ten times as likely as other women to have another set.

Twins may develop from one egg, in which case they are identical in sex, appearance, and mental capacity; or they may arise from the fertilization of two separate eggs, the more common type, in which case they may not necessarily be of the same sex and will resemble each other no more than ordinary siblings. Identical twins occur about 25 per cent of the time, while fraternal twins occur in 75 per cent of the cases.

Twins are frequently born early, 80 per cent within three weeks of term and less than 50 per cent reaching the ninth month. Although the size of each baby is apt to be smaller than that in a normal birth, the combined weight often considerably exceeds the weight of a singly born baby. An instance is reported of twins weighing a total of thirty-four pounds at birth.

Because complications of pregnancy occur more often with twins, women expecting multiple births should co-operate closely with their physicians as regards weight gain, frequent rest periods, and other hygienic measures.

birth certificate. The written, authenticated record required by law of the birth of a child, whether at home or at the hospital and reported by the doctor or the midwife to the local registrar or the Bureau of Vital Statistics. The birth is placed in a permanent record and a certificate is issued to the parents. A name for a boy or girl should be picked beforehand so

that the certificate is complete and accurate. If a child dies during birth, an immediate certificate is demanded. This certificate must contain not only a statement of the cause of death, but also any secondary causes which have been noted.

The birth certificate is of great importance on many occasions. Proof of parentage is required when a person applies for citizenship, a government position, passport, entrance to school or college, and on many other occasions. Therefore, a birth certificate or a certified copy should always be on hand. As the birth certificate is so significant throughout life, some certified copies should be made with the original. If a certificate is not received by the parents in due time, the delay should be checked with the local Board of Health.

birth date. To calculate the expected date of delivery of a baby, add seven days to the first day of the last menstrual period and count back three months.

birth injuries. Hazards to the well-being of an infant while it is still in the womb of the mother may result from an injury or disease during pregnancy. Certain viruses have now been proved to cause damage before birth. Other dangers may develop during the birth itself, or just after birth. The brain of the baby may remain undeveloped, or birth injuries may be of varying degree. In some instances, delivery is hastened to safeguard mother and child, or forceps applied to the baby's head before it appears at the opening of the birth canal, methods which can, in some cases, cause birth injuries.

Even a normal birth subjects the skull and brain of the baby to much possible trauma. In the case of premature births, the chance of injury is even greater. The softer bones of the premature baby do not protect the brain as well as the harder ones of the full-term infant; thus intracranial injuries are more frequent. So many factors are involved that physicians find it difficult to diagnose certain afflictions as being due to birth or postnatal injuries. Such traumas of the brain at birth are responsible for at least one-third of all infant fatalities during the first two weeks of life.

Bleeding into the brain is a frequent cause of immediate disturbances in the newborn infant, or even of death. A tendency to these intracranial hemorrhages in the newborn will increase the peril of even the slight injury to the baby as well as to the pregnant mother. While fractures of the skull of newborn babies are rare, pressure on the skull occurs with consequent contusions and cerebral injuries not accompanied by hemorrhages. Irreparable damage to the brain may be the result of a premature separation of the placenta, or twisting of the cord and an inadequate oxygen supply. Birth injuries may bring about chronic lesions or alterations of functional capacity. Varying in the degree of severity, they include congenital faulty development of the external gray layer of the brain, cysts, and hardening.

Birth injuries have various symptoms, such as suffocation, irregular and curtailed breathing, feeble cry, pallor or excessive redness, stupor, and inability to suck. Involuntary muscular spasms and convulsions may also be observed, as well as dilated eyes and irregular pupils because of bleeding of the retina. In some cases, positive symptoms from hemorrhages cannot be discerned. Diagnostic signs may be as obscure as lack of appetite, inability to gain weight, a slight increase of the size of the head, or one or perhaps a few convulsive seizures.

Persistent injuries of the brain, resulting from birth casualties, produce some types of neurological disturbances such as paralysis of one side of the body or of muscles and limbs with a characteristic rigidity. Birth injury is one of the causes of the paralysis, due to a lesion of the brain, commonly called cerebral palsy.

Difficulties during delivery are responsible, too, for damage of the spinal cord. As the tendons of the spinal column of the newborn baby are elastic, the slight twisting or stretching may result in serious dislocation. Damage to the skeleton may not be apparent and yet such injuries can have a direct effect on the spinal cord and its membranes. A complete breaking of the cord may follow in the wake of a severe mishap. Here, too, however, hemorrhages provide the most serious consequences. The damages of the spinal cord may be of different degrees of severity, and the neurological symptoms may thus vary in the few infants who survive such birth injuries. *See also* CEREBRAL PALSY.

birthmark (nevus). A congenital skin blemish or circumscribed area of pigmentation. Birthmarks include pigmented moles and skin discolorations brought about by blood vessels, as, for instance, "strawberry" marks. Some birthmarks develop years after birth, but the skin defect is there from the beginning, from the formation of the skin in the fetus. Nothing can be done to prevent birthmarks. Immediately after birth, these marks may be small and insignificant, but they may gradually grow larger and more prominent by the time the child is a few weeks or months old. Then they may stop growing or, in some cases, even disappear. Yet it is impossible to foresee whether or not a spot will cause symptoms.

The strawberry birthmark is produced by a mass of blood vessels which collect in a cluster near the surface of the skin. It may be deep scarlet color if deep below the skin, or bluish if more superficial. Pressure on such a birthmark makes it colorless, in proportion to the blood forced from the blood vessels. A survey made in 1955 by a surgeon proved that without surgery or other treatment ordinary strawberry birthmarks often disappeared or became inconspicuous as the person grew older.

Another type of birthmark, of a pale blue or gray color, is characterized by more cellular tissue and less fluid, and is less spongy than the strawberry blemish. Its color cannot be pressed out, since it contains a smaller amount of blood vessels.

The port-wine birthmark, another type of skin blemish, is a collection of small blood vessels with various amounts of pigment deposited from the blood into the skin. Not much can be done for these, but fortunately they rarely enlarge. Treatment with ultraviolet rays may, in some instances, effect complete disappearance. If the blemishes are large and unsightly, they can be covered with one of the several cosmetic preparations available.

Skin lesions of the birthmark type may be treated with the electric needle, frozen with carbon dioxide snow, cauterized chemically, removed surgically, or treated with radium. All these methods have merit when properly used in the right case.

Recently a "plastic planing" device has been successfully applied. The marks are actually scraped or planed away with a surgical device like an emery wheel, allowing the growth of smooth new skin. Another modern method is to inject the blood vessels in such growths with various chemical substances that cause a slight inflammatory reaction inside the blood vessels which eventually results in scarring and obliteration or disappearance of the birthmark. Such methods are exceedingly delicate, but in most instances successful when carried out under proper conditions by an experienced physician.

bismuth. One of the elementary chemicals. Its derivatives are used chiefly in medicine as contracting agents for the mucous membranes and as sedatives, antiseptics, and neutralizing substances for the stomach and the bowels.

Bismuth subcarbonate, for example, may be employed by the physician in food poisoning, in case of chronic gastritis, and for vomiting in indigestion.

blackwater fever. A tropical disease which occurs almost exclusively among members of the Caucasian race, and is limited in the United States to the South. Apparently produced by small intracellular parasites in the blood, it is infectious and often fatal. Among the symptoms are irregular fever, chills, vomiting, jaundice, and labored breathing, with nephritis as a complication.

bladder. Urinary, a hollow muscular organ which serves as a reservoir for urine. Its normal capacity is said to be about fourteen ounces.

bladder diseases. The term bladder designates two organs of the body; the urinary bladder, a sac which receives urine from the kidneys and holds it temporarily until voided; and the gall bladder, a similar structure which stores a supply of bile, manufactured by the liver for use in digestion. The term bladder used by itself usually refers to the urinary bladder.

The kidneys deposit urine in the bladder at the rate of about thirty drops a minute through two tubes, the ureters, each about a foot long and a fifth of an inch in diameter. The passage through which urine is excreted from the bladder and from the body is the urethra, a tube about eight inches long in the male and an inch and a half in the female.

The urinary bladder and the urethra are susceptible to a number of diseases and accidents. Either one may become inflamed or infected. New and abnormal growths may occur in or on the bladder, it may form stones, or it may be bruised or ruptured.

Inflammation of the bladder is known scientifically as cystitis. It can occur in either acute or chronic form and from many different causes. Cystitis is much more common in the female because the shortness of the urethra affords invasive organisms easier access than in the male. An inflamed bladder is almost always related to a previous infection, above or below the bladder, in the urinary tract, or to an obstruction. Infection in the bladder alone, without infection elsewhere, is a rarity.

A common source of infection is an obstruction of the normal flow of urine, such as tends to occur in elderly people or anyone of advanced years who is bedridden. An enlarged prostate gland may affect a male in a similar way. Sometimes the offending factor is bacteria introduced on a catheter which has not been properly cleaned. Older men who must be catheterized frequently, practically always develop some cystitis.

Symptoms of cystitis are undue frequency of urination, a burning sensation when voiding, and sometimes the appearance of blood in the urine. Persistent desire to void after retiring therefore calls for careful medical investigation. Bladder infection usually is not accompanied by fever, and a normal temperature is not an assurance that an infection may not be present.

Diagnosis of a bladder inflammation usually demands a number of tests which include examinations of the urine taken at various times over the full twenty-four-hour period, especially for the presence of bacteria, pus, or solids. Frequently dye stuffs are used to determine the body's ability to excrete fluid. In addition, the condition of the prostate gland will be sought.

One of the remarkable achievements of modern medicine is the development of an extraordinary instrument, the cystoscope, to aid in making such a diagnosis. Through this, the doctor can actually look at the inside of the bladder. The cystoscope, a long tube with a light at its end, is passed into the bladder through the urethra. Fluid is then injected into the bladder by way of the tube, distending its walls temporarily for purposes of the examination. The tube and its light then are turned in different directions and a system of mirrors which are part of the cystoscope are so focused as to enable the physician to see the presence of infection inside the organ. Sometimes inflammation is indicated by abnormal changes in the wall of the bladder and growth can usually be seen with this instrument. The cystoscope can be used to administer drugs and for other treatment of infections of the bladder.

New methods for combating bladder infection represent a vast advance over what was formerly available. These include penicillin and other antibiotic drugs, the sulfas, Mandelamine, Pyridium, Furadantin, and others. They are administered both by mouth and by injection, through which they reach the bladder by way of the bloodstream. Some drugs are injected into the bladder itself, for direct application to an affected area.

Cystitis in chronic form may result from an initial acute attack, but may be caused also by stones or tumors. Occasionally, older men contract it as the result of retaining urine in the bladder for a long time, especially if the urine decomposes.

The most critical infection that may affect the bladder is tuberculosis, which usually accompanies tuberculosis of the kidney.

Stones in the bladder, formed either within the bladder itself or passed into it from the kidney, although not uncommon, are not encountered as often as in the past. Men are twenty times more susceptible to stones than women. The stones may be tiny or range in size to that of an egg, and symptoms encountered are similar to those of cystitis. In women, often a stone may be extracted by dilating the relatively short urethra. *See also* URETHRA; URINATION; URINE.

blastomycosis. Or Gilchrist's disease, an infection caused by a yeastlike fungus. It is found chiefly in the central regions of North America, and is more common in men than in women.

bleeding. *See* HEMORRHAGE; WOUNDS.

blepharitis. A contagious inflammation of the edges of the eyelids that most often affects children, especially following an illness. Small infected blisters form at the roots of the lashes. These may lead to ulcers, then scars, which change the direction of the lashes, turning some of them inward against the eyeball. Sometimes the entire edge of the lid is distorted inward or outward. If not eliminated, the condition will eventually make the affected area red, thickened, and covered with scales.

Because faulty vision may prolong the disease, the eyes should be examined promptly so that glasses can be prescribed if necessary. The general health and sanitary habits of the child should also receive careful attention, not only for her own welfare but also to protect the rest of the family from infection through use of the same towels or bedding.

In severe cases, sulfa or penicillin drops may be prescribed by the physician. Recurrence frequently calls for repeated and persistent treatment.

blisters. Small, bladderlike cavities under the skin containing watery material. Blisters may be the result of an infection, such as eczema, herpes, impetigo, or chickenpox, or they may be caused by injuries, such as pinching, chafing, burning, or scalding.

Painful blisters may also result from sunburn. To prevent this, yellow petroleum jelly, olive oil, or cold cream may be applied to the skin before going out into the sun for any length of time. A number of commercial preparations are available which are designed to filter out some of the ultraviolet rays. If blisters occur as a result of exposure to the sun, they are treated as any other burn with soothing medications or creams. Severe sun-

burn can be dangerous as well as painful, and should be treated by a physician.

In time, most blisters dry up without special treatment. Those which burst should be washed with soap and water and covered with a sterile dressing. If a large blister is opened, this is done near the outer margin with a sterilized needle. After pressing gently to eject the fluid, a sterile dressing should be applied. *See also* BURNS.

bloating. A swelling or accumulation of fluid or air brought about by any cause.

blood. The opaque red fluid which flows through the blood vessels is the transport medium of the body, bringing to all the tissues the food and oxygen they need for growth and repair. It distributes the secretions, or hormones, manufactured by the important glands of the body, to the organs where they are needed to carry out their special functions. It removes the waste products from the tissues, transmits the carbon dioxide to the lungs where it is liberated and the remaining materials to the kidneys from which they are then eliminated from the body. Blood helps to maintain the body at a uniform temperature and keeps the other body fluids in a state of equilibrium. When the body is invaded by disease, the blood is the first line of defense against the infection by the action of its white cells and other substances, antibodies, which it transports to the involved site. Another of its functions is to prevent any increase in acidity or alkalinity within the body.

blood bank. Exactly what its name

implies; a depository for blood or blood derivatives. Blood storage has now become a significant adjunct to most hospitals. Blood of the various types, O, A, B, and AB, given by donors, is stored so that victims of accidents, patients after surgical operations, and sufferers from certain diseases can be quickly supplied with new additions of blood.

Blood plasma instead of liquid blood now also is widely stored. It keeps for long periods and does not require typing. By addition of water to the powder, plasma is promptly available. In a few diseases of the blood, however, plasma cannot be used. *See also* BLOOD TRANSFUSION.

blood poisoning. *See* BACTEREMIA.

blood pressure. Measured in two levels, it is the degree of pressure exerted by the heart and arteries to keep the blood circulating in the blood vessels throughout the body. The maximum level, the systolic pressure, records the force exerted in the arteries with each heartbeat or contraction to propel the blood out of the left ventricle of the heart into the aorta, the large artery. The minimum level, the diastolic pressure, records the relaxed phase of the heart, between beats. This pressure indicates to the doctor the condition of the small blood vessels or arterioles—that is, their ability to contract and keep the flow of blood constant throughout the body. This pressure is maintained at a constant level, since each heartbeat forces into the large artery an amount of blood equal to that which escapes more gradually from the arterioles into the capillaries. Blood pressure tends to rise during the last month

of pregnancy and to rise continuously during labor. *See also* BLOOD PRESSURE, HIGH; BLOOD PRESSURE, LOW; BLOOD PRESSURE, NORMAL; CIRCULATORY SYSTEM; HEART.

blood pressure, high (hypertension). The state of blood pressure beyond the normal limits. One cause of hypertension is the narrowing, or constriction, of the smallest branches of the arteries throughout the body. This tends to slow the flow of blood through the tiny vessels, and causes the heart to pump harder in order to keep the blood circulating throughout the body. Hypertensive disease affects about 5 per cent of the adult population.

A simple elevation of blood pressure may be due to a variety of causes, all of which increase the systolic pressure and are classified as systolic hypertension. A high systolic pressure is frequently the result of decreased elasticity of the arteries, as in some types of rheumatic heart disease, which causes heart block; in hyperthyroidism, which causes the thyroid gland to function excessively; and in arteriovenous aneurysms. These conditions are not considered true hypertension, but are significant as indications of an underlying disease.

True hypertension, or diastolic hypertension, due to a narrowing of the arterioles, is rare in persons under thirty-five years of age, and then usually is a hereditary manifestation. As a rule, hypertension is found in persons past forty, though many persons who first discover a mild hypertension at forty to fifty years of age may have had an elevated blood pressure for many years previously. The disease is more prevalent in persons between sixty and seventy years of age, and occurs more often in women but more seriously in men. Usually these cases follow a mild, uneventful pattern. Hypertension also is found more frequently in patients with diabetes mellitus.

Although the body build does not seem to be significant in hypertension, obesity does constitute a serious factor. Overweight increases the amount of work the heart must perform, and a loss of weight is often accompanied by a fall in blood pressure. The person with high blood pressure is frequently a high-strung person who reacts tensely to the everyday problems of living, and is apt to suppress hostilities, aggressions, and fears. These inner conflicts establish a nervous reaction which may become localized in the tiny blood vessels and eventually cause high blood pressure, just as tensions in some persons may cause ulcers of the stomach. Although hypertension is not a hereditary disease, the tendency or predisposition to the disease is stronger in some families than in others and, not infrequently, the condition will be found in more than one member of a family.

In true diastolic hypertension, the cause is definitely known in only a small percentage of cases and in these is generally attributed to kidney disease. Acute glomerulonephritis, a kidney disorder often seen in children and young people following a streptococcal infection, results in high blood pressure. Most of those affected recover completely. The toxemia of pregnancy, which usually occurs after the sixth month, involves the kidneys and is associated with high blood pressure.

Hypertension may also be caused by tumors of the endocrine glands, or by certain nerve cells. The adrenal glands, which are a part of the endocrine apparatus, are located over each kidney and secrete the hormone adrenaline into the bloodstream. Adrenaline raises the blood pressure and when a tumor develops in the adrenal area an excessive amount of adrenaline is secreted. Surgical removal of the tumor lowers the blood pressure to normal. A tumor of the pituitary gland, another endocrine gland, located just below the brain, may also induce hypertension. Occasionally tumors arising in certain nerve cells of the sympathetic nervous system will produce a sustained type of hypertension. Surgical removal of the tumors reduces hypertension. The increased occurrence of hypertension during the menopause in women and the climacteric in men is also attributed to endocrine causes, although the mechanism involved is not clearly understood.

Another form of true hypertension, a narrowing or stricture of the aorta, found in children and young people is coarctation of the aorta. Some children are born with the disorder, which results in a high blood pressure in the arms and a low pressure in the legs. This condition is cured by surgery.

The specific causes of high blood pressure are known in only about 20 per cent of all cases involving hypertensive disease. In these cases, high blood pressure is called "essential hypertension," which also has the characteristic narrowing of the arterioles throughout the body with the consequent resistance in these tiny vessels to the flow of blood, and the rise of blood pressure necessary to keep the blood circulating in the body. The course of essential hypertension and the complications that accompany it are practically identical with that of diastolic hypertensions due to known causes. When the ailment progresses slowly over many years, it is noted as benign, or mild.

Benign hypertension may exist for many years without any evidence to suggest its presence other than a moderate elevation of blood pressure. A person past forty may see a doctor because of headache, dizziness, failing vision, or noises in the head, expecting to be told that the discomfort is due to high blood pressure. Actually the elevation of blood pressure may not be great, and it may vary from one visit to the next; such changes are of little significance. In many instances, persons with high blood pressure remain well for years without showing any apparent change in health. The complaints are not due to the hypertension, but rather to some of the complications associated with hypertension.

Once the presence of the disease is definitely established, a thorough, inclusive examination is essential to evaluate the complications and determine the progress and severity of the hypertensive condition. These complications may not appear for years, but when they do, the organs most frequently affected are the heart, eyes, brain, and kidneys. The examination, therefore, is directed toward a search for signs that indicate an insufficient flow of blood to any of these organs, or that suggest the possibility of disease of any of these organs.

When the arteries which feed the heart, the coronary arteries, become narrowed, a person may experience a temporary pain, angina pectoris, on exertion. Or he may be subjected to a more serious attack, coronary thrombosis, which is accompanied by shortness of breath, particularly at night, and other manifestations of shock. Hypertension may also cause an enlargement of the heart which results from the exertion of the heart muscles pumping against the resistance of the arterioles. Eventually this disorder will also cause heart pain and shortness of breath.

When the arteries in the brain become hardened, personality changes appear, with emotional instability, failure to concentrate, and forgetfulness, especially of recent events. This is particularly true of older people who have developed cerebral arteriosclerosis. Temporary weakness, unsteadiness in walking, and noises in the ears are symptoms which may precede a cerebral hemorrhage or clot in one of the arteries, which causes a stroke or apoplexy. The less serious cases of stroke cause paralysis of one side of the body with, occasionally, an interference in speech. The paralysis usually disappears entirely or partially within a period of months.

High blood pressure is frequently accompanied by hardening, sclerosis, of the arteries throughout the body. This process is called arteriosclerosis, one of the commonest disorders of advanced age. Usually the first indication of its presence is a clotting of a larger artery, or thrombotic occlusion. This may develop into cerebral thrombosis, angina pectoris, or coronary thrombosis.

In cases of hypertension, both physical and psychological factors are significant. Most doctors feel that an overconsciousness of blood pressure makes some people lead lives of excessive concern and even semi-invalidism. While the prevention of anxiety may not alter the course of the hypertension itself, it makes a great difference in the person's attitude and outlook on life. Too often people have been invalided merely from overawareness of their high blood pressure rather than from the physical effects of the hypertension. Hence, the reeducation of those people with high blood pressure is essential so that they may carry on normal lives. They should learn to discuss themselves and their problems objectively, as individuals rather than as medical cases. This will not only permit a greater insight into the situation but will often result in relief from anxiety.

The general fear of hypertension is one of the great obstacles to minimizing an anxiety reaction. Yet this can be overcome when one knows how blood pressure normally var-

ies, not only from time to time but from person to person, with every exertion or emotional experience. That the definition of normal blood pressure has been broadened is significant and encouraging.

Many persons with milder degrees of hypertension need not even be subjected to dietary restriction unless they are obese. They can follow the activity pattern of normal living, avoiding only overwork, overexertion, and excesses.

Overweight in people with hypertension is a liability and the frequency of incidence of illness and death is directly proportional to the amount of extra weight. A suitable low-calorie diet, usually high in proteins and low in fats, starches, and carbohydrates, should be selected and continually supervised by a doctor.

The use of a low-salt diet for hypertension has been effective in reducing the blood pressure in many cases, often bringing it to normal levels.

New drugs for the treatment of hypertension are designed to inhibit the effects of the sympathetic nerves. Development of new drugs is making operation much less frequent.

blood pressure, low (hypotension). Approximately 25 to 30 per cent of the population has primary hypotension, arbitrarily described as pressures falling below 110 millimeters of mercury for the systolic level, and below 70 millimeters for the diastolic.

When a known cause cannot be found for the low pressure, it is called primary, or essential, hypotension. Many normal men and women have blood pressure in this range. Symptoms cannot be attributed to this type of low blood pressure, and actually it is compatible with a greater than average life expectancy.

Hypotension which sometimes develops in the course of a serious disease is known as secondary hypotension. Among such diseases are acute infections, heart failure, Addison's disease, malnutrition, Simmonds' disease, circulatory shock from hemorrhage, trauma, hyperinsulinism, or other causes. Persons with secondary hypotension are weak, tired, and occasionally complain of dizziness and faintness. In general, despite the drop in blood pressure in these cases, the body manages to maintain a sufficient blood supply for its needs. As recovery from the original cause progresses, the blood pressure becomes normal.

Another type of low blood pressure, postural hypotension, as the name implies, is associated with change of position. Usually, when a person stands up, the blood pressure rises, in response to the energy exerted for this motion. In some cases, however, the blood pressure drops and causes faintness. Many normal people feel a slight dizziness when they change position suddenly, because the flow of blood to the brain is thus suddenly slowed and the brain tissue is sensitive to a lack of blood and oxygen. However, in postural hypotension the change in position provokes blurred vision, weakness, and

fainting, and on lying down consciousness returns.

blood pressure, normal. People vary in their response to external stimuli such as heat or cold, and also in their blood pressures. Transient deviations from the normal in any person are caused by such everyday activities as digestion, change of posture, exercise, and emotional stimulation. The degree to which the pressure is raised depends on the intensity of the stimulus and the individual response.

At birth the blood pressure is about 75 millimeters systolic and 40 diastolic, or, as it is usually written, 75/40. This rises gradually and at adolescence is about 100/60, and between the ages of twenty and forty it is 120/80. The rise continues slowly and at the age of sixty is around 145/90. After that the diastolic pressure remains fairly stationary, although the systolic may become somewhat higher. However, these figures represent the average, and a difference of 10 per cent or more in either direction is still within normal limits.

Blood pressure gradually increases with age; at sixty-five most normal men may have a systolic pressure up to 170; and normal women, up to 175. The diastolic pressure may range between 100 and 110. In some cases a systolic pressure as high as 180 and a diastolic pressure of 110 seems to be normal. With an increase in weight there is a progressive increase in blood pressure, regardless of age or sex.

Wide variations exist in the so-called normal blood pressures at different ages. Blood pressure which falls in the outermost limits of normal does not in itself constitute a disease. Many factors combine to keep the blood pressure within normal limits—for instance, the exertion of the heart muscles as they pump the blood through the body, the degree of elasticity of the arterial walls as the blood flows through them, and the resistance encountered by the blood in the smaller blood vessels. Since all these may influence blood pressure, they must be carefully considered before an elevation of blood pressure is considered significant.

blood transfusion. The transfer of blood from a donor to a recipient; one of the most widely used procedures in medical treatment. When severe hemorrhage has resulted in a great loss of blood, a transfusion will restore the circulating blood volume and the red blood cells which provide oxygen and food to the body tissues. Blood transfusion is an invaluable supporting treatment for surgical shock, to replace an excessive loss of blood at childbirth, or in such conditions as leukemia. In some cases, even when the circulating blood volume is normal, transfusion is used to replace a deficiency in one of the constituents of the blood, thus providing red cells in cases of acute anemia, or in hemophilia, which is due to the lack of a specific clot-promoting factor in the blood plasma.

blood types. Blood is classified into four types—A, B, AB, and O.

Type O blood can give to all blood types, but can receive only from type O. AB blood type can give to only AB, but can receive from any group. Thus type O is sometimes called the universal donor and type AB the universal recipient. Type A can give to types A and AB and receive only from types A and O, and type B can give to types B and AB, and receive only from type B or O. The ideal blood transfusion utilizes the same type of donor and recipient blood. In the United States, 85 per cent of the population belong to groups A or O, and types B and AB are rare. The distribution of blood types varies considerably with geographical population. Blood types are inherited.

As a safety measure, before a patient receives a whole-blood transfusion, the compatibility of his blood with the donor blood is checked by a cross-match test. Small samples of red blood cells are combined and examined under a microscope for signs of incompatibility or clumping.

If incompatible bloods are mixed, the red cells of the donor blood are rapidly destroyed, liberating free hemoglobin into the patient's circulating blood. The free hemoglobin breaks down and may be excreted through the kidneys; if the urine is acid, the newly formed pigment which has resulted from the destruction of hemoglobin cannot be absorbed by the kidneys and is deposited on the tubular cells of that organ. This causes kidney failure, with eventual death. The practice of cross-matching bloods before transfusions has virtually eliminated deaths from transfusion.

Highly significant in transfusions

and obstetrics are Rh blood groups. The Rh factor, a substance present in red blood cells, was uncovered during experiments with rhesus monkeys; thus the name Rh for rhesus. Subsequently, this factor was related to unexplained accidents in transfusion, including hemolytic disease of newborn infants, characterized by disintegration of red blood cells. Eighty-five per cent of white persons have Rh positive factor, indicating that the red cells are agglutinated by antirhesus serum; the other 15 per cent are Rh negative, since their cells are not agglutinated by antirhesus serum.

When an Rh negative person receives Rh positive blood, he will develop particular antibodies. If the Rh negative person later again receives Rh positive blood, a hemolytic anemia may result. This anemia appears in newborn infants most frequently when the mother is Rh negative and the father is Rh positive. It will occur only when the mother has had previous direct contact with Rh positive blood such as in transfusion or by previously bearing an Rh positive child. Treatment involves giving the infant transfusions of Rh negative blood, and in severe cases the infant's blood is almost totally replaced by Rh negative blood of the correct type. Blood banks keep on hand large supplies of Rh negative blood.

Laboratory tests can reveal this sensitization, and the physician can then take measures to avoid or diminish accident to mother and child. A mother-to-be whose tests show she might give birth to an Rh positive child must receive careful medical attention. Only one in forty or fifty cases of mating between an Rh negative woman and an Rh positive man results in hemolytic anemia. *See also* ANEMIA; CROSS MATCHING OF BLOOD.

blue baby. A baby born with a congenital structural defect of the heart, which results in constant recirculation of some of the dark or venous blood without its prior passage through the lungs to pick up oxygen, thus giving the skin, lips, and nails a bluish look. Since 1945, many such infants have been saved by an operation developed by Drs. Alfred Blalock and Helen Taussig at Johns Hopkins University. Before that time, little could be done for the condition except to keep the child at rest and free of infection. Life expectancy was low.

Such defects occur frequently when the prenatal opening between the two pumping vessels of the baby's heart, the ventricles, which normally closes at birth, fails to close. In addition, distortion of the major artery leading away from the heart, and of the artery leading from the heart to the lungs, throws an abnormal load on one of the ventricles. Blood which has been oxygenated by the lungs and has taken on the characteristic color associated with arterial blood is mixed with the bluish blood from the veins, which should have gone to the lungs but did not.

By joining two arteries, the Blalock-Taussig operation increases the flow of blood to the lungs so that a greater proportion of the baby's blood receives oxygen. This ends the blueness of the skin and the breathlessness associated with the condition. Short of violent athletic competition, such children are thereafter able to live normally active lives. *See also* CYANOSIS.

blushing. *See* PIGMENTATION.

body lice. Small, wingless insects, ectoparasites, carriers of disease and producers of irritating dermatitis. The louse is one of the commonest of the insects that attack the hairy parts of the human body. Wherever large numbers of people congregate, as in the armed forces, concentration camps, or jails, delousing techniques have to be developed to cope with the pest. Not only must the body be rid of the louse, but its eggs (nits) must also be eliminated from clothing. For the latter purpose, live steam is generally used.

The louse is a carrier of typhus. It becomes infected by ingesting the blood of a diseased person.

To remove the nits, the hair must be wet thoroughly with hot vinegar, and a fine-toothed comb used. This should be repeated daily, making sure that the hair is thoroughly dry before the individual goes outdoors.

body odor (bromidrosis, or fetid perspiration). The excretion of sweat with an unpleasant odor. The eccrine and apocrine are the two types of sweat glands in the body. The apocrine glands are found only in certain sections of the body, such as under the arms, and they produce a secretion often regarded as unpleasant. Women have twice as many apocrine glands as men.

Sweat with the accompanying offensive odor is usually excreted from certain parts of the body such as the armpits, feet, and occasionally other regions. Persons who have bromidrosis must pay particular attention to personal cleanliness, and bathe once or even twice a day, using plenty of soap. Special soaps are available but they do not appear to be any more effective than ordinary soap. Deodorants and antiperspirants may be used on parts of the body where perspiration is likely to be excessive. Checking perspiration under the arms or other parts of the body is not harmful. After the lotion has been applied, an antiseptic dusting powder may be used on the skin.

Extra excretion of sweat may be associated with nervousness. Proper treatment will help control abnormal perspiration. In some instances, the application of X-ray by competent specialists has been found useful.

Boeck's sarcoid. A chronic disease characterized by benign tumors resembling flesh. It is usually an ailment of young adults, but sometimes of older people. Skin, eyes, lungs, and bones of the feet and hands are especially affected. The cause of Boeck's sarcoid is unknown, and a specific treatment has not as yet been found. Cortisone has been used with great success in treating the condition, but relapses are frequent.

boil. Scientifically called a furuncle, is a painful nodule with a hardened outside and a soft core of pus within.

bone bank. Bone banks have been established at many hospitals. Small chips for filling cavities, and larger bones are preserved in deep freeze, to be grafted, after thawing, in the operating room. They are taken originally from amputated limbs, from deceased people, or from those undergoing orthopedic surgery. The thawed bone which is grafted does not itself grow, but stimulates growth of the healthy bone to which it is united.

bones. The solid elements of the body. Without a bony skeleton, the human being would collapse into a heap of tissues and organs, be completely unable to move and extremely vulnerable to injury. In addition to acting as a framework, bones often play a crucial role in the protection of organs. The skull, for example, protects the soft tissue of the brain; the spinal column shields the spinal cord; the pelvic bones help guard the kidneys and other organs of the abdomen against damage; and the ribs help avert injury to the lungs and other organs of the chest. With the aid of muscles attached to them, bones also make movement possible.

Bones are a part of the connective tissue system, one of the most widespread systems of the body. Generally, this system consists of collagenous or fibrous tissue or both, but bone also contains mineral matter which gives it hardness.

Bone originates from small, irregularly shaped cells called osteoblasts, which are believed to come from the connective tissue system. During the early stages of bone formation, these cells manufacture a soft substance which forms around them and into which animal material, called ossein or gela-tin, and minerals, mainly calcium phosphate and calcium carbonate, are later deposited to impart the stony quality. About one-third of the weight of bone is the animal material; the rest is mineral. In the childhood disease rickets, which is caused by a deficiency of vitamin D, the bones lack adequate mineral material and are relatively soft. The long bones of the legs bend under the weight of the trunk, and other bone malformations occur, depending upon the degree of softening. Vitamin D is essential to the metabolism of calcium in the human body.

Bone difficulties can accompany old age. Osteoporosis is characterized by a general decrease in bone mass with resulting strains on the skeleton. Usually a thinning of the long bones in the legs develops, sometimes with spontaneous fractures. The cause is a reduction in osteoblast activity so that new bone is not laid down at a rate needed to replace worn bone. Osteoporosis may also occur earlier in life, as a result of metabolic disturbances such as diabetes, overactivity of the adrenal glands, or as a consequence of vitamin deficiencies, particularly vitamin C, or starvation.

The growth of bones in childhood and adolescence determines the height and body structure of the person. This is usually hereditary, but is often influenced by diet. Frequently, improved nutrition results in offspring who have attained heights several inches above those of their parents. In some instances, disturbance of the glands which regulate growth may cause either giantism or dwarfism. The anterior portion of the pituitary gland, a gland located at the base of the brain, is particularly involved with the growth of long bones, and may undersecrete, causing dwarfism, or oversecrete, producing giantism. Either condition should be treated by an endocrinologist, a physician who specializes in glands and their secretions. Dwarfism can be treated by the administration of pituitary extract. Undersecretion of the thyroid gland, which causes cretinism, in which the mental and physical growth of the child is stunted or slow, can be corrected by administration of thyroid extract.

The number of separate bones in the human body is generally given as 206. Up to the age of twenty-two, the number of bones in men differs from that in women, because of the changes that take place in the joining together of small bones to make up larger ones.

The cavities of all bones in the body are filled with marrow, which in the bones of the young and in spongy bones of adults is red. Red marrow is considered a valuable breeding place for red blood corpuscles. Marrow in adults generally is yellow. Marrow consists of connective tissue interlaced with a network of small blood vessels. In the meshes of this network are various kinds of cells, including red and white blood cells, connective tissue, and fat cells. An examination of bone marrow tissue has become an advantageous technique for the diagnosis of many disease conditions, pernicious and other anemias, and

ailments such as hypersplenism, leukemia, and lymphoma.

Bones sometimes become diseased as a result of infectious material being carried from other areas of the body through the blood vessels. Nerve cells, too, branch through these canals and produce sensations of pain in event of injury to the bone. Inflammation of the periosteum, or osteomyelitis, an inflammation of the deeper bone tissue, usually due to infection, also produces much pain. Growth, however, does not cause pain, and if a child complains of pain in the bones or joints, it should not be dismissed as "growing pains" but investigated by a physician.

Bone building does not end with maturity. Childhood is the period of the greatest growth in size, strength, and shape of bone, but bone building is a daily process which continues throughout a lifetime. The diet of everyone, not only young and growing children, should include ample mineral-containing foods, proteins, and vitamins. Children need a larger amount of calcium and phosphorus-containing foods, such as milk and cheese, and adequate vitamin D. Older people also require milk, though the period of intense bone growth is over, and a pint of milk daily is advisable. Necessary amounts of vitamin C, vital to connective tissue health, should be assured.

The types of injuries, outside of fractures, which are most likely to afflict bones and their joints involve tendons and ligaments. Tendons tie muscle to bone, and ligaments are tough bands of fibrous tissues that bind the articulating bones together. Sometimes ligaments form a circular band, a capsule, that surrounds the joint and attaches to the periosteum and the bone beneath. Ligaments do not have the ability to contract, but are slightly elastic and bear much of the brunt of injury in case of sprains and dislocations.

In a sprain, for instance, a tearing of the binding ligaments occurs with swelling caused by ruptured blood and lymph vessels and an increased secretion of synovial fluid. In a dislocation, however, the articulating ends of the bones are displaced. The ligaments are usually badly torn, the blood vessels at the joint severely injured, and the muscles around the joint are frequently in contraction because of the pain. This muscular contraction adds to the difficulties of getting the bones back into place. Injury to the nerves may also occur, and swelling and the degree of deformity in the joint will depend on the extent of the injury.

Crippling injuries to and malformations of the bones, joints, and muscles are cared for by medical specialists called orthopedic surgeons. These doctors can make bone grafts to replace damaged areas, transplant bony tissue, and create new sockets for the ends of bones which have been injured or destroyed by disease. A number of bone banks have now been established throughout the country, from which bone tissue can be drawn for grafting. *See also* CARTILAGE; OSTEITIS; OSTEOMYELITIS.

booster dose. "Shot" of vaccine given some time after the original immunization to maintain the immunity against certain diseases. The added injection of a particular vaccine will greatly stimulate the formation of antibodies at a time when the concentration of antibodies may be at a low level. *See also* IMMUNIZATION.

boric acid. A substance of colorless scales or crystals or a white crystalline powder, possessing the properties of a weak acid. Soluble in water, it is used externally as a mild antiseptic. For example, diapers may be rinsed in a saturated solution of boric acid in the case of intertrigo or "diaper rash." Because of its action in deterring the growth of germs, a small amount of boric acid is an ingredient of many protective and soothing dusting powders.

Boric acid eyewash soothes irritated membranes of the eye and inflammation of the eyelids, conjunctivitis. It is also extensively employed as an antiseptic first-aid dressing for burns, local inflammations of the scalp, in the care of babies' ears, and as a throat spray and mouthwash.

Taken internally, boric acid is poisonous and can cause death. It should always be plainly and distinctly marked in the medicine chest, and should be kept out of the reach of children.

botulism. The most severe and dangerous of all food poisonings. It occurs as a result of eating canned and preserved foods which have been contaminated by the germ *Clostridium botulinum.* This organism produces a toxin or poison of extraordinary power, so great that one part of it in ten million will kill a mouse. The symptoms occurring in human victims of the disease are due to the toxin rather than to the presence of the organism itself.

The toxin attacks the nerves, induces weakness and paralysis, including difficulty in swallowing, talking, and seeing. Death finally results from respiratory failure.

The bacillus *Clostridium* is an inhabitant of the soil in every country in the world and is therefore a potential contaminant of everything grown in soil where it exists. In the United States, the danger develops when contaminated farm products, especially string beans, corn, spinach, asparagus, beets, and apricots, are preserved and canned by inadequate methods, and the germ survives, produces its toxin, and poisons the food in the can or jar. The amount of toxin produced depends on the character and chemistry of the food in question, its acidity, the presence of sugar, and the quantity of heat applied to it. In Europe, preserved sausage meats and similar products, such as fish pastes, have been implicated most frequently.

The foremost problem about the bacillus *Clostridium* is that its reproductive spores survive treatment that ordinarily disposes of microorganisms. Six hours of boiling does not destroy them, nor does six minutes' exposure to steam pressure at fifteen pounds. The toxin itself is fortunately much less resistant and is rendered harmless by six minutes of boiling.

While ordinarily commercially canned foods are safe, and an outbreak of botulism from this source has not occurred for some time, the same cannot be said for home-preserved products, which are processed under less rigid standards. All home-canned foods should be boiled for six full minutes before being even tasted. One exception is those packed in brine, which renders a food reasonably safe. Cold salads of home-canned fruits or vegetables have been involved in several outbreaks of botulism, which could have been due to the use of containers or foods or both which were not sterilized under pressure. This omission permitted the survival of the spores.

Speed in summoning the doctor and securing treatment, which will consist primarily of administration of one or more antitoxins that have been developed, is a matter of life and death to the victim of botulism. Damage suffered from the toxin cannot be repaired. All that can be done is to arrest the progress of the poisoning, and assist with secondary measures. *See also* FOOD POISONING.

bowel. The portion of the digestive system which extends from the stomach to the anus, and includes small intestine, large intestine, and the rectum which is about six inches long.

brachial. A term relating to the arm. Brachial arteries, for example, extend along the inner side of the upper arm, and brachial glands are the lymphatic glands in the armpit.

brachydactyly. Based on the Greek

brachy meaning short, and *dactyly* meaning condition of fingers, a term denoting abnormally short fingers and toes.

brain. The human brain is a large mass of nerve tissues contained in the skull, connected to the spinal cord, and surrounded by three layers of tough membranes called the meninges. The brain cells, with the spinal cord, are interwoven into a complex relay system which collects, stores, and sends out sensations and information.

breast. One of the paired mammary glands on the front of the chest. They are composed of fatty tissue and glands capable of producing milk and are ordinarily much more developed in women than in men. At the center of each breast the milk glands fuse into a single outlet, the nipple, also more developed in the female. Since the growth of the breasts depends largely on production of female hormone, they may become larger in some young boys before puberty, and also in men who develop hormone-producing tumors. The female breast is usually much larger during pregnancy, because of heightened production of female hormone and increased production of milk glands. Some of the earliest suggestions of pregnancy—fullness, prickling, and tingling of the breasts—may be felt from the third week. The veins of the breast become visible, enlarged, and tense from the eighth week. After the twelfth week a clear fluid can be expressed from the nipple. A pigmented area, the areola, may also be seen around the nipple at this time.

Breast cancer is perhaps the most frequent female cancer and for this reason every woman should know how to detect early symptoms within her breasts. The most common sign is a small lump. Other symptoms are pain, bleeding from the nipple, or ulcerations which do not heal. Not all lumps in the breast are cancerous, however, and many, perhaps most, are due to small clumps of fibrous tissue called fibromas; to small cysts which are collections of fluid; or to harmless clusters of glandular tissue called adenomas. The nipple may bleed in cases of bruising or because of harmless glandular development. A doctor should be consulted in all cases, however. If the condition seems suspicious, a small piece of tissue is removed from the breast and thoroughly studied under a microscope by experts. This procedure, known as biopsy, is usually performed in a hospital.

Infection of the mother's breasts may occur after childbirth, and is characterized by high temperature, and redness and pain in the breast. This condition is successfully treated with penicillin or other similar drugs.

The nursing process after childbirth depends on hormones from the pituitary gland which help produce actively secreting glandular structures. Generally, milk begins to flow within a few days of birth, though it may begin sooner. At first, the milk, yellowish and cheesy, is a protein-rich substance known as colostrum. Finally this gives way to true milk, a thin, bluish-white secretion. Opinion favoring breast feeding fluctuates. However, it seems best for new mothers to try to breast feed their babies. Allergies are fewer in such babies and infants usually do much better in general on mother's milk. Some belief prevails, too, that breast cancer may be lower in women who nurse their babies.

The size and shape of a woman's breasts depend on fatty tissue rather than glands, and thus women with larger breasts do not find it easier to nurse their babies than do those with smaller breasts. Many products are sold to help women increase the size of their breasts. Hormones are used but in general are best avoided, because of the dangers of stimulating a cancerous process. There does not seem to be any completely safe or desirable way to increase the size of the breasts. *See also* CANCER; FEEDING, BREAST; MASTITIS; PREGNANCY.

breathing. The act of inhaling and exhaling air. The normal rate of breathing in women is 18 to 20 times a minute, in children 20 to 26 times a minute, in infants 30 to 35 times a minute. In men it is 16 to 18 per minute. In women and children, breathing is largely done from the chest, in men largely from the abdomen. Restricted abdominal breathing occurs during pregnancy. *See* ASPIRATION.

breech presentation. In childbirth, the arrival of the buttocks first, rather than the head. The danger is that the head of the infant has to be delivered through passages which may not be fully dilated.

bromides. Bromides of potassium, calcium, iron, ammonium, and so-

dium are used in medicine. Bromides generally have a sedative effect and allay nervous tension. Some people are as allergic to the basic bromine as they are to some other drugs and may develop skin rash, boils, inflammation of hair follicles, and other inexplicable symptoms during the course of a disease.

Taken over a long period, bromides have a cumulative effect. When the level gets too high, bromide intoxication, or bromism, occurs, with such symptoms as headache, coldness of the extremities, drowsiness, apathy, delirium, hallucinations, and pallor of the skin.

bronchial tubes. *See* BRONCHIECTASIS; BRONCHITIS; BRONCHOPNEUMONIA; PNEUMONIA.

bronchiectasis. A chronic enlargement of the major or minor passages which carry air to and from the lungs; it usually produces an accumulation of infected mucus, consequent violent coughing, and markedly offensive breath. The cause may be an acute infection such as tuberculosis, pneumonia, or bronchitis, a protracted asthmatic condition, or a foreign body in the main air passages.

bronchitis. The condition caused when the bronchial tubes become inflamed or infected. The bronchial tubes are large delicate tubes that carry air into the tiny branches and smaller cells of the lungs after this air has passed through the mouth, nasal passages, and windpipe, or trachea. Usually inflammation or infection begins as a cold which persists and leads to chronic cough. The bronchial tubes may become infected after measles, whooping cough, or influenza, or during infection with any of the germs that infect the nose and throat. Viruses may also cause bronchitis. Bronchial irritation from excessive smoking, inhaling noxious gases or fumes and irritating dusts may lead to inflammation and bronchitis. Frequently, chronic irritation from these substances will weaken the resistance of the lining of the bronchioles and they become more susceptible to infection by germs.

bronchopneumonia. A type of inflammation of the lungs, caused by germs such as the pneumococci, streptococci, Friedländer's bacillus, or by a number of others. In children under three, pneumococci are usually responsible. Bronchopneumonia is a hazard to life all year round, and its various forms claim their victims at every period of life.

In contrast to lobar pneumonia, in which one or more lobes or large divisions of the lobes are affected, bronchopneumonia is caused by scattered pus forming patches of inflammation in the lung. In most instances, bronchopneumonia begins with an infection of the nose, throat, or bronchial tubes, or as a complication of another disease such as whooping cough, measles, influenza, or a common bronchitis. As a secondary disease brought about by a variety of organisms, it may affect all age groups, but as a primary disorder bronchopneumonia occurs only in children under three years of age.

The aged often become victims of bronchopneumonia because of their tendency to accumulate mucous material in the lungs. As the power of the lungs to repair themselves has diminished, small areas of degenerated tissue are affected and the accumulating material must be expelled from the lungs. The continued inhalation and coughing results in disturbances such as bronchopneumonia.

The disease may not start as abruptly as other types of pneumonia. Symptoms like fever, coughing, and shortness of breath gradually become worse. The temperature lowers step by step with recovery.

Such drugs as the sulfanilamides and antibiotics are most frequently used in the treatment, and the response is best if the invading organisms are susceptible to them. *See also* PNEUMONIA.

brucellosis. *See* UNDULANT FEVER.

bruises. Injuries, sufficiently severe, to the surface of the body which do not break the skin. If the skin breaks and bleeds, the wound is called a laceration. Bruises are usually caused by bumping against hard or sharp surfaces, by falls, or by blows.

bubo. A painful inflammation or swelling of a lymphatic gland, which usually develops in the groin, especially after venereal infections. An abscess caused by injury or irritation, not by infection, is a "sympathetic" bubo. *See also* LYMPHOGRANULOMA VENEREUM.

bubonic plague. An acute infectious disease caused by bacteria transmitted by the rat flea. It is characterized by enlargement of the lymphatic glands and toxic symptoms of great severity. The mortality rate is high.

bulbar. In medicine, a term pertaining to the medulla of the brain. Formerly the medulla oblongata, the lower part of the brain stem, was called a bulb.

bulbar poliomyelitis. *See* POLIOMYELITIS.

bunion. A painful swelling and overgrowth of bone on the foot. The deformity usually affects the large toe, the joint becoming swollen while the tip of the toe is forced inward against the other toes. Occasionally a bunion will occur on the top of the foot. The skin is usually thickened.

Bunions are often caused by poorly fitted footwear; and properly fitted shoes, perhaps padded, will usually help to relieve the discomfort. Complete relief, however, is brought about only by surgical removal of the bunion together with a part of the overgrown bone beneath it.

burns. A burn is a searing of the flesh which can be caused by many agents—from hot steam to the sun's rays. Each year over 6000 fatal burns occur in the United States and burns are a common cause of death in young children. Burns involving over one-third to one-half of the body are often fatal, especially in children.

bursa. A small fluid-filled sac which serves as a cushion against friction among joints that move upon each other. For example, a bursa lies between the heelbone and the Achilles' tendon. *See also* BURSITIS.

bursitis. An inflammation of a bursa; one of the most frequent rheumatic ailments. A bursa is a small sac situated between joints that move on each other, a kind of lubricating part around them. An inflamed bursa contains calcium deposits in a semisolid state. Bursae in any of the joints may become inflamed. Most frequently, however, the shoulder is affected; bursitis of the elbow and above the knee is less frequent.

Ordinarily, bursitis is extremely painful in both the acute or chronic form. It may appear suddenly, following chilling, strains, blows, or infection. Frequently, bursitis results fom excessive use of a joint, as, for example, in playing tennis, or prolonged standing or stretching. Chronic bursitis may be a consequence of acute bursitis or it may be a chronic manifestation from the beginning.

The symptoms of acute bursitis are always a sharp pain and discoloration at the spot where the inflammation is located. In some cases, limited swelling is present and the inflamed bursa can be felt. In chronic bursitis, swelling and tenderness fluctuate and progress with intermittent pain, brought on perhaps by changes of weather or excessive use of the joint.

Sometimes acute bursitis heals without any treatment. The inflamed bursa may drain itself, through rupture. Resting the afflicted part, however, is always imperative. Hot or cold applications, whichever the patient prefers, are often soothing, and exposure to the sun may help relieve chronic recurrent pains. Most physicians do not recommend massage under any circumstances. If the pain does not subside with such usual palliatives as aspirin, analgesic drugs, or even codeine, morphine or other narcotics may be prescribed by a physician. Sometimes he will irrigate the bursal cavity by needle or by incision and drainage.

Cortisone and ACTH have been successful in relieving severe cases of bursitis, but these drugs must be used for long periods. Deep X-ray therapy often brings good results. *See also* BURSA.

buttocks. The two fleshy parts of the posterior part of the body on which one sits; they are formed by the glutei, or buttock, muscles.

Butyn. A trade name for butacaine sulfate, a substitute for cocaine as a surface local anesthetic for mucous membranes and eyes.

cachexia. A state of malnutrition, wasting, constant pain. Associated with toxemia of pregnancy, as well as malignant disease.

calamine. Zinc carbonate, pulverized and cleansed. In compounds it is used externally as an astringent and dusting powder. As a soothing protection, calamine lotion is applied in cases of sunburn, insect bites, acne, and other skin irritations.

calcium. A silver-white, soft metal which occurs only in combination with other elements. It is present in spring and river waters and in plants and the bodies of man and animals.

The body of the average person contains significant amounts of thirteen minerals. Of them all, calcium is present in the largest amount and is one of the most essential. It is present in and vital to the health of every known tissue and cell in the body. It is a significant element in building strong bones and teeth.

A calcium deficiency may be involved in the cause of so-called degenerative diseases—those diseases involving a loss in the power of functioning of any part of the body —such as hardening of the arteries, some allergies, disorders of the heart, kidney, and blood vessels. The U.S. Department of Agriculture publishes lists of foods rated as excellent or good in calcium richness, which can be used as a guide in helping to assure an adequate supply of calcium in the diet. Listed as excellent are: broccoli, buttermilk, cabbage, chard, Cheddar and Swiss cheese, clams, dandelion greens, kale, milk in all its forms—whole, skimmed, evaporated, condensed, and dried—molasses, mustard and turnip greens, watercress, and yeast. Listed as good are: almonds, artichokes, all kinds of beans including dried, kidney, string, and snap, carrots, celery, cottage cheese, crabs, cream, eggs, endive or escarole, dried figs, lettuce, lobsters, maple syrup, oysters.

If foods were listed in the order of their significance, milk in its various forms, excepting butter, would lead the list, followed by green, leafy vegetables.

To insure a good supply of calcium during pregnancy and eliminate leg cramps, physicians frequently prescribe calcium in different compounds as a dietary supplement. *See also* VITAMINS.

calcium-phosphorus ratio. A particular balance between calcium and phosphorus must be maintained within the body so that healthy tissue evolves from strong bone cells. Therefore, both calcium and phosphorus are essential in the diet.

calculus. A stone, or concretion of mineral salts, which forms most frequently in the cavities of the body which act as reservoirs for fluids. Often the stone takes its name from the cavity in which it grows—for example, kidney stone or gallstone. Calculi may develop in any tissue in which calcium or other minerals are deposited. *See also* BLADDER DISEASES; COLIC; GALLSTONES; KIDNEYS.

callus. Generally any area of hardened, thickened skin caused by friction, pressure, or other irritation. It is also new tissue which forms where a fractured bone heals.

Most calluses—for example, those on the palm of the hand—do not cause trouble and do not require medical attention. But in other locations calluses may cause pain. For instance, when pressure is exerted on a heavily thickened callus on the foot at a point where it is caught between the shoe and the prominent bones beneath the ball of the foot, treatment may be necessary. Paring off the outer layers of the hardened skin with a sharp knife or file is the usual way, but chemicals also are sometimes used. In severe cases, relief is secured by inserting a protective device within the shoe or by changing the area of weight bearing.

Great care must be taken not to damage the delicate tissue beneath the callus by cutting too deeply. Di-abetics and persons suffering from any arterial disease must never try to treat corns or calluses themselves. It is better to prevent calluses by making certain that shoes are properly fitted, by avoiding continued pressure irritation, and by taking sensible care of the feet. *See also* FEET.

calorie. The unit by which the energy value of food is measured. Specifically it is equivalent to the amount of heat required to raise one cubic centimeter of water one degree Centigrade. Foods vary widely in their caloric contents. For instance, a pound of butter will supply a vastly larger number of calories than a pound of lettuce. By checking the number of calories consumed against the energy output charted for a person's age, height, weight, and occupation, the doctor can determine whether the person eats too many, too few, or sufficient calories for his daily needs. If too many, the excess is stored as fat in specially provided cells in the body. If too few, the body draws either upon its fat deposits or tissues to make up the deficit and the person will show a weight loss. If caloric intake and energy output balance, weight tends to remain stable.

camphor. A volatile oil with a characteristic aromatic smell. It is a mild irritant and cooling antiseptic when applied to the mucous membranes and the skin. Camphorized ointments and oils aid the relief of nasal congestion, but must not be used for infants or small children. In acute inflammations of glands, camphor has been beneficial as a

cooling pain reliever. *See also* POI-
SONING.

cancer. A disease characterized by
abnormal and often unpredictable
growth of cells. Cancerous growths
are also disposed to invade normal
healthy tissues and destroy or
even replace them by wild growth
of the cancerous cells. Nerves may
be affected, causing pain; blood vessels may be broken open by the
invading growth, causing hemorrhage; and structures such as lung
tissues, the arteries, kidneys, or
bladder may be obstructed by in-
filtration of cancer tissue. Every
part of the body is susceptible to
cancerous growths, though some
organs, such as stomach, bowel,
lung, and the sexual organs, seem
more frequently involved.

Accumulations of rapidly growing
cells may form a lump known as a
tumor, but not all tumors are cancerous or dangerous. Many, such
as fibromas, clumps of scar-type
tissue; adenomas, clumps of harmless glandular tissue; warts, fatty
tumors, or lipomas do not invade
normal tissue and do not lead to
serious consequences. They are benign or harmless growths or tumors. Groups of cells which invade
normal tissue and destroy healthy
cells are malignant. Growth may be
rapid or slow, but usually is progressive.

Some cancers remain in one location; others tend to spread through
the bloodstream or lymphatic
stream throughout the body. These
"pilgrim-type" growths, metastases,
in general represent a more serious
type of cancer.

The exact cause of cancer is unknown. Some scientists believe that
persons are born with abnormal
cells and that these remain quiescent throughout life or until some
factor starts them growing. Others
believe that chronic irritation of a
certain group of cells may lead to
cancerous changes. Cancer of the
lip is common in pipe smokers and
lung cancer in cigarette smokers.
Some specialists feel that irritation
from the sun may lead to skin cancers, common in farmers and outdoor workers. Chemicals also may
induce cancer. The sex hormones
are related to cancer development,
especially of the breast or reproductive system. Because wives of
circumcised men rarely develop
cancer of the cervix, some experts
believe that the uncircumcised male
may harbor a cancer-producing secretion under the foreskin. A relationship may exist between failure
to breast feed and breast cancer.
Heredity is probably significant, but
just how is not yet known. Cancer
is probably not contagious; nevertheless, experiments utilizing our
knowledge of viruses are being
made to confirm this.

Doctors classify cancer according
to many factors: the type of tissue
involved; the speed of its growth;
the portion of the body involved;
and sometimes even according to
the chemical changes that take
place within the tumor.

Some cancers are easily seen or
felt, such as breast and skin cancers; some can be detected or
suspected by rectal or vaginal examination, by introduction of instruments into the stomach, by
X-ray, blood, or urine tests, and

other techniques. Certain cancers —for instance, breast cancers—are found predominantly in women. Lung and mouth cancers are more common in men.

The symptoms of early cancers are often barely noticeable; therefore, a complete and thorough medical checkup is desirable at least once a year, and oftener if abnormal symptoms occur. Lives are needlessly lost because cancer is diagnosed much too late for the doctor to achieve successful treatment. Often the symptoms are caused by a harmless condition, but delay in treatment can be hazardous.

Any of the following symptoms should be checked promptly by a competent physician:

Mouth. Any sore in the mouth, or anywhere for that matter, that lasts more than a few days without healing should be reported.

Larynx. Hoarseness that persists for more than a week, and for three weeks at the most, should be suspected. By examination of the vocal cords, the doctor can determine whether or not they are inflamed or irritated, or affected by tumors of a benign or malignant nature. Removal of the growths and examination of the specimen under the microscope will aid in making the diagnosis.

Breast. Any discomfort, pain, thickening, dimpling, or lump in a breast of a man or woman that does not disappear within a week, and any discharge from the nipple, bloody or otherwise, demand immediate attention. Delay can be perilous. If the doctor demands surgical removal of the lump for expert examination, this should be done without delay as only by microscopic examination of tissue can definite diagnosis be made.

Stomach. Stomach cancer seldom causes pain. Ordinarily, early signs include loss of appetite, diarrhea, appearance of black material in the stools, regurgitation, or difficulty in swallowing food. Generally these symptoms point to conditions less serious than cancer, and the doctor can make correct diagnosis by using X-ray and other techniques.

Among women, prolonged, irregular, or unusual bleeding, especially after the age of thirty-five or between periods, should always be investigated promptly.

Cancer may be diagnosed in many different ways, some simple, others complicated. Most significant is a detailed history of the onset and nature of the patient's symptoms, followed by a thorough examination. When suspicious growths are noted on the skin, in the breasts, or within the reproductive organs, the doctor may take a piece of tissue for examination under the microscope. This is known as biopsy. The cancer cell, when viewed under the microscope, is different from the normal cell. In some cases, changes in the cells may be difficult to detect, even by experts.

The Papanicolaou test for cancer is widely used. In this test, scrapings taken from the surface of the cervix of the uterus or from the walls of the vagina are treated with certain chemicals. The tissues are then placed under the microscope, where careful examination can usually rule out or indicate the presence of early cancer changes. The test can be used on the sputum of presumed lung cancer, and also on stomach secretion when cancer in that organ is suspected.

Tissue from within the body can be removed for analysis by curettage, as in the uterus when the uterus wall is scraped. Investigation may be performed by bronchoscopy, in which a long tube is inserted into the lung structure to remove tissue; by gastroscopy, done with a stomach tube; or proctoscopy, in which a long telescopelike instrument is inserted into the rectum. These instruments used for detecting cancer are often provided with a light so that the operator can actually look into the organs.

X-ray is invaluable in detecting cancer. To aid in finding stomach or rectal cancer, barium, a white substance, is introduced into these organs and helps X-rays detect any tumors by outlining them. Occasionally, substances may be injected into the bloodstream to outline the kidneys or other organs.

Blood tests for the detection of cancer, except for cancer of the blood, are being studied extensively, but as yet none of the tests has been accepted.

Some scientists are convinced that some cancers are caused by a virus, a form of living growth too small to be seen under the microscope.

Hormones, particularly sex hormones, may stimulate cancer growth. These include the female hormone estrogen, and the male hormone testosterone. Estrogen in excessive amounts may stimulate growth of breast cancers while it may delay growth of male cancers, notably prostate cancers. The male hormone may actually help to stop the growth of female breast cancer, and conversely stimulate prostate cancer.

Is cancer hereditary? Studies on animals indicate that the tendency to develop cancer seems stronger in some families than in others, although there does not seem to be a true inheritance. In some families, cancer apparently will develop in certain circumstances. Therefore, when any cancer is common in one family, members of the family should avoid taking sex hormones and overexposure to X-rays or to other chemicals or irritants.

Cancer-stimulating substances are thought to include coal tars, X-rays, excessive exposure to the sun, viruses, and hormones. Mechanical irritation, such as tight girdles or collars and friction on a mole on the skin may be harmful. Rough teeth and improperly fitted dentures may, by causing irritation, lead to cancer of the mouth, as may pipe and cigarette smoking.

Cancer of the blood usually manifests itself by anemia, fatigue, loss of weight, and shortness of breath. The diagnosis is made by examining the blood and a specimen of tissue taken from the bone marrow.

Surgery has always been one of the most effective ways to remove cancers. By the removal of localized growths, the patient may be completely cured. Approach to treatment may be varied, and may not, in some cases, even include surgery. X-ray, or radium treatment is employed successfully in many types of pelvic cancer. Chemical therapy includes hormone treatments of breast and prostate cancer, and also drug management of the leukemias, blood cancers. Often a combination of surgery, X-ray, and drugs is used.

Most exciting of recent approaches to treatment is the use of radioactive isotopes. The isotopes are chemicals having radioactivity combined with a chemical element. Since these chemicals are likely to go directly to one tissue of the body, they concentrate in that organ and destroy abnormal tissues there. Cancer of the thyroid has been successfully treated by using radioactive iodine. Iron, sodium, potassium, chlorine, bromine, calcium, strontium, sulfur, carbon, and hydrogen have all been subjected to experiments in controlling growths in various parts of the body. Radioactive phosphorus has also been applied externally to warts, moles, and other growths on the surface of the body, and in some instances with apparent success.

The nitrogen mustard chemicals, developed for use in warfare, have been helpful in destroying cancer cells. These drugs are used effectively in Hodgkin's disease, chronic leukemia, and in other tumors.

canker sore. Usually a small ulceration on the inside of the mouth, lip, or cheek, which may appear from a variety of causes. Sometimes the cause stems from the nervous system; often the sore is a manifestation of a sensitivity to certain substances taken into the body; and frequently it is due to a virus infection such as a cold. Whenever canker sores appear persistently, a medical study should be made for some functional disturbance, including an examination of the blood to determine the status of the clotting elements in the bloodstream. Tests should also be made for sensitivity to various foods, and the fillings in the patient's teeth examined, since it has been shown that dissimilar metals used as fillings in the same mouth may create electrical currents sometimes associated with the appearance of cankers in the mouth.

cantharides. Popularly called Spanish fly, a bitter-tasting powder made from an insect known scientifically as *Cantharis vesicatoria*. The active principle in the drug is cantharidin, which is marketed in many forms, such as cantharidin plaster, blistering fluid, cantharidin ointment, and tincture of cantharidin.

The drug should be used only when prescribed by a doctor, and the utmost precaution should be taken to prevent it from entering the mouth, the eyes, or other sensitive areas.

Cantharidin is never used before the condition of the patient's kidneys has been checked, since the drug is easily absorbed through the skin. It must not be applied to any part of the body on which the patient is likely to lie, since the heat and perspiration result in blistering. Furthermore, it is dangerous when applied to paralyzed arms or legs. Such reputation as it has as a stimulant to sexual desire is without any good evidence.

Cantharides is intensely irritating to the kidneys and should never be taken internally. In the treatment of children, the aged, or the weak it should never be used, even externally, for any purpose.

Symptoms of cantharidin poisoning may be intense pain in the alimentary canal, in the stomach and kidneys, or in the urinary organs. Vomiting and diarrhea ordinarily occur, and a persistent desire to urinate is noticeable. The pulse is usually weak and slow and collapse is not unlikely. *See also* BLISTERS.

capillaries. The smallest branches of the arterial tree; fine, filamentlike vessels through which blood pumped by the heart through increasingly smaller branches of the arterial tree finally passes by osmosis, an exchange of substances, to the cells of body organs and tissues. They are the minute structural elements which connect arterial circulation with venous circulation and carry deoxygenated blood back to the heart. *See also* BLOOD; CIRCULATORY SYSTEM.

carbohydrates. Organic substances which contain carbon, hydrogen, and oxygen and are stable, easily digestible sources of calories or nutritional energy. They belong to the class of nutriments represented by sugars, starches, celluloses, and gums. Foods with large carbohydrate content are sugars, jams, jellies, preserves, syrups, molasses, honey, cocoa, chocolate, candy, grains, grain products, and farinaceous substances. Nuts, although they contain a larger proportion per weight of protein, and an even greater proportion of fats, are also substantial in carbohydrate content. All dairy products, fruits, and vegetables have carbohydrates in varying amounts. Dates and figs are especially rich in this nutriment, and potatoes, parsnips, and most lentils are also plentifully supplied with carbohydrates.

carbon dioxide. A colorless, odorless gas, a molecule of which consists of one atom of carbon in combination with two atoms of oxygen. It is one of the end products of the cellular metabolism of proteins, carbohydrates, and fats, all of which are carbon-containing compounds. It is given off by the body during that phase of respiration known as exhalation.

carbon monoxide. A colorless, odorless gas, a product of the incomplete combustion of carbon. It is extremely poisonous. It burns with a pale blue flame to form carbon dioxide. Carbon monoxide may develop when coal oil, charcoal, gas, or kerosene is burned in a poorly ventilated room. A frequent source of carbon monoxide is the exhausts of automobiles. In the open air, the gas quickly becomes carbon dioxide, but in a closed garage a running motor may produce enough carbon monoxide to kill in a matter of minutes.

Carbon monoxide invades the bloodstream through the lungs, unites with the hemoglobin in the red blood corpuscles so that they cannot carry oxygen to the cells of the body, and asphyxiation ensues. The blood of victims of carbon-monoxide poisoning is a bright cherry red.

Early symptoms of carbon-monoxide poisoning include yawning, headache, nausea, dizziness, ringing in the ears, and abdominal pains. Gaspy breathing and unconsciousness quickly follow. The victim should get fresh air immediately, and he should be kept lying down and warm. A physician should be called promptly, and inhalations of oxygen or of oxygen-carbon-dioxide mixture administered. Pure oxygen accelerates the release of carbon monoxide and frees it from the blood about four times faster than simple inhalation of air. If the breathing of the victim is gasping or has stopped, artificial respiration should be given at once.

If the carbon-monoxide poisoning is serious, the victim should be taken to the hospital as soon as possible for treatment which may include blood transfusions. Since the nerve cells are involved in the poisoning, temporary or permanent damage can be done to the brain, with serious disturbances of vision, hearing, speech, and memory.

Because carbon monoxide cannot be seen or smelled, danger of poisoning is especially insidious. Care should be taken that rooms in which fuels capable of producing carbon monoxide are being burned are properly ventilated, and that a car motor is not kept running in a closed garage.

carbuncles. Painful infections of the skin layer below the surface, accompanied by the production and discharge of pus and dead tissue, and tending to affect the general health. A carbuncle may be distinguished from a boil by its greater severity and depth and especially by its having several openings instead of one.

The first symptom of a carbuncle is a painful, hard lump which develops under a tight and reddening skin. Several pus-discharging openings later appear in this surface. Eventually the entire mass will tend to separate itself, leaving an open sore.

Carbuncles appear most frequently on the face, neck, and shoulders. They particularly afflict persons who suffer from diabetes or Bright's disease. In such people, resistance to invasive microorganisms which set up infection is lowered.

carcinogens. Substances or agents that cause the development of cancer of any type—for example, certain tar or coal products.

carcinoma. A technical word for cancer.

cardiac. Related to the heart. A person referred to as a "cardiac" is one afflicted with heart disease.

carditis. An inflammation of the heart, a manifestation and significant part of rheumatic fever. Internal carditis or endocarditis is the inflammation of the valves of the heart and membranes which line it. Pericarditis is the inflammation of the sac which encloses the heart. *See also* BACTERIAL ENDOCARDITIS; ENDOCARDITIS; PERICARDITIS.

carminative. An agent which relieves flatulence and colic.

carotene. A chemical precursor of vitamin A, is a yellow pigment found in green and yellow vegetables such as carrots, sweet potatoes, yellow corn, and string beans. It is converted in the animal body into vitamin A. *See also* VITAMINS.

carpal bones. The eight bones of the wrist. On the back of the hand, five metacarpal bones connect the fingers with the wrist.

carrier of disease. The agent which transmits a communicable disease. It can be any of a vast number of things—air and dust, nose and throat secretions, sputum, clothing, insects. For example, certain mosquitoes carry malaria, dengue, and filariasis. Disease-producing bacteria cannot penetrate unbroken skin and must enter by means of wounds, scratches, abrasions, or a natural opening of the body. *See also* BACTERIA.

car sickness. *See* MOTION SICKNESS.

cartilage. A white, semi-opaque connective tissue characterized by extreme smoothness, elasticity, and toughness. It covers the ends of the bones where they meet to become joints.

cascara. Because of its effective action on the colon, cascara is widely used as a laxative. Usually cascara is prescribed in the form of an aromatic extract. Cascara sagrada, the bark of California buckthorn, is especially useful in cases of chronic constipation.

casein. The principal protein in milk. In milk, a liquid precursor, caseinogen, is present rather than casein itself. Converted into solid casein, for instance by rennet, a ferment in the stomach, it is the basis of curds or cheese. When milk is drunk slowly, its casein content becomes a light, flaky mass of curds in the stomach, rather than an indigestible dense body. This action is significant for children, older persons, or invalids.

castor oil. An effective and prompt purgative and one of the oldest household remedies for constipation. It is likely, however, to be followed by costiveness and is therefore seldom used in chronic constipation. Castor oil is also used to counteract the effects of acid splashed in the eye.

castration. The removal of one or both testes or ovaries, with a consequent deficiency of the endocrine hormones. It is one of the oldest surgical operations and was well known in earliest antiquity. Male foreign captives were castrated to prevent a mixing with foreign blood. Castration was sometimes a ritual which eliminated sexual desire so that an ascetic life could more easily be led.

In women, castration consists in removing the ovaries, and is medically termed an oophorectomy.

cataract. Opacity producing loss of transparency of the lens of the eye; if the lens becomes entirely opaque, sight is lost. A cataract may be present at birth, and in young people it may appear as a result of injury. However, most cataracts occur in persons between the ages of fifty and seventy and are due to the gradual degeneration of the tissues of the lenses. To some extent, a tendency to this degeneration may be hereditary. Although the disease may show itself at first in only one eye, in almost all instances it will eventually appear in the other also. The process is gradual and "ripeness" or full opacity may take two years to develop.

Among the earliest symptoms of cataract are red eyelids, unexplainable daytime headaches, small specks seen constantly before the eyes, and other gradually developing symptoms which should be called promptly to the attention of a physician skilled in treatment of eye disorders. Temporary eyesight can be maintained by frequent changes of glasses.

Physicians generally agree, however, that the only effective treatment for a cataract itself is an operation. Such an operation restores good vision to approximately ninety-seven persons out of a hundred. The surgery, relatively simple, is followed by the prescription of so-called cataract glasses, which contain biconvex lenses to replace the clouded natural lenses that are removed. *See also* EYE.

catarrh. A term which was formerly used for inflammations of mucous membranes, especially those of the nose, throat, and the air passages. A cold with secretions—as a "running nose," for example—was popularly called a catarrh.

cathartics. Drugs or medicinal preparations to relieve constipation and cause an evacuation of the bowels. Cathartics stimulate the muscular activity of the intestines and promote the flow of liquid to the bowels, thus flushing the alimentary canal. If the cathartic is especially strong, it is called a purgative. If it is mild, it is called a laxative.

Elimination of waste is a natural process, assisted by coarse foods, water, exercise, and laxative material in the diet such as fruit juices, vegetables, whole wheat, honey, and oatmeal. Most people can eliminate waste materials without artificial stimuli. The frequency of defecation—emptying the bowel—is not significant in most cases. If the use of cathartics appears to be frequently necessary, a physician should be consulted. The habitual use of cathartics irritates the bowels, weakens their normal movement, and results in irregularity of elimination. The incidence of hemorrhoids, for example, is high among those who habitually use cathartics. In obesity, the prolonged use of cathartics is not only ineffectual but harmful.

Cathartics of any kind should never be taken when abdominal pain is present. This pain may be the first sign of a beginning appendicitis, and if an abdominal pain persists or appears to be exceedingly severe, medical treatment is imperative. When the appendix is inflamed, cathartics may increase the irritation and peritonitis may occur as a result. In many cases, such inflammation of the membrane which lines the interior of the abdominal cavity is fatal.

Mineral oil and mineral oil modified with various substances are among the mildest of the cathartics currently used.

Other methods of relieving constipation are glycerin suppositories, enemas, and castor oil, an old household remedy. A tablespoon or two of milk of magnesia taken occasionally is considered a safe cathartic. Saline cathartics such as Epsom salt (magnesium sulfate), sodium sulfate, etc., are active cathartics, especially useful in inflammatory infections and as blood purifiers in cases of poisoning. *See also* CONSTIPATION; MEDICINE CHEST; and names of specific cathartics.

catheter. A flexible or rigid tube used to drain fluid from various cavities of the body, especially when the normal outlets do not function properly. The tube may be passed gently through the nose to the Eustachian tube which communicates with the ear, for example, or into the urethra which connects with the urinary bladder. A catheter should never be forced into or through any cavity.

caul at birth. Caul is a popular term for the sac in which the child lies during pregnancy. Part or all of this fetal membrane may be brought forth in labor, preceding the child. A caul at birth has sometimes been considered by superstitious people to be a sign of good luck.

causalgia. A sharp, burning pain, sometimes a symptom of injuries of the nerves, particularly the sensory nerves supplying the palms and soles. The disturbance may be associated with many vasomotor, digestive, and dermal changes in the affected parts.

cavities. *See* DENTAL CARIES.

cecum. A portion of the bowel on the lower right side of the abdomen. The appendix branches off the cecum.

celiac disease. An ailment which affects children under five years of age, most frequently between the ages of two and three. In celiac disease, the child is unable to digest and utilize fats, starches, and sometimes sugars. Sensitivity to gluten from wheat or rye grains was recently established as the cause of this inability. The child becomes weak and undernourished, anemic, and his growth is stunted. Sometimes the stomach is swollen, as in starvation. Since the child is not well, he may be irritable, sullen, and behavior problems result as a consequence. Usually he has little appetite and even when obviously hungry will often refuse food. Conversely he may eat voraciously, with no gain in weight. Severe diarrhea is almost always the most telling symptom and stomach cramps may accompany it. Most of these symptoms are common to other conditions, and only a doctor can determine if celiac disease is the cause.

Celiac disease is ordinarily treated by a special diet. Fats, such as butter, cream, fried foods, and ice cream, and foods containing wheat or rye grains are excluded from the diet. Sugar tends to increase the amount of gas and to provoke diarrhea, and natural sugars, as are found in fresh fruits, are best tolerated. Protein foods can usually be eaten without ill effect, and so milk protein, egg white, lean meat, fish, liver, and protein-rich vegetables constitute part of the diet. Of special benefit is a milk preparation which is high in protein but low in milk sugar and fat. For a time bananas were considered beneficial and banana diets were prescribed. However, now it is felt that any benefit derived from bananas is due to the fact that bananas replace gluten in the child's diet. Vitamin B complex supplements are also given.

cell. A mass of protoplasm containing a nucleus; it constitutes the basic unit of life. *See also* BLOOD.

cellulitis. Usually refers to a diffuse inflammation of connective tissue. However, any inflammation of the cells of the body, at any point, can be called cellulitis. This disease may be caused by various bacilli, such as streptococci, staphylococci, or pneumococci.

cerebral. Denotes anything that is related to the cerebrum, the chief portion of the brain. For example, the cerebral cortex, also called "gray matter," is the outer part of the cerebrum where most of the cell bodies are located. The cerebrum is divided by a deep groove into two cerebral hemispheres. These cerebral hemispheres are representative of approximately 70 per cent of the nervous system.

Illnesses associated with brain injuries are denoted by the addition of the word "cerebral" as, for example, cerebral dysrhythmia, which is epilepsy, and cerebral palsy or paralysis due to hemorrhage. *See also* BRAIN.

cerebral arteriosclerosis. *See* SENILITY.

cerebral hemorrhage. *See* APOPLEXY.

cerebral palsy. A long-term neuromuscular disease of the central nervous system. It is usually caused by damage to the brain. Once injured, the brain does not heal without scar tissue and areas are destroyed and cannot function. Thus far cerebral palsy cannot be prevented or cured, but research in causes and prevention has progressed greatly, and much can now be done for the afflicted child if treatment and training are begun early.

The crippling that results from cerebral palsy is a physical complication, but its cause lies in the original brain damage, with different degrees of physical disability, impairment, and mental retardation. Spasms, lack of co-ordination, weakness, tremors, rigidity, and difficulty in seeing, hearing, and speaking can be observed in the patient.

While cerebral palsy is not synonymous with mental deficiency, a large proportion of afflicted children, estimated at 50 to 70 per cent, are mentally retarded to some extent, and the disease is significant in an overall consideration of the problem of mental deficiency. The brain of the child with cerebral palsy may be damaged before birth or during infancy. Various factors may cause the brain damage, such as faulty brain-cell development of the child in the mother's womb, disorders such as kidney disease, convulsions in the mother, incompatibility of the Rh blood factors of mother and child, or childhood infections with accompanying high temperatures.

Weight at birth seems to be involved in cerebral palsy incidence, because of more protracted and difficult labor. As older women generally have heavier babies and boys are frequently heavier at birth than girls, the disease occurs more frequently in male babies born to older mothers. The risks are particularly great in premature babies since the skull of a premature baby is so mobile that damage to the brain can easily occur. Since a greater number of premature babies now survive than formerly, the incidence of cerebral palsy is steadily increasing.

Treatment varies according to the cause and severity of the disease. In mild cases, the child may receive muscle training and other special treatment and live a relatively normal life. Braces are employed to support weak muscles and prevent their shortening. Training in muscular movements, relaxation, and speech therapy is also essential. Any treatment of cerebral palsy requires great patience and must be supplemented by common-sense management of individual cases. *See also* BIRTH INJURIES.

cerebrospinal fluid. A clear, watery fluid secreted by the capillary blood vessels in the small cavities of the brain. The cerebrospinal fluid acts as a cushion for the brain and spinal cord, as well as a conveyor of the waste of metabolism.

cerebrospinal meningitis. Meningitis, as such, is not a definite disease but an inflammation of the meninges, the membranes of the brain and the spinal column. The invasion of the cerebrospinal column by micro-organisms such as pneumococcus, staphylococcus, or streptococcus is usually responsible, but various viruses also cause meningitis.

Cerebrospinal meningitis, also called spotted fever and cerebrospinal fever, is a sporadic or epidemic form of meningitis caused by a germ, the meningococcus. This disease is characterized by inflammation of the cerebrospinal meninges.

While the cause of cerebrospinal meningitis is not yet fully established, medical scientists believe that it is spread by contact with germ-laden droplets, produced by coughing and sneezing, from the nose and throat of infected carriers. The incidence of the disease, which most frequently affects children and adolescents, is highest in winter and early spring. In its epidemic form, cerebrospinal meningitis sometimes occurs in overcrowded, unsanitary surroundings. Epidemics in schools are much less frequent than generally believed.

The onset of cerebrospinal meningitis is sudden, and has many characteristics of the common cold, such as chills, headaches, and pains in the neck and limbs, often accompanied by vomiting and prostration. Stiff neck is one of the most characteristic symptoms of cerebral meningitis. It develops within thirty-six hours and renders movement of the head extremely painful. The victim ordinarily will be sensitive to noise and light and his face may be either pale or cyanotic.

Fatalities from cerebrospinal meningitis have been greatly reduced by chemi- and bio-therapeutics, including sulfa drugs and penicillin. Thus, while still serious, it is no longer feared as it was in the past. The duration of cerebrospinal meningitis is variable, but recovery is now usually rapid. However, in some cases, consequences such as behavior changes, muscular weakness, and disturbances in vision and hearing may develop.

Anyone who suspects that she has come in contact with a person infected with this disease should be examined by a physician immediately so that sulfa and antibiotic treatment can be given, if necessary. *See also* MENINGITIS.

cerebrum. The frontal and upper part of the brain, consisting of two separate halves or hemispheres. The nerve endings believed to control thought and judgment are centered here. In human beings this organ is by far the largest part of the entire brain. Because of its vital functions, the word "cerebrum" is often used as a synonym for the brain itself. This term should not be confused with cerebellum, the smaller rear portion of the brain which governs muscular movements. *See also* BRAIN.

cervix. The entrance or mouth of the womb. It is situated deep within the female sexual passageway and resembles a small hollow cylinder about two inches long and one inch wide. Following ejaculation by the male, the spermatozoa travel through the canal of the cervix into the uterus and Fallopian tubes, where fertilization may take place should an ovum be present. At the beginning of labor, the "bloody show" heralds the onset of labor in most women. During labor, the opening in the cervix, normally the width of a pencil, is gradually stretched to permit the child to pass through. This is known as dilatation and is accompanied by the familiar labor pains. After delivery, the cervix quickly shrinks to its normal dimensions.

The cervix is one of the most significant tissues in a woman's body. It may be affected by infections, inflammations, or cancer. Fortunately the physician is able to see this tiny organ clearly with the aid of a small instrument known as a speculum which separates the walls and tissues of the vagina. Early treatment of disorders of the cervix is always essential. Ailments of the cervix are described under the general name of "cervicitis."

Infections of the glands within the cervix are especially common after childbirth. Symptoms include profuse irritating discharge from the vagina and occasionally oozing of blood, especially after sexual relations. These infections may be treated with vaginal creams and suppositories, by painless treatment in the doctor's office, or with douches of prescribed medications. Sometimes a badly infected cervix may require surgery or cauterization. Cauterization involves burning away infected tissue with chemicals or electrical current.

Raw areas, erosions, may occur after delivery, and cause oozing of blood and irritating discharge. Their treatment is similar to that of infections. Treatments should be continued until the cervical infection or erosion is completely cured, for cancer may develop in later years unless irritations of the cervix are entirely eradicated.

Fleshy warts which often grow on the cervix and sometimes cause bleeding are best removed by simple surgical measures. Cysts on the cervix may provoke bleeding or watery discharge. Treatment varies.

Cancer can occur on the cervix and constitutes one of the most common types of cancer affecting women, especially after forty. Symptoms vary from none at all to bloody or irritating discharge. To verify his diagnosis, the doctor will take a small bit of suspicious tissue from the cervix for examination under the microscope. Should cancer be present, treatment includes complete surgical removal of all the internal female structures, and often the use of X-ray and radium. Only the doctor can decide which combination is best. Results in early cases are excellent. For this reason, all women over thirty-five years of age should have an internal examination every six months. *See also* CANCER.

Cesarean section. The surgical operation by which childbirth is accomplished when normal delivery is either dangerous or impossible. Each year, approximately 150,000 births occur in this manner, comprising 4 per cent of all deliveries. The operation was done in early times, and received its name from a law in the days of the Caesars stating that all pregnant women dying before giving birth be so delivered in hopes of saving the unborn child. Tradition has it that Julius Caesar was delivered this way, but this is refuted by the fact that Caesar's mother lived years after his birth.

Formerly, because of uncontrollable hemorrhage and infection, the operation was extremely hazardous, but today, in skilled hands, the risk is about the same as that in simple appendectomy. The technique of Cesarean section consists of entering by incision the abdomen and uterus in which the child develops during pregnancy. Once a woman has had one Cesarean section, future pregnancies are usually delivered by this operation, but occasionally normal delivery is possible.

chafing. The irritation which results when two delicate skin surfaces persistently rub against each other, or when a foreign substance rubs the skin. The skin becomes red and painful and is often raw and moist. Chafing occurs most frequently in the armpits, in the groin, between the buttocks, below the breasts, in the folds of the skin, and also between the fingers and toes where it may be mistaken for a finger infection. Such an irritated area is a fertile place for germs or fungi.

For simple chafing, the treatment may consist of drying the skin thoroughly after bathing and applying a suitable dusting powder, zinc ointment, or cold cream, or one of the newer protective ointments. Cleanliness is important. Primarily essential, however, is the removal of the irritant which originally produced the lesion. This may mean more carefully fitted shoes, a larger, looser garment, or possibly a loss of weight. Sometimes a flat gauze bag filled with talcum powder and placed between the rubbing surfaces is soothing. *See also* ECZEMA.

chancre. The first visible symptom of syphilis is a sore, known as a chancre or hard chancre. The chancre usually develops from three to five weeks after exposure. It appears at the point where the spirochete has entered the body, which is ordinarily on the genital organs. Since it is possible, however, to contract syphilis without sexual contact, the chancre may occasionally appear in some other area, such as the mouth. If syphilis is treated in the primary, or chancre, stage, it can be cured with the use of antibiotics.

The term "soft chancre," also known as chancroid, designates an inflammation of the genitals caused by an entirely different micro-organism from that responsible for syphilis. The soft chancre, a yellow sore, discharging pus, appears a day or so after exposure. Unless the person is confined to his bed, so that his movements can be restricted to a minimum, the soft chancre may become an abscess. Swelling may also develop in the glands of the groin. Chancroid yields readily to treatment with proper hygiene and the use of antiseptics. Since syphilis may be involved, a physician should always be consulted. *See also* CHANCROID; SYPHILIS.

chancroid. A lesion in which the chancre, or sore, is soft, in contrast with the syphilitic chancre which is hard. It involves the genitalia and is usually of venereal origin. Early English writers sometimes referred to the disease, calling it the "groyne bump" or "Winchester goose," a name derived from the city of Winchester, where the disease was apparently widespread, and from the awkward gooselike walk of the victim.

The disease starts with an ache in the groin and inflamed glands. These swollen glands gradually gather into a painful poison-filled mass, called a bubo. Eventually the bubo bursts and the poison drains out. In many cases, the bubo remains open for weeks, and during this period the person may experience so much pain and discomfort that he is unable to walk.

Chancroid is caused by a streptobacillus and its incubation period is two to fourteen days after sexual intercourse. Treatment varies from washes and salves to caustics, electric cautery, and surgery. Sulfonamides are now an effective treatment, and antibiotics like streptomycin have also been successfully used.

chapped skin. A roughened, reddened, irritable condition caused by loss of the natural oils in the skin. It occurs especially when the air is dry or when the skin is exposed to irritants such as cold hard water and harsh soap. Some persons are particularly susceptible to chapping because their skin glands do not respond to climate changes.

To prevent painful irritation of the skin, the use of soap and water during the winter months should be kept to a minimum. For personal use, mild oils may occasionally be used instead of soap and water, and fats in the skin replenished with cold creams, or lotions and creams, which increase the moisture content of the skin. Rubber gloves or similar protective gloves may be used for household tasks.

The use of harsh soaps should be avoided. Hard water may be softened with washing soda or borax.

A soft towel should be used to dry the hands; never a hot fire or an electric air drier. Lips, especially vulnerable to chapping because their sensitive surface is frequently moistened, may develop ugly, painful breaks in the skin which are easily infected. A precautionary measure is to apply cold cream or petroleum jelly to the lips before going out into the cold. Chapped skin can be minimized if the home is properly heated, and overheat and excessive dryness avoided. A pan of water kept on the floor in each room will add moisture to the air through evaporation.

Despite all precautions, some chapping of the skin will occasionally occur. When this happens, the affected area should be protected from infection just as a wound is protected. Cracks in the skin may be treated with a mild ointment such as cold cream and then covered with clean gauze. If the irritation is prolonged, a physician should be consulted. *See also* CHILBLAINS.

chemotherapy. The prevention or treatment of certain infectious diseases by various chemical agents which act as antiseptics in the body or inhibit invading parasites without producing serious toxic effects on the patient.

chest, or thorax. Starts just above a dome-shaped muscle called the diaphragm, ends at the shoulder blades, the clavicles, and is surrounded by a cage of flexible bones, the thoracic cage. This cage is formed by twelve pairs of flat bones, the ribs, which are attached to twelve pairs of spinal vertebrae in the rear.

chickenpox. One of the most common as well as one of the most acute contagious diseases of childhood. It is characterized by a superficial eruption of flat transparent blisters which appear in successive crops on different parts of the body. Chickenpox develops most often in winter and spring, and the age group five to six is particularly susceptible. The condition is seldom seen in persons over twenty.

Chickenpox is caused by a virus, and is medically known as varicella because its rash resembles the rash in mild cases of smallpox, or variola. The infection is spread in the air, from the patient's nose, mouth, and blisters, and by contact. The contagious period is usually about fourteen days, starting about two days before the rash appears. One attack of chickenpox normally confers permanent immunity.

The infection usually begins with a slight fever, headache, listlessness, and loss of appetite. In a day or two, tiny red patches, about the size of a pinhead, appear on the back and chest. Within a few hours, blisters filled with clear liquid begin to develop in the center of the pocks, surrounded by a reddened area of skin, and continue to appear for three or four days. The rash may spread to the face, scalp, hands, and feet. The fluid turns yellow in a day or so, then a crust forms. The crust begins to peel off in the next five to twenty days. During this period, troublesome itching develops, and the chief difficulty is to restrain the child from scratching and incurring further infection.

Chickenpox is usually mild and

does not require special treatment. If itching is severe, the doctor may prescribe a calamine lotion or some other drug to relieve it. The child's fingernails should be cut short, and the fingertips and nails scrubbed often and thoroughly with soap, water, and alcohol. As long as fever is present and new blisters continue to appear, the child should be kept in bed and isolated, especially if other young children who have not had the disease are in the house.

As with other virus diseases, body resistance is lowered, and the child should be protected against possible complications, especially secondary infection. The scabs should be kept clean and free from irritation, and should be allowed to loosen and fall off naturally. Forcible removal of crusts may leave permanent scars. Diet should be especially nourishing, to build up the body and encourage more rapid healing.

chiggers. The larvae, or young, of certain types of mites. Depending for survival on other organisms, they frequently attach themselves to the skin of human beings. Although they do not actually burrow under the surface, they do introduce into the skin a substance which produces severe itching. Red blotches develop on the skin and are soon followed by blisters.

Anyone who plans to enter a tropical or wooded area should protect himself against this pest by sprinkling flour of sulfur on his undergarments and stockings, or by rubbing sulfur foam on the skin. Leggings are also a useful protection against chiggers.

Those who encounter chiggers should wash the skin carefully with soap and water. This treatment is more effective if the lather is left on the skin about ten minutes. Thereafter one of the many anti-itch preparations can be applied. This treatment will lessen the discomfort from itching until the lesions have gradually healed.

chilblains. An inflammation of the skin and of the tissues under the skin caused by cold; appears most often on the toes, fingers, ears, or nose.

The initial inflammation is followed by a burning or itching sensation, after which the area ordinarily becomes swollen and dark red. This color, as well as the characteristic chilled feeling, is due to a reduced circulation of blood in the area.

Those susceptible to chilblains should take protective measures. Warm clothing and carefully fitted warm shoes and gloves should always be worn during the winter months. Regular and vigorous exercise, such as walking and skating, is also advisable. Vulnerable areas of the body should be briskly massaged every day to encourage circulation of the blood. Regular doses of cod liver oil, as well as a healthful diet, are helpful, and general good health should be maintained.

Treatment of chilblains often includes painting the inflamed areas with a tincture of iodine. Zinc ointment is also beneficial. If blisters form, every effort should be exerted to prevent them from bursting, since healing is likely to be slow because of the condition of the affected area. If they do break, a stimulating ointment should be applied. A lotion composed of hydrogen peroxide and warm water in equal parts is useful for washing the sores, especially if they are discharging pus.

childbirth. *See* PREGNANCY AND PRENATAL CARE.

child care. At birth, girls generally weigh about half a pound less than boys. The average infant weighs about seven pounds. It is not unusual or abnormal for a child to weigh eight or even ten pounds. Babies born weighing less than five and a half pounds are classified as premature, regardless of how long the pregnancy has lasted, and require special care. Most babies will double their birth weight at six months of age and triple it at a year.

Length at birth is generally between nineteen and twenty-one inches and by the end of the first year the baby will have grown an additional ten inches. The baby's head and chest circumference should be equal at birth. Thereafter, the head size grows rapidly, increasing two and a half inches in circumference by the end of the first year. The bones of the skull are soft at birth and often the skull is misshapen from the effect of labor and may be molded right after delivery. An odd-shaped head should not cause alarm; within a few weeks the skull will assume a normal contour. Since the bones of the baby's skull are soft and easily molded into an incorrect shape, infants should not lie in one position too long during the first year. They

should lie on the left side after one feeding, on the right side after another, and be encouraged to sleep on both stomach and back. Fontanelles, the two soft spots in the skull, are places where the skull bones have not yet fused. The spot toward the back of the head usually fills in by the fourth month, and the spot in the front by the eighteenth month. Special care of the spots is not necessary, but they should not be disturbed.

Some children will begin to creep about the seventh month, while others sometimes wait until as late as the tenth or eleventh month. By the end of the first year children should easily be able to pull themselves into the standing position and to walk holding on to something. Usually they can walk at about eleven months if someone holds their hand. Walking unaided usually starts at about twelve to sixteen months. Of course, some children progress faster than others, but about 40 per cent of children can walk at a year, and 67 per cent at fourteen months. Occasionally, if the child is fat or has been ill, she may not walk until the end of the second year. Sometimes a slippery floor or crowded play area, or ill-fitting shoes discourage the child from walking. Occasionally muscle disease, rickets, or nerve damage may be involved but this is rare. Parents should be patient with the child who is reluctant to start walking. Urging her to walk before she is ready can only make her insecure. Letting the child play with other toddlers will encourage her to imitate them and try to walk herself. At birth, babies can distinguish between light and dark, but they are not able to fix their attention on any object until about two weeks of age when the eyes can focus on light. Usually, at four weeks, the baby can look at something and at two months follow a moving object with her eyes. During the first few months, difficulty in focusing correctly the delicate eye muscles may cause the eyes to look crossed. Parents should not be alarmed since this difficulty normally disappears soon.

Babies recognize noises and voices soon after birth, but are unable to distinguish specific sounds for two or three months. An infant of two or three months enjoys listening to music and often will stop crying if the radio or phonograph is turned on softly.

Babies do not have a developed sense of taste as a rule and can usually distinguish only between sweet and sour foods.

Physiologists recognize the value of crying for the new baby. Crying helps ventilate the baby's lungs, forcing out old air and replacing it with fresh air. The thrashing about of arms and legs associated with crying helps develop the body musculature. Also, crying is the only way a baby can indicate her needs, whether it be food, sleep, a change of diapers, or love, to those around her.

Most of the time a baby cries because she is uncomfortable, and parents should check for wet or soiled diapers or an open safety pin. The child may be too hot or cold. Often crying may indicate fear or anger. A new baby enjoys being in command and if she learns that she can control adults by crying she will continue to do so. Always be sure when the baby cries that she is comfortable, dry, and has had enough to eat.

Practically all babies, some more than others, suck their thumbs. In moderation, thumb sucking does not do any harm and interference with the eruption of teeth will ordinarily not happen unless the habit continues past two years of age. Thumb sucking may indicate that the child is hungry or unhappy. It frequently occurs among babies who are weaned too soon, thus depriving them of the pleasurable, satisfying practice of sucking. Artificial devices to prevent thumb sucking, such as arm splints or bitter preparations on the thumb, should not be used. It is better to try to find out the reason why the baby sucks her thumb. She may need more love and security. Her hand should not be pulled out of her mouth, and the parents should avoid appearing upset about the habit. Ordinarily the child will discontinue sucking her thumb before the habit is prolonged enough to harm her.

Children usually learn bladder control during the end of the second year. Nighttime control may not occur until the third or even fourth year; but ordinarily it is accomplished by the end of the third year. If persistent bed wetting continues beyond four years of age, consult the doctor.

Bed wetting may arise from emotional reasons, such as insecurity or jealousy of a new baby in the family. It can also occur if parents are too vigorous and rigid in insisting on early toilet training. Best results are obtained if the parents are understanding, patient, and do not push day or night toilet training and do not make a fuss about occasional accidents.

When the child is young, the bladder empties automatically, without any control from the brain. Gradually the brain becomes involved so that the child is able to control her urine when awake. Nighttime control does not require much help from parents and if they are patient the child will eventually discipline herself.

Bowel control is easier to teach than bladder control. The following points will help the child learn to control her bowels. (1) Do not begin bowel training until the child can sit comfortably by herself, at about the age of eight or nine months, although some authorities suggest much later. (2) The child may be placed on the toilet two or three times during the day at about the time she usually moves her bowels. This may be following meals and just before bedtime. (3) Soiled diapers should be promptly changed. (4) Do not leave the child on the toilet seat for more than a few minutes at a time, and do not permit the child to play with toys while on the seat. (5) Undue fuss should not be made over moving her bowels, or failing to do so.

Many mothers, because of excessive modesty, teach the child all sorts of tricks to indicate that she wishes to go to the toilet. Often strange gestures and queer words are used. The child should learn from the beginning the commonly accepted words used for this normal function.

Babies need exercise as much as adults do, though often of a different kind. Kicking and moving about vigorously is really strenuous exercise for a baby and time should be allowed every day for unrestrained activity. All her clothes should be removed, the child placed on the bed or a thick blanket on the floor in a warm room and then permitted to kick and move about freely. Someone should play with the baby.

Exercise is essential in all stages of childhood, but violent play is to be avoided, especially just before eating. Be sure the child is dressed suitably for the temperature with clothing that is loose and unconfining.

When exercising the small baby care should be taken not to push her into activity for which her body is not ready. The baby will indicate when her muscles are ready to perform such actions as sitting or standing. Playpens are good places for babies to learn to stand and move about without danger when they cannot be closely watched.

The best possible food for the infant is its mother's milk, particularly during the earlier months of life. For unknown reasons, many women today are unsuccessful in nursing their babies, but fortunately many excellent substitutes are now commercially prepared which resemble mother's milk. The new mother should not feel disturbed or guilty if she is unable to nurse her baby.

Babies can derive benefit from breast feeding for about six months, or even as long as nine months. When the baby cannot get at least half its food supply from its mother's breast, it is advisable to begin weaning. Most babies require weaning by the fourth to sixth month.

All mothers should make every effort to breast feed their babies, since breast-fed infants have a much lower incidence of infection, and seem to develop a little faster. In only rare instances does the milk of the mother fail to agree with the child. Occasionally diarrhea occurs if some element in the mother's diet disagrees with the child, but this can easily be detected and corrected in most cases. The diet for a nursing mother is little different from that of any healthy adult woman, with about an extra quart of fluid, half of which is whole milk, each day. The diet should be about 2500 to 3000 calories, which usually does not lead to any increase in the mother's weight. The nursing mother should avoid taking substances such as strong laxatives which deplete her body's fluid resources, or excessive amounts of coffee or tea, which stimulate the kidneys.

The theory that a nursing mother should avoid gassy or sour foods such as cabbage, salads, and raw fruits is also without foundation, unless, of course, she herself is allergic to a particular food. Fried foods may be eaten when a woman is nursing, but it is best to avoid chocolate since many people are sensitive to it. The best flow of milk results from regular nursing of the baby because the sucking action actually stimulates the formation of milk in the mother.

The diet of the nursing mother should contain about one quart of milk each day, some butter, four eggs a week, two green vegetables daily, and fresh fruit every morning, particularly oranges or tomatoes which are rich in vitamin C. Butter provides vitamins A and D; to provide a full supply of these vitamins the mother may take cod liver oil as directed by her doctor. The milk drunk daily may be whole, or non-fat dry milk if she is overweight. If she doesn't wish to drink milk, it may be used in food such as ice cream, custards, or cocoa drinks.

Mothers often worry about taking medicine, fearing that it will appear in the breast milk and harm the baby. Actually few drugs will do this, but if in doubt consult the doctor.

Secretion of milk begins a few days after the baby is born. In some cases, the breast may leak fluid during the last few weeks of pregnancy. During the first few days, the flow is usually scanty but becomes more profuse by the end of the first week if nursing is frequent and the child is hungry enough so that she sucks vigorously. The first secretion of milk is actually not milk, but a cheesy, protein-rich substance known as colostrum which appears about the third day and is nourishing for the baby.

Later the true milk begins and is pale bluish white in color, resembling skim milk. This color is normal and does not mean that the milk is weak.

By the end of the first week, the average mother should have no difficulty secreting a pint of milk daily. This gradually increases and by the sixth month she is producing a quart of milk daily. The amount produced usually parallels the demands of the baby. Complete emptying of the breasts at nursing time is desirable to encourage good milk production. Nursing from both breasts at each feeding is recommended until maximum production is established. Then alternate the breasts to avoid overproduction.

Breast milk is considerably sweeter than cow's milk, though somewhat lower in protein. It is also much more digestible and breast-fed babies are less apt to regurgitate or have gastrointestinal upsets. Through the mother's milk they also receive protective antibodies against disease which are not found in cow's milk. If the mother's diet is insufficient, the milk will be poor in quality. Vitamins should be taken by the nursing mother to enrich the milk.

Smoking does not affect the milk, and alcohol may be taken in moderation while the mother is nursing since it does not pass into the milk except in small amounts.

The size of the breasts does not seem to be linked to supply of milk and women with smaller breasts often produce the most milk. Determining in advance whether or not a mother will be able to nurse her baby is not possible. Certain women should not nurse, however. These include those women who are not in good health, those who have active tuberculosis or other infections, those who have had arduous labors, and those who have previously had tumors of the breast or breast infection. If the breasts become infected while nursing, it should be discontinued.

Premature babies thrive on mother's milk, but often their sucking power does not permit nursing. In some hospitals the mother's milk is drawn off by a breast pump and then fed to the baby with an eye dropper or small tube until it is strong enough to nurse by itself.

If the baby begins vomiting or fails to gain weight, the mother probably should stop nursing. However, she should consult the doctor first. Failure to nurse one child need not imply that future attempts will be unsuccessful.

If the baby seems fretful after nursing, mother's milk may be insufficient. In such cases, the doctor will prescribe a supplementary formula to be given after the regular nursing period.

Most babies stop nursing when they have had enough and seldom does a nursing baby overfeed. Occasionally, however, a baby getting too much milk too fast may vomit or regurgitate, or have an upset stomach afterward, but this is rare. If it does occur, the nursing time should be shortened.

When preparing the formula, all equipment needed should be washed thoroughly and boiled daily. The top of the bottle or can containing the milk must be washed with hot water and soap and rinsed thoroughly. Mix and measure the ingredients in sterilized containers, wash and boil the bottles to contain the formula, and close with sterilized rubber nipples. Individual bottles for each feeding are preferable to one large bottle from which the milk is measured. To provide for accidents, such as breakage or contamination, make one extra bottle. It is usually easier to make the whole day's supply in advance, preferably in the morning. After the feedings are prepared, the formula should be placed in the refrigerator. Nipples should be made of thin rubber, washed and boiled daily, and rinsed after use to extend their life.

Recently it has been reported that babies do not need their formula served at body temperature. The baby will do just as well with formula at room temperature or even at icebox chill. This was established after an experiment with premature babies who thrived on formula just out of the refrigerator.

Also new is instant, ready-made formula in a container that is completely disposable. This eliminates formula preparation, or refrigeration, and sterilization of bottle and nipple.

Cleanliness in the care of the baby's feedings is essential when she is young to protect her against serious infection. Sterilization is not essential after six to nine months, but the equipment should be carefully cleaned before use.

Changes in the formula should be made only on the advice of the doc-tor because the baby's stomach and digestive system are extremely sensitive. If the baby seems healthy and continues to gain weight, there is ordinarily no need to change the formula. If she fails to gain weight, of if diarrhea or constipation occurs, the doctor may prescribe a new formula with an increase or decrease or adding or elimination of some ingredient.

A baby's weight gain is not always continuous. If she drinks greedily and rapidly, cries for more, or gets fretful long before feeding time, she probably needs more food. But the baby may be crying for other reasons and the mother should be sure that underfeeding is the reason before increasing her food, or overweight may occur. At one time, fat babies were considered the healthiest babies but this idea has been disproved and in fact the opposite may be true. The baby should never be deliberately overfed. She can handle so much food a day and beyond her limit will become upset and nauseated.

chill. A sensation of cold, accompanied by shivering and usually with teeth chattering, throbbing, and trembling; frequently a prominent early symptom of acute infection. Any severe chill during a fever is a danger signal and a doctor should be called at once.

chiropractic. A therapeutic system based on the theory that the bones of the spinal column, by pressing on the spinal nerves, cause an interruption of the normal function of the nerves.

chloasma. *See* LIVER SPOTS.

chloroform. A heavy, colorless liquid

with a typical ether smell. Chloroform is best known as an anesthetic. It became fashionable as an anesthetic in childbirth when Queen Victoria permitted its administration during the delivery of her seventh child.

Chloromycetin, also called chloramphenicol. A recent antibiotic effective in, among other diseases, undulant fever, urinary infections, bacillary dysentery, whooping cough, and virus pneumonia.

chlorosis. A form of anemia, characterized by a large reduction of hemoglobin in the blood, but with only a slight diminution in the number of red cells. Some decades ago, chlorosis, or "green sickness," was common among girls and young women, but today it has almost completely disappeared because of increased knowledge of the place of iron in the diet. The symptoms of this iron deficiency are a greenish color to the skin, and menstrual and gastric disturbances.

chlorpromazine. One of the recent tranquilizing agents. Effective in the prevention of vomiting, the inhibition of temperamental disturbance, and general sedation without drowsiness or reduction in consciousness.

cholecystitis. The scientific name for inflammation of the gall bladder. *See also* GALL BLADDER.

cholecystography. Roentgenography, X-ray diagnosis, of the gall bladder after it has been made visual by substances not transparent to the X-ray. Gallstone attacks have characteristic symptoms, yet differences in related symptoms and severity of pain often make a definite distinction from other diseases diffi-

cult. The introduction of cholecystography has been a great advance in the diagnosis of gallstones.

cholelithiasis. A condition associated with calculi, stones in the gall bladder or in a bile duct. *See also* GALL BLADDER.

cholera. An acute infection which chiefly involves the small intestine. The main symptoms are severe, constantly flowing diarrhea, vomiting, collapse, cramps in the muscles, and suppression of the flow of urine from the kidneys.

cholesterol. A fatty substance, a basis for hundreds of chemical processes in the body. Animal meat, cream, butter, and eggs contain large amounts of cholesterol. Cholesterol in excess amounts in the bloodstream is believed by many medical investigators to be responsible for a type of arterial hardening known as atherosclerosis. In this disease, cholesterol plaques in the inside wall of an artery causes the wall to thicken and roughen. Ultimately the flow of blood through that portion of the artery is restricted, or a piece of the roughened wall may tear away and block the flow of blood to those tissues served by the artery. When this occurs in the arteries that supply the heart muscle with blood, the condition is called coronary thrombosis.

Medical investigators have produced atherosclerosis in animals by feeding them diets high in cholesterol. Certain heart specialists advocate a low-fat, low-cholesterol diet to prevent or control coronary heart disease, but others believe that since the body produces its own cholesterol, dietary restriction of it will not help appreciably. Investigations indicate that factors other than the existence of excess cholesterol may be responsible for arterial hardening. These may involve the body's ability to metabolize the cholesterol, or its ratio to other substances, such as protein and phosphatides, in the bloodstream, the size and number of the cholesterol molecules, and the effect of exercise on the amount of circulating cholesterol. In one experiment, Dr. Frederick J. Stare of Harvard University's School of Public Health reports a definite correlation between exercise and a reduction in certain types of cholesterol molecules. In 1964, the American Heart Association, which had advocated a low cholesterol diet, concentrating on polyunsaturated fats, for high-risk heart attack subjects, suggested that such a diet was advisable for all the general public over forty.

Later in the year, the New York Department of Public Health reported the results of a seven-year experiment in which men over forty who had followed a low cholesterol diet had a significantly lower incidence of heart attacks.

chorea. More familiarly known as St. Vitus' dance, a disease of the nervous system which causes involuntary twitching of various parts of the body. Children prior to puberty are most often affected. Unlike many diseases of the nervous system, St. Vitus' dance normally lasts a relatively short time, often no more than twelve weeks. Sometimes relapses occur, and in other instances the disease may endure for one or two years, although not usually.

Chorea is believed to be the result of a general streptococcus infection which in some apparently indirect way, perhaps through toxic substances developed by the germs of the infection, strikes at the brain and the nervous system. Children may develop a temporary, habitual twitch from imitating the movements of other people, but this is completely different in origin and in character from the involuntary twitching that is seen in St. Vitus' dance.

The onset of the disease, which often accompanies rheumatic fever, may appear as a generalized illness with fever, vomiting, and headache, along with dizziness and weakness. The first disturbances of bodily movement are often mistaken for clumsiness of the child. However, the true nature of the ailment soon becomes apparent.

When fully developed, the movements are rapid, of short duration, and distinctive; none exactly duplicates any that preceded. Muscular co-ordination becomes difficult and approximately 25 per cent of the cases are so severe as to disturb the speech function. The child becomes irritable and restless, and his memory, attention span, and emotions may be mildly disturbed.

The treatment of chorea, a disease implicating the whole system and not just isolated parts, begins with prolonged bed rest of three to six weeks at least. Because of the close relationship to streptococcus infection, the child should be kept under close observation. Any infection of the throat, in the tonsils or adenoids, in the teeth or elsewhere should be eliminated quickly and the child kept in bed. Both in streptococcus infections and in chorea attention must be given the heart, which may be particularly affected. The use of penicillin or sulfa is recommended by the American Heart Association to prevent streptococcal infection and to protect against a recurrence of rheumatic fever.

Baths and sedative drugs directed at alleviating the symptoms of chorea are frequently quite helpful. Both heat and drugs striking at the infection itself are often beneficial, but neither is specifically effective.

Convalescence of the patient with chorea should be gradual, with a nutritional diet assuring plenty of vitamins and minerals. Exercise and play should be resumed in moderation and under supervision, but the child must relax and not overdo. *See also* ATAXIA.

chorion. The outermost of the fetal membranes which covers, nourishes, and protects the developing ovum. Later it becomes the fetal part of the placenta.

chronic. Long-continued or of long duration. A chronic disease is prolonged, often slowly progressing and never completely cured—as, for example, chronic bronchitis or chronic arthritis.

chrysarobin. An orange powder used to treat psoriasis, and is also effective in fungus infections called dhobie itch and gym or jockey itch, involving the skin of the groin, perineum, and perianal regions.

cilia. Fine, hairlike appendages which cover the surface of mucous membranes, the moist, sensitive lining of the respiratory tract. The cilia are filtering organisms, a protective measure to keep harmful particles out of the lung. They move upward and downward, and through the more pronounced upward movement, mucus, dust, and other infectious particles are swept and propelled toward the mouth, so that they are not breathed into the lungs. Eyelashes are also cilia, and protect the eyes from foreign particles.

circulatory system. The heart pumps the blood through a "pipeline" of closed tubes or vessels. This pipeline forms two major circular routes in the body, the systemic circulation and the pulmonary circulation, with the heart acting as a central pump. The circulatory system, with its major and minor routes, reaches every cell in the body, bringing the blood with its life-sustaining products from the organs where they are manufactured to the tissues where they are needed. It also carries away the waste products to other organs in the body, where they are broken down and either converted to be used again or excreted as waste. In addition, the circulatory system takes care of the more active organs by bringing them an increased flow of blood, whereas those organs which are less active, or temporarily at rest, receive less blood. *See also* CORONARY THROMBOSIS; EMBOLISM; HEART; LYMPHATIC SYSTEM.

circumcision. The surgical removal of the loose fold of the skin, the foreskin, which covers the head of the penis.

The operation is recommended by many doctors as a routine hygienic measure, or to diminish the possibility of contracting venereal diseases. The best time for the operation is before the infant is ten days old, when it represents a minor procedure. Circumcision should always be done under strictest surgical or aseptic conditions. Proper repair of the tissues after the extra skin has been removed is essential. If the doctor's instructions regarding protection and cleansing of the wound are carefully followed, complications are rare.

Circumcision is recommended when the foreskin is unusually long so that it retains urine which might cause infection. Inflammation and irritation under the foreskin are also associated with various nervous manifestations.

cirrhosis. A chronic, progressive disease, essentially inflammatory, with a pathological hardening of tissue brought about by an increase of connective tissue elements. The lungs, ovaries, heart, or stomach may be affected with cirrhosis, but it occurs more often in the kidney and liver.

Cirrhosis of the kidney, chronic interstitial nephritis, is a chronic inflammation of the connective tissue elements of the kidney. Cirrhosis of the liver, the most frequent type, is usually a disease of adults but may occasionally occur in younger people, and is three times more common among men than women. It involves a scarring or hardening of the liver, produced by an over-

growth of the connective tissue elements to the neglect of the true hepatic cells.

Heavy consumers of alcohol are often victims of cirrhosis, but moderate drinkers may become affected. The disease may also be caused by bacterial infection, particularly from bacteria of the colon, infectious cirrhosis. *See also* LIVER.

citric acid. A tribasic acid occurring in the juice of many fruits and in various animal tissues. It appears as an acid flavoring and in effervescent drinks. Citric acid has an alkalizing effect, but is without vitamin value and is not an effective substitute for citrus fruits.

claustrophobia. An intense fear of being in a confined area. *See also* AGORAPHOBIA.

clavicle. "Collarbone," the curved bone which extends from the top of the breastbone out to each of the shoulders. Because the two clavicles are thin and small and support much weight, they are frequently and easily broken. While mending, a small bony disfigurement is likely to occur, unless the person will lie motionless on her back, without a pillow, so that the two parts can remain in perfect adjustment to each other until they have completely grown together.

cleft palate. A congenital defect, due to failure in fusion of embryonic facial processes, which results in a fissure through the palate. This cleavage, starting in the soft palate, may extend forward all the way across the bony roof of the mouth and even reach to the upper lip, resulting in harelip.

A person with this deformity is abnormally susceptible to inflammations in the area of the palate. Speech is difficult, as well as sucking, drinking, and chewing. Food being swallowed will frequently go through the roof of the mouth into the nostrils, and special feeding techniques are necessary.

A cleft palate can usually be corrected by an operation in which the tissues in the roof of the mouth are loosened and then fitted together. This operation is sometimes performed as early as the third month, or as late as the third year. If done before the child begins to talk, undesirable speech habits can be prevented. Even after a successful operation, however, some physical defect may remain. New techniques employing braces or plate or other prosthetic devices, along with intensive training, can significantly benefit persons with cleft palate. *See also* HARELIP; LIPS; PALATE.

climate. The average weather condition of an area over a period of years, as indicated by the temperature, rainfall, barometer, and other measurements. The connection between climate and health is a subject which has interested people for centuries. Greek and Roman physicians recognized that malaria affected persons living in low, marshy areas, but they believed the cause of malaria was sleeping in night air. Hippocrates, the father of medicine, who lived in the third century B.C., wrote, "If there be no rivers and the water that the people drink be marshy and stagnant, the physique of the people must show protruding bellies and enlarged spleens." He did not know that the protruding belly and enlarged spleen are results of malaria, prevalent in marshy areas. In his book, *Air, Water and Places,* he notes that ". . . the inhabitants of a region that is mountainous, rugged, high and watered, where the changes of the seasons exhibit strong contrasts, are likely to be of big physique, with a nature well adapted for endurance and courage." This is the first recorded recognition that the Temperate Zone is a region conducive to human well-being.

More recently, persons with "consumption," or tuberculosis, went to dry, high-altitude areas in an attempt to cure their illness. However, today climate is not considered important in treating tuberculosis, and emphasis is placed on drugs such as isoniazid, food, rest, and competent medical care.

Persons with rheumatic conditions frequently feel better when they are not exposed to cold and dampness. Research on rheumatism has shown that changes occur in the composition of the body tissues, including the blood, when there are changes in barometric pressure. Changes in blood supply to the joints are associated with sudden changes in temperature. While climate cannot cause rheumatic conditions, it may lower the resistance so that a rheumatic inflammation results.

For years the belief has been prevalent that dampness, cold, and drafts are associated with colds and pneumonia. However, statistics seem to indicate that, unless a person has a tendency to respiratory ailments, inclement weather does not cause such illness. For example, students at Stanford University at Palo Alto, California, have about as many coughs and colds as students at Harvard University in Massachusetts, despite the fact that the California climate is mild and the Massachusetts climate rigorous. However, persons whose resistance is generally low will be more susceptible to inflammation of the nose, throat, and sinuses during cold weather, and will benefit by a change to a warm, dry climate.

Persons with heart disease do not do well at high altitudes, because of increased difficulty in getting oxygen for circulation.

Generally a mild climate is most beneficial to those persons with chronic diseases, and a specialist may propose that a change of climate be made to relieve their symptoms. But it is wise to check with a physician before assuming that another climate will be more beneficial.

Clinitest. A commercially available kit by means of which persons having or suspecting a diabetic tendency may check the extent of sugar in the urine. *See also* DIABETES.

clitoris. The organ in women which resembles, in miniature form, the penis of the male. This small, tube-like body is located in the angle at the top of the vulva, the external sex organ of women. Like the penis, the clitoris is composed of tissue which becomes engorged with blood, and hard and erect during sexual excitement. *See also* REPRODUCTION SYSTEM.

clubfoot. A deformity of the foot, present at birth or caused subse-

quently by muscle paralysis or injury, in which the heel or the ball of the foot or one edge of it does not touch the ground.

In three-fourths of the cases noted at birth, the heel and inner edge of the foot are raised. This condition occurs once in every thousand births, and considerably more than half of those affected are male children. Also, in more than half the deformity occurs on only one side.

Treatment must be started at the earliest possible moment. The later therapy begins, the longer it will take to remedy the deformity. Children under a year can be treated in twenty-three weeks, whereas those of six years or more require about forty-two weeks. One of the signal achievements of modern medical science has been the development of treatment for clubfoot.

The doctor, usually an orthopedist, will outline a routine of the manipulations of the parts involved to get them into the correct position and then make the position secure with one or more of the devices designed especially for the purpose, such as adhesive bindings, plaster casts, or braces and splints. After the proper position has been firmly established, special exercises, shoes, massage, and other measures which may be beneficial will be prescribed. Active treatment often continues for several months, and followup supervision is necessary for years.

Manipulation alone may not be satisfactory. Then surgical rearrangement of the affected tissues and parts becomes necessary.

The cause of clubfoot is unknown. Heredity is suspected by some persons, because approximately 5 per cent of cases occur in families in which the deformity has appeared previously; others believe that an incorrect position of the child before birth is responsible.

coagulation. The formation of a coagulum, clot, or curd as in blood or milk. When bleeding is present, threadlike fibers called fibrin are produced by a substance in the blood, the fibrinogen. These fibers trap white and red blood corpuscles which form a clot. Contraction of the fibrin squeezes out the liquid portion of the blood, the serum, and a crust develops. The system of clotting is counteracted by agents, including heparin and other anticoagulants, which keep the blood fluid. The power of coagulation of the blood varies with different persons. In people with hemophilia, a hereditary disease, the clotting is so retarded that they bleed profusely from minor wounds and may even bleed to death.

Formation of a blood clot in a coronary artery may obstruct the flow of blood to the heart muscle and produce coronary thrombosis. The incidence of clotting may be increased when the person is under stress. A blood clot blocking an artery of the brain, usually where a weak spot has resulted through arteriosclerosis, is able to produce some conditions of rheumatic heart disease. Coagulation of blood in the lower body regions can cause serious complications if particles of the blood clot reach the lungs and obstruct the major blood vessels.

See also CORONARY THROMBOSIS; DYSMENORRHEA; EMBOLISM; HEMOPHILIA.

cocaine. An alkaloid derived from the coca bush, in use for centuries. Inca priests in Peru, for example, were aware of its anesthetic effect and chewed coca leaves in an attempt to improve their physical endurance.

Cocaine is habit-forming and poisonous, and should never be used in any way except when prescribed and administered by a physician. The amount of cocaine required to poison varies greatly; some people react unfavorably even to small doses. New synthetic compounds have been developed which are similar to cocaine but less toxic.

coccidioidomycosis. Also know as desert fever, San Joaquin fever, valley fever, or the bumps, a disease with pulmonary symptoms caused by one of the fungi, *Coccidioides immitis,* which thrives in the dry, dusty areas of the San Joaquin Valley and in the southwestern states.

The first symptoms, which resemble the symptoms of tuberculosis, are generally chills, fever, headache, general malaise, night sweats, and coughing. These symptoms usually subside after a week or two and small bumps may then appear under the skin, which also disappear in time. In severe cases, X-rays show changes in the lungs and occasionally thin-walled cavities which may persist for years.

Recovery from a simple lung infection is usually rapid and complete even without treatment, but in cases where deep lung cavities have developed, surgery may be indicated.

The growing prevalence of coccidioidomycosis has made it a public health concern. About 90 per cent of the people living in these arid regions have had the infection within a ten-year period as a result of inhaling the spores of the fungus. Droughts in this area add to the disease hazards. Residents or visitors who show signs of a chronic infection resembling any of the serious respiratory diseases should have chest X-rays and skin and blood tests.

coccyx. From the Greek meaning, "shaped like the bill of a cuckoo," the last bone at the lowermost end of the spine.

codeine. An alkaloid derived from opium and closely allied in chemical constitution to morphine. Though weaker, its action is similar to that of morphine, and it is used medically to diminish sensitivity to pain.

cod liver oil. The partially fixed oil from which stearoids have been removed, obtained from the fresh livers of cod. The liver of the cod (and also of the halibut) is one of the richest sources of vitamins A and D, and cod liver oil has been known for many years as an effective treatment for malnutrition. Mild cases of rickets improve quickly with cod liver oil. Diets which do not contain enough fat-soluble vitamins are a basic factor of sinusitis in children, and cod liver oil is recommended by many physicians as an effective preventive measure against this infection. Every growing baby and child should have cod liver oil or its equivalent in vitamins A and D, and nursing mothers are advised by physicians to take it regularly. The amount of cod liver oil usually recommended is a teaspoonful daily of the more concentrated preparations, or two teaspoonfuls of the less concentrated. However, since today more and more foods are being vitamin-enriched, the diet usually does not need to be supplemented by cod liver oil. *See also* CHILD CARE.

coffee. A beverage made by an infusion or decoction from the roasted and ground or pounded seeds of a shrub, small tree, or other species of the madder family. Although coffee has no nutritional value, taken in moderation it does have some distinct pharmacological worth. It has been described as a mild "psychic energizer."

An average cup of coffee contains about one grain of caffeine, an alkaloid which stimulates the brain, kidney, and circulation. It increases the force and beat of the heart and the flow of urine and thus helps cleanse the body of metabolic endproducts. This action has made coffee valuable in cases of edema or dropsy, conditions in which fluid accumulates excessively in the tissues. In these cases, it is vital to increase the heart rate so that more blood is pumped into the blood vessels, thus promoting greater flow through the kidneys with elimination of fluid.

Generally a cup of coffee after dinner may have a good effect on the digestion since it increases the gastric juice. However, an excess of coffee can easily have toxic effects, such as rapid pulse, nervousness, irritability, and insomnia. In some persons, too much coffee may even bring on attacks of dizziness and faintness, or palpitation from an overaccelerated heart rate and force. The amount of coffee that can safely be drunk varies among people.

Tests made by the American Medical Association established that a cup of regular ground coffee has almost twice as much caffeine as a cup of instant coffee, and a cup of regular decaffeinated coffee has about one-third the amount of caffeine as a cup of regular ground coffee.

colchicine. A water-soluble, pale brownish alkaloid, derived from the meadow saffron, which has been used as an efficient pain reliever in gout for more than a hundred years. However, it has proved of little value in other types of arthritis and rheumatism. *See also* GOUT.

cold. *See* COMMON COLD.

cold cream. A mixture in an ointment of petrolatum, lanolin, and rosewater, which is useful for soothing dry, inflamed, or irritated skin, and also for removing cosmetics. *See also* COSMETICS.

cold sore. *See* HERPES SIMPLEX.

colic. The abnormal and violent contraction of certain internal muscular tissues. Intestinal colic is caused by a sudden contraction of the intestine. When the bile ducts contract abnormally, biliary colic results, and renal colic is caused by a tightening of the tube, the ureter, which passes between the kidney and bladder. Alternate contraction

and relaxation is the normal behavior of these organs, and pain occurs only when this contraction becomes spasmodic.

Intestinal colic is the most common. The pain is noticed usually around the navel, and is often accompanied by a clogging or loosening of the bowels. If the cause of pain is doubtful, cathartics and laxatives should be avoided but an enema may be given if necessary. A simple chill, infected food, or a nervous condition are a few of the many possible causes of colic. Colic may be easily confused with a serious disorder, such as appendicitis. If the pain does not respond promptly to simple treatment, such as an electric pad or a hot-water bottle, or bicarbonate of soda, a physician should be called.

Intestinal colic, produced by gas, is commonly seen in infants. Often this condition results from the air taken in with the child's milk or food. Occasionally, however, it may be generated by the fermentation of food in the bowels. Regardless of the source, this gas can often be relieved simply by placing the baby across one's shoulder after every feeding and tapping it lightly on the back until it "burps." If the pain persists or is severe, a doctor should be consulted.

A special type of stomach colic, afflicting adults, which involves spasmodic contractions of the large bowel, is known as mucous colic. The pain occurs characteristically after meals, and is located chiefly in the right section of the lower abdomen. Such symptoms should be carefully investigated by a specialist who may take X-rays, inspect stools, and study the person's diet. Occasionally psychiatric observation may be necessary.

Renal colic, distress after meals and in the lower right abdomen, is usually caused by a stone in the kidney trying to descend to the bladder. The pain almost always starts in the kidney area and moves to the abdomen, leg, and genitals. Nausea and a frequent desire to urinate appear. In attempting to walk, the person will experience a pronounced tendency to tip her body to the side affected, depending on which of the kidney areas is affected. The pain may fluctuate and may even be severe enough to induce delirium. Renal colic can be subdued by proper drugs. The pain will sometimes persist for days, but usually is limited to twelve hours or less. The stone is sometimes passed spontaneously in the urine, but frequently surgical treatment is required. *See also* CONSTIPATION; DIARRHEA; INDIGESTION.

colitis. Inflammation of the colon, the part of the large intestine extending from the cecum to the rectum. Various forms of colitis can occur. Simple colitis is an acute irritation or infection of the colon, accompanied by diarrhea. Some types of colitis are caused by infection of the colon by specific organisms.

Mucous colitis is a condition in which the mucous membrane of the colon is inflamed, with symptoms of colicky pain, and constipation or diarrhea. It would seem to be primarily a psychosomatic ailment, which frequently becomes chronic.

Another form which is probably usually mental in origin is ulcerative colitis, characterized by ulceration of the mucous membrane of the colon. The symptoms may range from only painless excretion of blood in stools to dysentery, fever, and death as a result of exhaustion, perforation of the colon, and general peritonitis. Less critical cases usually recover completely, although frequently there are periods of relapse. Sometimes the disease becomes chronic, but without producing any severe disability. The entire length of the colon becomes scarred and thickened with ulcerations, and at this stage such complications as perforation, malignant disease, nutritional deficiency, and intestinal obstruction frequently occur.

Treatment of ulcerative colitis requires medical care, including bed rest, proper diet, sedatives, control of infection, and, if necessary, blood transfusions. Cortisone and ACTH have been used in treatment. Occasionally surgical removal of the colon is advised; and when emotional factors are thought to be involved in any way, psychotherapy is recommended.

collarbone. The common name for clavicle. *See also* CLAVICLE.

colostomy. A surgical operation, usually on the left side of the lower abdomen, creating a more or less permanent opening in the colon to permit evacuation after the normal rectal and anal opening is lost.

common cold. An acute inflammation of the upper respiratory tract, involving the nose and throat. Its specific cause is little understood.

Susceptibility to colds is almost universal, particularly among children. The cold is highly contagious, especially indoors, and places where groups of people congregate are excellent transmission spots for the infection.

In large urban communities where the climate is temperate, the general population averages about three colds a year. This median is higher among susceptible adults and children. The incidence is lowest in the summer, rises in the autumn, reaching its peak in midwinter, and declines in the spring. Several peak periods occur in smaller urban communities. The first is in early autumn when schools reopen and children are brought into greater proximity indoors. In addition to the winter rise in incidence of colds, a smaller rise often appears in the spring.

Colds are definitely communicable and are transmitted either by direct contact or by spread of the infected droplets of discharge. A practical method to control the spread of colds has not yet been developed. The common cold may be due to one or more viruses. Scientists believe that the virus is generally present in the throat but it becomes active only when the body resistance is lowered. When the cold virus attacks the mucous membranes of the nose and throat, these tissues are weakened and become susceptible to infection by bacteria which are also generally found in the body. The bacteria are secondary invaders and the virus paves the way for their entry into the mucous membranes. Although they are not responsible for the common cold, the bacteria may initiate a secondary infection which either intensifies the local inflammation present, prolonging the cold, or causes new complications such as purulent sinusitis or otitis, an inflammation of the ear. Infants and young children appear to be more susceptible to these secondary infections than adults.

A cold usually begins abruptly, with a sense of soreness and dryness in the nose or back of the throat. Within a few hours the nasal passages feel congested, sneezing develops and a colorless watery discharge comes from the nose. After forty-eight hours the cold is usually at its peak, and is accompanied by excessive watering of the eyes, huskiness of the voice, and difficulty in breathing as the congestion spreads. The nasal discharge becomes thick and sticky and some coughing may develop. The cough does not usually bring up much discharge unless the person has a tendency to chronic bronchitis. Frequently a headache, a sense of lethargy and malaise, and vague pains in the back and limbs accompany a cold. A fever is rarely present, although in children a temperature of 102° or even higher often develops.

The uncomplicated cold generally lasts from one to two weeks and terminates without special treatment. Colds which persist or recur repeatedly, or in which there is a steady, prolonged fever or chills, particularly in children or susceptible adults, may indicate complications and a physician should be consulted. As yet, a specific agent has not been developed to control the common cold and treatment is confined to relief of symptoms and control of complications. Treatment of the cold is not much different today from the treatment used by past generations. Bed rest should be enforced whenever possible and as much isolation as is practical. Plenty of liquids, hot or cold, a light diet, and keeping warm promote greater comfort. Aspirin in small, repeated doses generally gives relief as does gargling in cases of sore throat. An aspirin tablet or a teaspoon of salt dissolved in hot water is beneficial for gargling. In the latter stages of a cold, when the discharge has thickened, an atomizer or nose drops or inhaler helps clear the nasal passages. They should not be used more than once in four hours and if the person has a tendency to nasal inflammation should be employed sparingly.

Cold vaccines, which are suspensions of dead bacteria collected from the discharge of a cold, have not been found to be significantly effective either when taken by mouth or when given as an injection or nasal spray. However, continued research is being done. The routine use of sulfonamides or antibiotics for colds is definitely discouraged. These drugs should be given only in cases with a definite bacterial secondary infection—for example, in bronchopneumonia, sinusitis, or otitis media. Persons who have a consistent history of recurrent colds with accompanying complications may use antibiotics or sulfonamides, but only on the advice of a physician.

Although little is known about curing a cold, measures can be taken to ward off the infection and decrease its incidence. A well-balanced diet, sufficient rest, proper dress both indoors and out, all help to keep the body resistance high. Undue exposure to sharp changes in temperature should be avoided. Proper ventilation of rooms, with sufficient humidity in the air, helps to keep the mucous membranes in healthy condition. If humidifiers are not used, adequate moisture can be maintained by keeping a pan of water on a radiator or stove. Particular care should be taken to avoid contact with persons who have colds. Simple hygienic measures like washing the hands before eating or covering a sneeze all help to decrease the occurrence of colds. *See also* BRONCHOPNEUMONIA; CHILD CARE; OTITIS; SINUSES.

communicable diseases. Those which are transmissible from one person to another. The difference, often disregarded, between infectious and communicable contagious diseases is that while infectious diseases are caused by the invasion of an infective agent like a fungus, bacillus, or virus, the agents are not necessarily transmitted by a person.

compound fracture. The breaking of a bone is a fracture. In a compound fracture, the point of the fracture is in contact with the outer surface of the body—for example, through a wound. If the break is covered by the skin, it is a simple fracture. *See also* BONES.

compress. A piece of folded gauze,

cloth, or a soft pad which is applied firmly to a part of the body to relieve inflammations, produce pressure, or prevent hemorrhage. It may be wet or dry, hot or cold, and is sometimes perforated for drainage or observation of the underlying skin.

compulsion. Defined in psychology as an irresistible, irrational desire to repeat certain acts. For example, a person may have the compulsion to wash her hands every few minutes, or to avoid stepping on the cracks in the sidewalk.

conception. The union of sperm and ovum, the male and female sex cells, leading to the development of a new life. Conception is sometimes called fertilization, impregnation, or fecundation, and should be distinguished from the term copulation, which refers to the act of sexual union between the male and female.

Since the egg cell of the female lives for only about twelve hours out of every month, the male seed must be deposited within the female genital tract during these few hours, or within two or three days of release of an egg. The sperm cells live about two to five days after ejaculation.

Conception usually takes place within the Fallopian tubes adjacent to the uterus and ovaries, and may occur within an hour of intercourse. Following union of the male and female sex cells, development is rapid, and eight to fourteen days later the product embeds itself in the lining of the uterus where it remains until birth. *See also* REPRODUCTION SYSTEM.

concussion. A shock, severe shaking or jarring of a part of the body, usually resulting from a fall or blow. It also refers to the morbid state resulting from such a jarring. A concussion of the brain is actually a paralysis of its function, and symptoms are not due to any fracture or laceration. Signs of hemorrhage or loss of blood from the coverings around the brain may be present. Sometimes disturbances occur in the circulation of spinal fluid through the brain, and occasionally part of the soft white material of the brain is crushed or the connection cords between different portions of the brain are damaged or destroyed. *See also* SHOCK.

conditioning. The development of a better physiological condition through physical exercise and training.

condom. A rubber sheath used to cover the penis during sexual intercourse to prevent the male sperm from reaching and fertilizing the female egg cell. The device prevents infection as well as conception. *See also* CONTRACEPTION.

conjunctivitis. Inflammation of the conjunctiva, the mucous membrane covering the globe and lids of the eye. Many types of conjunctivitis exist, including allergic conjunctivitis, catarrhal conjunctivitis, the most common form of which usually results from irritation of a cold, and acute contagious conjunctivitis or pinkeye. *See also* EYE; PINKEYE.

constipation. The retention of solid waste material within the bowel for an unusually long time, or undue difficulty in its evacuation.

The excretion of undigested residue is the final step in the process of digestion. The waste material enters the colon as a loose, moist mass and there the excess water is absorbed by the body. The relatively solid mass of waste material then moves on into the rectum, where it normally prompts the desire for a movement of the bowels.

Evacuation ordinarily occurs once or twice every twenty-four hours, with a wide range of variation among individuals. With some persons greater frequency is common, while with others an interval of several days may often pass without ill effect. A fixed schedule for this function for all persons is unknown. Most doctors believe that the nature of the action, which should occur with some regularity and should produce well-formed stools, neither too moist and loose nor too dry and hard, is more desirable than the frequency.

Babies normally have three or four bowel movements a day, but the child who has less than three is not necessarily constipated. If the infant remains well and continues to gain weight, his digestion and elimination are probably normal for him. When constipation does occur, insufficient water, underfeeding, or an excessive amount of fat in the diet may be causative. Children who are weak or who have rickets may have difficulty in performing the necessary muscular actions associated with elimination.

Constipation is often the result of faulty habits and improper training. The habitual failure to respond promptly to the body's signal is often a basic cause. A lazy attitude, poorly developed habits, false modesty, or other extraneous factors often create a situation in which the signal is at first ignored and later not even felt. When such a pattern has been established by a person, she may develop chronic constipation, which, as an adult, she will usually attribute not to the bad habits which are actually basic but to non-existent organic causes, which she will attempt to remedy by laxatives, enemas, and irrigations. These in turn may disrupt and interfere with the normal process of elimination and thus intensify her problem still further.

This type of constipation is commonly complicated even more by intricate chains of habits and misconceptions. Some constipated persons develop elaborate and mistaken notions about the shape, color, frequency, time, and consistency of the evacuation. A first step in overcoming constipation of this sort is to correct these mistaken beliefs. Thereafter, new habit patterns can be encouraged. A baby can be trained so that the simple act of placing it on the pot causes evacuation. With adults the pattern becomes much more elaborate, and can include getting up, bathing, having breakfast, even having the right magazine and a cigarette. The principle nevertheless remains the same and the development of an effective habit pattern is often the most successful treatment for chronic constipation.

The symptoms of constipation vary from few or none at all to a condition resembling a wasting disease. Loss of appetite comes early and halitosis is likely. The person becomes depressed and dull without apparent cause, tires easily, cannot cope with her responsibilities as usual, and may look pale and unwell. Frequent indigestion and discomfort or pain in the digestive system are common.

In most cases of dyschezia, or constipation involving largely the lower end of the digestive tract, actual re-education is necessary to start regularity and reliance on natural processes. Often, however, enemas, suppositories, or mild laxatives may be used to get new habits under way. Regular exercise is frequently advisable, especially for a sedentary person. A walk before breakfast or daily exercise of the abdominal muscles may be desirable.

Along with re-education, an adequately varied diet is probably more significant than any other factor. The major constituents of a normal diet—proteins, carbohydrates, fats, mineral salts, vitamins, and sufficient indigestible bulk—should all be assured. Fruit, especially stewed prunes and apples, are recommended for breakfast, and green vegetables and salad at both luncheon and the evening meal. Bran should be considered as a medicinal food, to be used only on the physician's advice, because it seems to accomplish little more than other bulk foods and may be irritating to the bowel.

Many drugs are available for treating various kinds of constipation. Vegetable and salt cathartics, organic and mineral medicines, substances which act mechanically, and water in various forms are among the most common. Cathartics of both the mineral and vegetable types irritate the bowel and are not advised for long use. They include the strong salts, cascara, jalap, senna, rhubarb, and aloes. Among the substances that act mechanically are mineral oil, bran, agar-agar, flax seeds, and psyllium seeds which lubricate the digestive tract or work by pushing its contents before them. Mixtures of mineral oil and such materials as agar-agar or flax seeds form a mucilaginous mass. Caution is necessary in using mineral oil because it absorbs vitamin A and may lead to a deficiency of that vitamin, and also because of a tendency of mineral oil to leak out of the bowel. Phenolphthalein is the chief ingredient of many widely used laxative combinations.

contact dermatitis. An inflammation of the skin due to a sensitization to a substance with which it comes in contact. As a permanent injury to health, contact dermatitis is not a serious disturbance, but this minor allergy is persistent and often exceedingly annoying. It affects all age groups from infants to old people.

Whenever the skin is exposed to allergens, substances to which a person is sensitive, rashes, hives, cracks, burning, sores, and other irritations may develop. A good example is poison ivy in which an itchy rash is produced on the skin through contact with an oil in the poison ivy plant.

The substances to which a sensitive person may react on touch are numerous and include plants, wood, fur, silk, wool, dye, resin, plastic, rubber, metal, and many more. Some women have cosmetic contact dermatitis and cannot use ordinary beauty products such as soap, bleaches, deodorants, or powder.

contact lenses. Eyeglasses that fit directly over the eyeball and fully aid the vision. A mold of the eye is made, exactly as one makes a cast of the inside of the mouth when it is necessary to have false teeth on plates. From this fragile mold a permanent one is made with dental plastic; then the glass is modeled to fit the mold. The inner surface of the contact lens must fit the eyeball so that it will not injure the sensitive tissues or interfere with the circulation of the blood. Before the mold has been prepared, it is necessary to fit the contact lenses. This means that the eye must be studied by all of the usual methods in order to determine the difficulties of vision so that the lens will meet its needs.

In fitting the contact lens to be worn, the eye is anesthetized and the contact lens shell is filled with a salt solution of the same density as the blood. The lids of the eye are then separated by the thumb and forefinger of the left hand, and the contact lens, held with a little rubber suction bulb, is inserted between the eyelids and the eyeball, first beneath the lower eyelid and then beneath the upper eyelid. This bulb must be gently released from the glass and should not be pulled in removing it. Otherwise the fluid will be lost from beneath the contact lens. If there are any bubbles under the lens they must be removed and the procedure repeated until the lens fits closely and no bubbles are in the fluid. Once the lens is fitted correctly the person is given instructions in setting and removing the contact lens, and practices, seated by a low, cloth-covered table with a mirror before her.

Experiments have shown that the average person learns to insert lenses in approximately nine minutes. At first, these lenses are worn only an hour or two at a time, but many who become well accustomed to them wear their lenses six to eight hours. Several months may be required, in some cases, before the person becomes sufficiently used to contact lenses to be able to wear them a long time without removing them with fluid, and also without resting the eyes.

contraception. The use of a device, substance, or method to prevent conception during sexual intercourse.

Perhaps the commonest of the various methods of contraception are the use of the sheath or condom of rubber worn by the man and, alternatively, the pessary or diaphragm worn by the woman. Chemicals especially fixed in thick creams, which destroy or immobilize the sperm cell, are also used. The American Medical Association has listed a number of such creams by name as acceptable when prescribed by the doctor.

The physician's advice as to the proper use of such devices, materials, and methods is desirable, since not all are of equal effectiveness. The combination of pessary and cream, for instance, is probably 90 per cent or more effective; none is 100 per cent reliable. The pessary must be prescribed and fitted for a woman by the physician; otherwise, at best, its use will be haphazard protection. Creams and other chemicals are safe only on the advice of a physician. The use of douches is also common, but if they are to be effective and safe, should be employed only with medical advice. Many cleansing or sterilizing agents are dangerous to the body, or may alter normal bacterial growth undesirably in the parts where they are used.

Another method of avoiding conception is the so-called rhythm technique. The basis for this theory is the regular monthly cycle of ovulation. An egg cell or ovum passes from the ovary once every month, and consequently during the month the woman is more likely to conceive at one time than another. These intervals are commonly referred to respectively as the fertile and the safe periods. For the woman who menstruates regularly every twenty-eight days, the safe period is calculated as approximately a week before and a week after menstruation. More exactly, the first nine days of the cycle, beginning the first day of menstruation, are safe. The fertile period, which normally is a maximum of eight days, follows, and then the next eleven days are again safe. When the menstrual interval is shorter or longer than this, or is irregular, the physician's advice is desirable. One new oral hormone is now available which apparently makes menstrual cycles quite regu-

lar and will, therefore, make it possible to practice the rhythm method with considerably more confidence.

Another way of identifying the fertile period is to record the body temperature in the morning, before any food is eaten or water or other fluids are drunk. Ovulation brings with it a fall in temperature, then a rise. Abstinence is practiced during the period of ovulation, and for three days before and the three days after.

The latest development is a number of oral contraceptives which inhibit ovulation. Their action is two-way in nature. While being taken, pregnancy is not possible but upon stopping the dosage, fertility is increased. Side effects are rare and, though the pills have been tested for a number of years, no long-term reactions have been discovered. In fact, among women using oral contraceptives, a significant reduction in the incidence of cancer of the cervix has been found.

contusion. A superficial injury or bruise, produced by impact, in which breaking of the skin does not occur. If the skin is punctured also, the term "contused wound" is used. *See also* BRUISES.

convalescence. The period of gradual restoration to health following disease, injury, or operation.

convulsion. An involuntary general attack of muscle contraction. In a tonic convulsion, the contractions occur without relaxation; and in a clonic convulsion, alternate contractions of opposing groups of muscles take place. The convulsion may or may not be accompanied by unconsciousness. The word "fit" commonly denotes an attack of convulsions.

Convulsions may appear, together with subsequent coma, as a disturbance of late pregnancy. Convulsion in infants is sometimes a reflex action connected with teething, indigestion, rickets, worms, diarrhea, breath holding, an emotional habit which some children develop, and, in particular, high fever, as in tonsillitis. When the convulsion is not brought on by high fever, it may be longer and more serious. Infant mortality rate from convulsions has dropped sharply; in 1900, 1 out of 1000 births resulted in death from convulsions; in 1948, the figure had been reduced to 1 in 10,000, due mainly to advances in the care of infants.

Although convulsions are often frightening, especially in children, a convulsion itself is not fatal. The patient should be prevented from injuring herself, but any use of force kept to an absolute minimum. A piece of wood placed between the teeth will keep the patient from biting herself. Her clothes should be loosened, especially around the neck and across the chest, and she should be placed on her back, unless she vomits, in which case she is placed on her side. As the patient recovers, an effort should be made to communicate with her and to reassure her. *See also* CHILD CARE; ECLAMPSIA; EPILEPSY.

copulation. A technical term for sexual intercourse. *See also* REPRODUCTION SYSTEM.

cornea. The tough transparent membrane in front of the eyeball. It occupies about one-sixth of the circumference of the globe of the eye and acts as a kind of magnifying and protective lens for the eye. Various disorders of the cornea result in serious visual defects.

corneal transplantation. An operation in which a section of clear transparent cornea is substituted in places where opaque cornea has been removed. Corneal tissue is removed from the healthy eyes of persons immediately after death and shipped by air to "eye banks," where doctors can use the tissue as needed. The tissue must be used within thirty-six hours after its removal.

coronary thrombosis. A rather loose term for a condition more accurately described as acute coronary occlusion or blocking of a coronary artery of the heart. This means that a clot of blood has formed within the heart or blood vessels, usually due to a slowing of the circulation or to alteration of the blood or vessel walls. The ability of the heart to function efficiently depends primarily on the state of the heart muscle, or myocardium; thus, life itself depends largely on the state of the blood vessels which bring nourishment to the myocardium. These blood vessels are known as the coronary arteries.

cortisone. A highly complex chemical which is a constituent of adrenal cortical extract. Its formula is known, but the chief available basic source is the gall bladder juice of cattle. ACTH, not a synthetic like cortisone, is secreted by the pituitary glands of hogs.

Hydrocortisone, a derivative, has been found more effective than cortisone for local applications, such as to the skin or for direct injections into joint cavities. These drugs are not a cure for disease; they only relieve and suppress its manifestations.

New preparations have been developed more effective than cortisone without such side effects as disturbance of the water-salt balance. Among them are prednisolene, Meticorten, Kenacort, Aristocort, Decadron, and others.

Cortisone, quickly absorbed in the alimentary canal, is converted into hydrocortisone in the body and is thus a substitute for the natural hormone. It is used in certain acute conditions such as the collagen diseases including rheumatic fever, rheumatoid arthritis, and polyarteritis. Corticotrophin (ACTH) stimulates the adrenal cortex to increase hydrocortisone production. An intact adrenal cortex must be present for ACTH to take effect. *See also* ACTH.

coryza. An inflammation of the mucous membranes of the nose, characterized by sneezing, discharge of watery mucus, and watering of the eyes. Translated from its original Greek, coryza means a "running at the nose." The term is used as a synonym for head cold, and hay fever is also called allergic coryza.

cosmetics. Preparations intended to beautify the skin, hair, and face.

Women of today employ a wide range of cosmetic products and treatments. Face powder is used by most American women. Its practical purpose is to protect the skin against the weather, absorb moisture, cool, relieve irritation, and provide a faint, pleasant odor. Esthetically it eliminates the shiny appearance of the skin which women regard unfavorably.

In the past, face powder has been composed of various ingredients; vegetable powders of rice, wheat, and corn flour, acacia and tragacanth; mineral powders of chalk, talc, kaolin, magnesium carbonate, bismuth nitrate, or carbonate and zinc oxide, with orris root frequently used to fix them. Today most face powder on the market is a combination of finely pulverized chalky minerals, fatty acids, and soaps blended with perfume and coloring matter. Face powder is more absorbent and adheres more evenly to the skin's surface than toilet powders which contain a large proportion of inert substances such as talcum, boric acid, zinc stearate, and perfume and are designed primarily to absorb moisture and perfume the body. For example, talcum powder, developed in this country in the 1890s as a protection against the weather, is magnesium silicate, slightly perfumed. Rouge is merely powder to which coloring matter and binders have been added. In the cream rouges, the coloring is in the waxes and oils.

Powder and rouge do coat the pores, but if used reasonably should not cause any particular enlargement. Pores are openings which are normally almost closed and occasionally open. With the passage of years, some elasticity is lost in these structures and they fail to close as completely as they once did, so that some enlargement of the pores is noted. The danger, although slight, in the use of face powder may be an allergic reaction to some substance in the powder. Some people are especially sensitive to orris root, now rarely used, and the use of face powders with this ingredient may cause sneezing, eruptions, eye inflammations, asthma, or hay fever.

Creams and lotions are another part of the modern woman's toilette. The creams usually consist of mineral or vegetable oil, water in an emulsion brought about by the action of beeswax and borax, triethylamine, alkali stearates, or a lanolin alcohol such as cholesterol. At one time some creams contained dangerous salts of lead or mercury.

Most dermatologists, or skin specialists, feel that creams are beneficial in cases of exceedingly dry skin and may help protect against chapping, cracking, and roughness, or soften lines and wrinkles, but not, however, prevent or eliminate them. In the application of cream, the face is usually massaged and, especially if heat is applied, a temporary swelling of the skin surface may occur with an ostensible closure of the pores; as a result, the skin may feel temporarily smoother and softer. Since the skin is a living tissue with certain automatic powers of regeneration, any improvement in its circulation will improve its condition. Proper diet and hygiene is the best way to encourage circulation and a good skin condition. Wrinkling is essentially due to a gradual loss of the elasticity of the connective tissues underlying the skin, which creams and lotions

cannot correct. No method has been found for restoring elasticity to connective tissue. Face lifting does not do this; all that it accomplishes is a temporary smoothing by removal of a portion of the sagging skin, a process similar to taking a tuck in a loose dress.

Face creams can be useful as cleansing agents, but creams advertised as "skin foods" and "tissue builders" have no proven value. There is no evidence that vitamins can be absorbed into the skin to nourish it. The skin, like all other tissue in the body, must be nourished by food eaten, digested, and absorbed into the circulation.

Weight-reducing creams are also worthless for the purpose claimed, and creams promising to "rejuvenate" the skin are no better than any other cream. Hormone face creams, which contain estrogen, the female sex hormone, have been the subject of much discussion. Actually, if there is enough estrogen in the cream to restore elasticity to the skin, its use may be dangerous; if there is not enough to produce such an effect, the preparation is misleading. So far it would appear that the creams available supply insignificant quantities of the hormone in comparison with medically recognized therapeutic doses. As yet there is no conclusive evidence that harm has resulted from their use although large doses of estrogen may disturb the menstrual cycle.

Vanishing creams are not entirely greaseless and usually contain potassium or sodium stearate and a little glycerin, plus some lanolin and mineral oil. The value of these creams is that as rubbed into the face they serve as a slight massage which increases the blood supply to the face and produces a temporary filling-out effect.

Particularly dangerous are removers for wrinkles, freckles, moles, and warts, and bleaches and skin peels. Astringent substances produce a slight and temporary contraction of the cells around the pores but cannot remove wrinkles. Moreover, strong astringents should not be applied to the face. Eggwhite preparations have been made which stiffen the skin and give the impression that the skin is being straightened although actually it isn't.

Bleach creams have contained ammoniated mercury which acts as an irritant and speeds the peeling of the outer layer of the skin. They may have some bleaching effect, but cannot affect skin blemishes of internal origin. Furthermore, such bleaches can be injurious if applied excessively, too often, or to broken skin surfaces. Liver spots cannot be removed by bleach creams.

Freckles are pigmented areas of skin and freckle removers are designed to peel the skin slowly. The danger is that any preparation strong enough to remove this pigmentation may be strong enough to affect underlying tissues. Skin peels cannot remove skin blemishes of internal origin, and in addition often contain salicylic acid, resorcin, arsenic, and carbolic acid, any one of which may be dangerous to tender skin. Mole removers also generally contain a caustic which again, if strong enough to destroy a mole, can also damage surrounding tissue. The primary danger here is that every mole is a potential site of skin cancer which an irritant, such as a mole-remover preparation, can excite to malignancy. The only wise course in treating skin blemishes of any kind is to consult a physician, preferably a skin specialist, or dermatologist. In the interim, harmless preparations are available which can be applied as a cover or a base for powder to diminish or conceal the defect.

Although occasionally women may be sensitive to dyes in rouges, lipsticks, or creams, more commonly a sensitivity prevails to dyes for hair, eyelashes, and eyebrows. Practically all effective dyes contain ingredients that may be poisonous to some people, and may have effects ranging from serious eye injuries, skin inflammation, infection, chronic poisoning, and ulceration to baldness, fragility of hair, and loss of hair luster. Dyes which are completely harmless, the vegetable dyes such as henna or indigo, are also relatively ineffective. The metallic salts used in metallic dyes vary greatly in harmfulness. Bismuth and mercury are highly toxic. Dyes of the lead sulfur type may be poisonous and should not be used if there is a break in the scalp. Caution should also be taken against oral contact. Dyes containing a large proportion of copper salts can be poisonous, although dyes in current use contain only a minute amount of copper salts. Silver nitrate is less dangerous, but dyes containing it can produce skin irritations or blackened skin patches. Dyes containing pyrogallol, with metallic salts such as the sulfates of copper or iron, can irritate or poison. Metallic dyes act slowly, and do not penetrate the hair shaft but deposit a coating on the outside of the hair. For this reason, such preparations have sometimes been advertised as "hair-color restorers," but in general they reduce the tensile strength of the hair and tend to rub off, sometimes staining the scalp.

Hormone creams to offset the effects of aging are now being offered on the market but there is no scientific evidence that they live up to the claims of their advertisers.

Aniline-derivative dyes, organic chemicals made from coal tar, act quickly and penetrate within the hair, and do not rub off or stain the scalp. Their danger is a tendency to produce dermatitis in some sensitive people and pave the way for serious infection. Some aniline-derivative dyes are safe as they are essentially non-toxic and non-sensitizing, but as a precaution a preliminary patch test is advisable before using them. This test should be repeated before each application since a person can be insensitive at one time and sensitive at another.

Dye should never be used for eyelashes and eyebrows. Mascaras or colorings with a carbon-black base are harmless but preparations of aniline origin or metallic salt, particularly the former, can cause serious injury to the eyes if carelessly applied.

Chemical depilatories should be used with great caution since any substance capable of dissolving hair can also injure or irritate the skin. Even though a substance is safe for most people, there may be a few who are sensitive to it.

If reactions to cosmetics are apparent, a physician may diagnose the condition as allergic and try to discover the causative agent. Often this involves a patch test, the application of preparations to a sensitive part of the skin which is then covered with gauze. At the end of twenty-four hours, if no irritation or eruption is evident, the cosmetic can probably be used safely. Cosmetic manufacturers now produce a complete line of preparations designed for sensitive and allergic people. *See* DEPILATORY.

costive. Constipated.

cough. A sudden violent expulsion of air after deep inspiration and closure of the glottis, the free margins of the vocal cords. It is a symptom rather than a disease itself. The most common cause of cough is irritation or inflammation of the delicate lining of the bronchial tubes or other parts of the respiratory apparatus. A foreign substance, allergy from inhaled substances, tumors of the lungs, or nervous disease may all cause a cough. The purpose of the cough is protective. The body tries by coughing to remove the irritation or obstruction from the breathing passages. Since coughing may spread germs it is advisable to cover the mouth and nose with a tissue or handkerchief when coughing. Coughing may occur in an asthmatic attack when the passageways of the lungs are constricted or narrowed.

crab lice. The body lice which attach themselves to the hair of the groin and also to underarm hair, eyelashes, and eyebrows. They are square in shape with legs well developed and adapted to clinging. This parasite feeds from the skin near the hair to which it clings, leaving pinpoint marks on the skin and causing severe itching. *Phthirius pubis,* the species which infests man, is ordinarily limited to the pubic region and is usually spread by direct personal contact. The female of the species, considerably larger than the male, lays eggs, ten to fifteen at a time, attaching them to hair at the site of contagion, and continues to lay eggs for fourteen days or until her death. The eggs hatch in about a week and there are three moultings in a period of about two weeks. Formerly difficult to eradicate, crab lice now succumb quickly to applications of DDT and other chemicals and ointments in a form suitable for application to the pubic area. These are obtainable by prescription. The venerable standard blue ointment is also satisfactory.

cramps. Sudden involuntary contraction of a muscle, or of a group of muscles.

When stomach cramps occur during the first day of a woman's menstrual period, the application of heat will often afford relief. Various drugs beneficial in relieving these cramps are now available. A woman who suffers persistently and severely from this type of cramp, however, should consult her doctor.

Cramps in the calf of the leg, occurring especially during sleep, are frequent. They may be relieved by forcibly bending the knee as far as it will go, so that the muscular contraction can be released. The muscle should then be vigorously rubbed.

Nocturnal leg cramps in anemic girls sometimes occur because the leg is not receiving sufficient blood. However, the flow of blood to the legs will be increased if the person affected will get out of bed and stand up briefly until the pain departs.

Cramps of the stomach are much more painful and common than leg cramps. Application of heat is often beneficial and sometimes a drug to expel the gas from the stomach may be helpful. One teaspoon of bicarbonate of soda mixed with soda water, peppermint water, or plain water may be used for this purpose. The possibility of appendicitis should always be considered with abdominal cramps. If the cramps are not relieved within a reasonable time, a physician should be called. *See also* ABDOMINAL PAIN; APPENDICITIS; COLIC; DYSMENORRHEA.

cretinism. A condition originating during fetal life or early infancy in which mental and physical development are stunted due to a severe thyroid deficiency.

The cretin may appear normal at birth, but her mental and physical deficiency usually becomes quite obvious during the first year. Characteristic symptoms of cretinism are rough, dry skin, a distended abdomen, a protruding, swollen tongue, apathy, and stolidity. In many cases, regular administration of thyroid extract in early life has helped to improve the condition, but the treatment must be prolonged or even permanent. Cretinism is more common in regions where endemic goiter is severe; otherwise it occurs sporadically.

cross matching of blood. The technique used to determine before a transfusion whether or not the blood to be given to a patient will mix safely with her own blood. Not all human blood is the same and death can occur if cross matching is not accurately done.

Cross matching of blood deals specifically with the oxygen-carrying cells in the bloodstream which are the erythrocytes, or red blood cells. A deficiency of red blood cells causes anemia when hemorrhage occurs and is dangerous because the body does not have enough cells to carry oxygen to primary structures such as the brain and kidneys. *See also* BLOOD TRANSFUSION; BLOOD TYPES.

croup. A disease scientifically known as acute obstructive laryngitis, diphtheria, or occasionally streptococcus sore throat. Croup really refers to a single symptom of throat infection since it is used to describe any condition characterized by a harsh, brassy cough and difficult respiration with a spasm of the larynx and a wheezing sound. Often caused by viruses, croup may be a secondary infection in cases of lowered resistance or other bacterial infections. Although it can affect adults, croup usually occurs in small children between one and six years of age. This age group is probably affected because it cannot easily cough up the bacteria-laden mucus which drips down the throat. The shorter channel to the larynx also permits easier infection.

In croup, the laryngeal, or vocal, cords are inflamed and swollen so that breathing has a wheezy sound. The child coughs constantly, endeavoring to get rid of the obstruction. In spasmodic croup, spasm of the cords occurs which makes them red and pulls them toward each other without the presence of any obvious infection. A form of spasmodic croup in small children is laryngismus stridulus or "false croup." The infant breathes laboriously and respiration may even stop; the face flushes and then turns blue. However, after a short time, relaxation of the spasm sets in. During a crying spell, breathing will become normal again.

The most significant step in croup is to determine exactly what is wrong. The most serious form of the throat infection is that due to the diphtheria germ. In diphtheria, a thick, adherent membrane forms in the throat. In severe forms of streptococcus of the throat, a membrane also forms, but usually is less thick and white. In the worst forms of croup, the fever is high, breathing excessively labored, and the child is exceedingly ill. In simpler cases of croup, the doctor usually advises that the child be put to bed promptly and given plenty of fluids. Steam inhalations, which may or may not be medicated with benzoin or other soothing oils, according to the doctor, usually provide noticeable relief. In cases of high fever, cool moist air may be preferred to hot steam. If coughing is severe, the doctor may prescribe sedatives which will relieve the spasms. An ice bag is sometimes used to relieve a sore throat.

The seriously dangerous cases of croup are those in which there is complete obstruction to breathing, and immediate medical attention is urgent. In these cases, the doctor may have oxygen supplied to the child through a small tube inserted into the opening remaining in the throat. A tube, known as an intubation tube, may be put into the throat to assure the passage of air through the larynx. In the most severe cases, a tracheotomy is performed; an opening is made directly into the windpipe from the outside which permits the patient to continue breathing while the inflammation is healing. Any case with severe swelling in the throat and difficulty in breathing should be regarded as serious, since stoppage of breathing for even a few minutes may be fatal.

curettage. The scraping of a body cavity with an instrument, such as a curette. The purpose is to remove a small amount of tissue and secretion for diagnosis.

Cushing's syndrome. A group of symptoms associated with Cushing's disease, which was first described in 1932 by Dr. Harvey Williams Cushing, famous American brain surgeon.

The disease, which seems to affect women primarily, is due to a tumor in the pituitary gland. Among its symptoms are excessive obesity of the abdomen and buttocks, color changes of face and hands which make the skin looked bruised and stretched, brittleness of bones, and disturbance of sexual functions. Diabetes often is a complication. Women with Cushing's disease develop excessive hair growth, such as mustaches and beards.

cutaneous senses. The four senses associated with the skin: touch, heat, cold, and pain. The sense of pain is especially well distributed over the surface of the body. The senses of heat, cold, and touch are responsive to lighter stimulation than the sense of pain. Pain develops as a sensation from stronger stimulation, and if the stimulus producing a sensation of touch, heat, or cold is increased, the sensation becomes pain.

cuts. Gashes in the skin made by a sharp-edged object such as a knife or broken glass. All cuts, even very small ones, must be carefully treated to avoid infection. They should be thoroughly cleansed with soap and water, and then covered with a clean piece of linen or sterile gauze. If the cut bleeds profusely, as it often does when blood vessels have been severed, pressure must be applied to control the flow of blood. Strong antiseptics should be avoided, but tincture of iodine, Metaphen, and other mild antiseptics can be applied to destroy surface bacteria.

cyanosis. A condition which may occur during the course of certain disorders of the respiratory, nervous, brain, and circulatory systems. The face, lips, and skin may acquire a bluish tinge. Cyanosis is caused by defects in the oxidation of the blood and may also be a side effect of sulfonamides and other drugs which influence oxidation.

cyclopropane. A saturated cyclic hydrocarbon gas which has the odor of petroleum benzene. It is a potent but relatively non-irritating and non-toxic drug employed as an inhalation anesthetic—for example, to lessen intense labor pains. Cyclopropane works rapidly and rarely leaves aftereffects.

cyst. Literally a bladder containing fluid. In medicine it denotes a sac which contains fluids or other semisolid morbid substances. Cysts develop in many parts of the body and are of all sizes and degrees of severity. While their cause cannot always be determined, cysts are apt to form lumpy swellings beneath the mucous membranes or beneath the skin. A cyst is ordinarily movable, while a tumor, a new growth of cells and tissues, is firmly rooted in the tissues.

Some harmless or benign forms of cysts do not require medical attention; others do. The most frequent location of cysts which demand surgery are in the skin and glands. Whenever the opening of the glandular cell or organ is blocked, the accumulation of fluid produces a cyst. Cysts are also quite frequent in various parts of the female reproductive organs and in breasts with cracked nipples, due to nursing.

Among other substances, cysts may enclose foreign bodies (adventitious cysts), gas (air cysts), jellylike substances (colloid cysts), and others.

cystitis. Inflammation of the bladder, acute or chronic, incited through infection by various bacilli to which the bladder is susceptible. It occurs more frequently in women than men, and pregnant women are especially vulnerable. Women are often predisposed to infections of the vagina or adjacent organs which spread to the bladder.

Male inclination to cystitis is increased by the presence of stones or malignant growths.

One of the common symptoms of cystitis is a frequent urge to urinate, which is increased by standing or moving. In many cases, pus is found in the urine, and painful spasms during urination radiate into the upper parts of the body. In men, pains from the lower abdomen or rectum may spread into the penis and thighs. Frequently a low fever is present and in more severe cases a rapid pulse, chills, and urinary retention.

Bed rest, hot sitz baths, consumption of large quantities of fluid, evacuation of bowels, and a soft diet without spices, condiments, alcohol, and other stimulants are the first steps in treatment. Under professional supervision, cystitis responds well to antibiotics and sulfa drugs. Among the new preparations used are Furadantin and Mandelamine. Irrigation of the bladder and elimination of acid in the urine are helpful, and severe pain has been relieved by prescribed suppositories. Should the symptoms of acute cystitis persist, the condition may become chronic. As the kidneys may be damaged, it is advisable to have an X-ray examination to determine the extent of the infection.

cystoscope. An instrument used in diagnosis and treatment of lesions of the urinary bladder, ureter, and kidney. It is inserted into the female urethra, or the opening of the male penis, and permits the physician to look directly into the bladder. The outer sheath of a cystoscope incorporates a lighting system and room for the passage of operative devices.

deafness. The complete or nearly complete loss of hearing due to a variety of conditions which may affect the functions of the ear. Deafness is congenital or acquired. It may be caused by an infection in one or both ears; result from another infection in the body such as meningitis, scarlet fever, measles, whooping cough, or pneumonia; or be due to damage to the eardrum from a blow or accident. It is sometimes caused by hysteria. If the ear is subjected to incessant loud noise over a long period of time, hearing may be impaired, and a sudden violent explosion can cause instantaneous deafness.

defecation. The act of elimination from the bowel. *See also* CONSTIPATION.

deficiency diseases. Abnormal conditions or diseases caused by the absence in the diet of certain necessary substances, such as vitamins, proteins, amino acids, minerals, usually supplied by food. Some of the deficiency diseases are rickets, due to a lack of vitamin D; scurvy, due to a lack of vitamin C; pellagra, associated for the most part with a lack of nicotinic acid, one of the B complex vitamins; xerophthalmia and night blindness, coming from a deficiency of vitamin A; beriberi, caused by thiamine deficiency; and goiter, related to a lack of iodine.

defloration. The destruction of the hymen (or maidenhead) during coitus, by accident, or vaginal examination.

degenerative diseases. The deterioration or breakdown of important organs of the body, such as the heart, liver, and kidneys, leads to disorders called degenerative diseases. A group of degenerative diseases of the nervous system, such as various forms of sclerosis, both hereditary and non-hereditary, produces serious paralysis in various parts of the body.

delirium. A severe mental disturbance in which the sufferer is confused and disturbed by delusions and hallucinations. Extreme restlessness and excitement generally accompany delirium. The chief cause of a delirious state may be high fever, but it may result from mental disease or disorder as well as a variety of conditions stemming from structural damage of the brain.

delirium tremens. An acute disorder of the mind and body which results from alcoholism. Visual and auditory hallucinations as well as the physical symptoms of delirium tremens may follow abstinence after prolonged addiction, or may occur at any point in a long debauch.

Ordinarily an attack of delirium tremens lasts from two to ten days. The mind wanders and sensations of pain, itching, burning, and prickling of the skin torment the victim. Her hearing and vision are disturbed and she may imagine she sees animals and loathsome insects of magnified size. In short, she has "the horrors." Muttering and muscular tremors are also characteristic of this state.

The control of delirium tremens is difficult. The mental aspects are important. The lack of food during a long drinking bout brings on deficiencies of such vital elements in the diet as thiamine and nicotinic acid which are important to replace in order to eliminate some of the nervous and muscular manifestations. Therefore, concentrated feeding of vitamins is essential in the treatment. Rest, too, is essential and if drugs and sleep producers are used these should be administered under most careful medical supervision.

Proper circulation of the blood must be maintained. Until recently the victims were often placed in strait jackets or otherwise forcibly restrained and the resulting blocking of proper circulation by tight straps frequently brought on collapse of the heart and even death. In present-day treatment rest, nourishment, and a more positive approach to the total problem of the alcoholic yield better results.

delivery. Expulsion of the child, with placenta and membranes, from the mother at birth. A precipitate delivery is one that occurs under non-aseptic conditions and when the physician is not present.

delusions. False beliefs manifested by victims of mental disturbances. A common type of delusion, occurring in melancholia, is one in which the person thinks that certain organs are missing. Frequently a delusion is the first sign of mental disorder, and calls for prompt professional attention rather than futile attempts at reasoning with the unfortunate person.

dementia. Loss or deterioration of mental faculties and is characterized by confusion, lack of contact with reality, and apathy.

dementia praecox. The old word, no longer used, for schizophrenia. *See* SCHIZOPHRENIA.

Demerol. A synthetic drug with an action similar to that of morphine.

dental caries. Another name for tooth decay, a process in which bacteria form on the surface of the teeth and act upon carbohydrates to produce acids which gradually break down the enamel and dentine. Focal infection and ultimate decay and destruction of the teeth may result. To keep the teeth healthy, both preventive and corrective measures are necessary.

Prevention of tooth decay begins with proper diet. A balanced diet that includes meat, milk, eggs, fruit, and vegetables is essential for mouth health. Sweets, starches, and carbohydrates, such as candy, bread, and potatoes, which tend to cause acid formation should be limited. Regular brushing of the teeth and use of dental floss is important. The dentist can demonstrate the correct way to brush the teeth. Teeth cleaning is most effective when it follows eating. Experiments in adding fluorine to the water supply have resulted in a significant drop in tooth decay. Another advance has been the discovery of a relationship between dental caries and vitamin C deficiency.

Fluorine in the form of sodium fluoride added to supplies of drinking water has been tested and found effective in reducing tooth decay, and increasing tests further corroborate this. Similarly sodium fluoride in a diluted solution can be directly applied to the teeth by the dentist. Fluorides have also been added to vitamin pills so that parents can be sure that children get fluorine in their systems in those communities which do not add it to the drinking water.

Although there is still no means of preventing tooth decay, certain precautionary measures can be taken by everyone. Thorough brushing of the teeth morning and evening, and preferably also after heavy consumption of sugary things such as candy, is a deterrent to decay. A good balanced diet, containing adequate amounts of proteins, carbohydrates, minerals, and vitamins, particularly A, C, and D, and calcium is an important protective measure for the health of the teeth as well as of the entire body. According to studies cited by the *Journal of the American Dental Association,* reduction of sugar intake will decrease dental caries in about 90 per cent of the people. Although some carbohydrate is essential in the diet, most people can benefit by a reduction of sugar-containing foods. *See also* FLUORIDATION; VINCENT'S ANGINA.

dentine. The major portion of a tooth, the chalky part, found under the enamel and under the cement of the root. Specifically it resembles bone, except that it is harder and denser and differs in structure. Dentine contains numerous tiny tube-like passages which not only branch outward toward the surface of the tooth but also contain the same pulplike material which is found in the center of the tooth. *See also* DENTAL CARIES; TEETH.

denture. An artificial restoration of several teeth.

depilatory. An agent to remove hair. The hair-removing agent may be a chemical paste, a wax, razor, abrasive, or electric current. When a chemical-paste depilatory is used, the paste is placed on the skin for a short time and the hair comes off when the paste is removed. Care should be taken to leave the paste on for only the necessary time since it might be injurious to the skin if left on longer. The skin should be washed as soon as the paste has been removed, and a cold cream may be applied to soothe the skin. In the wax method, liquid wax is applied to the skin and allowed to harden. The hair comes off when the layer of wax is removed from the skin. Here the primary precaution is that the wax be applied at the proper temperature to avoid burning the skin. Electrolysis attacks the hair root, and if done by a skilled operator when the hair is still fine and thin, the hair may be permanently destroyed, leaving no mark on the skin. *See also* COSMETICS.

dermoid cyst. A saclike growth found, for example, in the ovary or in the chest, and containing such startling elements as hair, skin, and teeth. This type of cyst, probably prenatal in origin, grows slowly and does not spread through the body. As the person grows older, however, the dermoid cyst may irritate parts of the body. Therefore its removal, by surgery, is usually recommended. Dermoid cysts do not tend to recur. *See also* CANCER; CYST.

diabetes. The ordinary designation for the condition in which the body cannot utilize sugar normally, causing unusually high sugar levels in blood and urine. Properly speaking, however, the medical term is diabetes mellitus, and is entirely unrelated to a completely different disease, diabetes insipidus.

The essential factor in diabetes mellitus is insufficiency of insulin, which is secreted by specialized cells in the pancreas. This lack has a profound effect on the body. Sugar is produced by the intestinal digestion of carbohydrate foods. It is then transported in the blood to the liver where it is converted into glycogen which can be stored in the liver and muscles and be readily converted to sugar for fuel when the muscles need it. When insulin is lacking, the body is unable to transform sugar into glycogen. Then the sugar remains in the blood, is excreted in the urine, and is unavailable to the tissues and organs that require it.

The diagnostic test for diabetes has traditionally been a urine test but recently it has been discovered that this is not sufficiently accurate and a blood sugar test is now preferred to find the many "hidden diabetics" unaware of their condition.

Diabetes insipidus is characterized by excessive overactivity of the kidneys and overexcretion of urine. Its source is uncertain, but it is believed to be related to some disorder in the central nervous system that involves the area of the brain with which the pituitary gland is associated.

Until the early 1920s, diabetes mellitus was an extremely serious disease. All diabetics died young and a diabetic child had a short life expectancy. The discovery of insulin and its proper use in restoring order to the disrupted sugar metabolism of the diabetic has removed fear of this disease. Although diabetes requires constant attention and skillful management, even diabetic children grow up to live active lives, marry, and become parents. In 1900 patients averaged a life span of approximately five years. Today they can expect to live out their normal life expectancy.

Diabetes today is less menacing than a major infection. The discovery and use of insulin have made the control of diabetes possible. But insulin does not cure the condition. It can only substitute for a critical deficiency. If this outside source is discontinued, the body will be in as dangerous a condition as before.

The basic concept of diabetes is that a disorder, such as an infection or a hereditary tendency, affects the pancreas or the insulin-producing parts of it. Excessive eating over a long time or emotional stress or mental shock can incite temporary attacks of diabetes. Studies now suggest that more may be involved than pancreatic disease alone. The pituitary and adrenal glands may be implicated and the whole diabetic process more complex than was formerly believed.

Without treatment, the diabetic, although eating and drinking in an endeavor to satisfy a perpetual hunger and thirst because of the sugar circulating in her blood, loses weight, becomes weak, and is susceptible to nervous complications. She is far more prone to infection than others, especially to tuberculosis, and is disposed to gangrene and skin damage. The characteristic terminal stage of the disease, when untreated, is a typical coma. Poisoned by acidosis, which results from disturbance of body chemistry, the diabetic person loses consciousness and dies without regaining it. Coma is also a threat to those treated. Therefore, careful regulation of the condition with insulin must be properly observed.

Diabetic coma results when the blood sugar level becomes high, and acid products of the incomplete breakdown of carbohydrates accumulate in the blood. It may occur when insulin dosage is missed or is inadequate to balance food intake, or under other circumstances, upsetting the necessary balance between the sugar and the insulin in the system.

Diabetic coma is apt to be preceded by nausea and vomiting and, before these, by gradually increasing fatigue, weakness, and irritability. The physician should be consulted promptly on appearance of any of these symptoms. The patient should go to bed as a precaution against coma until the physician arrives.

Despite its slow onset, diabetic coma moves swiftly and may be critical. Once unconscious, the patient requires constant attendance by a doctor and, if possible, a nurse until she regains consciousness and during the following week or two of recuperation.

Diabetic patients need never suffer coma, according to Dr. Joslin, if they adhere to the prescribed diet, keep a check on their output of sugar, and maintain the schedule of insulin injections scupulously. They should also know that extra insulin is needed to offset the effects of infection, which increases the severity of the condition.

During 1956, discoveries were announced of products which can be taken by mouth and which have an action like that of insulin in controlling metabolism of sugar. They should never be used unless prescribed by a physician. The drug works best in moderate cases of diabetes and in middle-aged persons.

Diabetes in pregnancy used to be disastrous. Now with insulin and the oral products it can be handled if the physician is on the lookout for it. A pregnant woman should tell her doctor if there is any family history of diabetes or, of course, if she has it herself. There is a high level of stillbirths among diabetic women and many oversize babies. Special care must be taken during pregnancy and at childbirth.

Untreated diabetes in young persons strikes with greater force and results in death more quickly than in older persons. In the latter, it may be quite mild and exist for years without serious effect. Diabetes does not usually appear in younger people. Two-thirds of all cases start after the person has passed the age of forty.

Overweight is one of the most significant factors associated with the development of diabetes, and modern living, with more eating and less labor of the kind necessary to burn up what is consumed, makes that condition a constantly greater problem. People become overweight, and diabetes is a price that many of them pay.

Although a hereditary tendency for diabetes does occur, it is a recessive characteristic, which means that unless reinforced by the addition of new diabetes-prone members, a family will tend to breed it out. The marriage likeliest to produce diabetic children is that in which both parents are not only diabetic but also come from demonstrably diabetic predecessors. All the children may well have the disorder. But the diabetic who marries a non-diabetic of non-diabetic stock has much less reason to fear that the children will be affected. In a marriage of two non-diabetics whose family records show a substantial number of cases, one of four children may manifest the tendency, though not inevitably.

Today control of the diet is an indispensable part of treatment. Unless it is co-ordinated with administration of insulin in the most rigorously careful manner, complications may occur. The phenomenon involved is not a single process and if one portion is disrupted the whole network is. *See also*

CLINITEST; DIABETES INSIPIDUS; INSULIN.

diabetes insipidus. A disorder of the urinary system in which large amounts of urine are excreted. The urine is itself normal and sugar is not present as in diabetes mellitus. The origin of diabetes insipidus is not yet definitely established. In a specific case damage to the pituitary gland, because of hemorrhage, infection, or a tumor, may be responsible. A disorder of the pituitary is probably accountable.

diaper rash. A roughness and irritation of the skin in the area of the baby's diaper. Ordinarily infection is not involved and the rash is caused by the rubbing of the skin against a wet diaper. The irritation is aggravated if the diapers have been washed with a harsh soap, such as a soap with a high alkali content, and then carelessly rinsed. The rash is also intensified if a high degree of ammonia has been permitted to form in the diaper itself. This ammonia is produced when bacteria come in contact with urine which has soaked into the diaper.

A zinc ointment may be applied to relieve diaper rash. To prevent a recurrence of the rash, the diapers should be carefully washed with a mild soap and thoroughly rinsed. After laundering, the diapers may be soaked in a boric acid solution and hung in the sun. The presence of the boric acid will help prevent the formation of ammonia. These measures, plus careful attention to see that the baby's skin is kept dry and clean, ordinarily will bring good results. Protective lotions are available, such as silica preparations and Diaperine. *See also* INTERTRIGO.

diaphragm. A wide muscle which separates the abdominal and chest cavities of the body, contracts and expands with breathing, and is significant both to the breathing process and to the circulatory system.

Hernia or rupture of the diaphragm may be caused by an injury, by a deformity before birth, or by a part of the stomach passing upward through the opening of the diaphragm at the esophagus. A child born with a large diaphragmatic hernia may also have what has been called an "upside-down stomach." Unless this condition is detected promptly and corrected surgically, the infant may not survive.

diaphragm. Popular name for a contraceptive frequently used by women which blocks the entrance of sperm into the uterus.

diarrhea. Excessively frequent and moist or liquid evacuations from the bowels of the residual wastes from digestion; a symptom and not a disease. It may result from a tremendous range of different disorders, from indigestion to an acute infection or a cancer.

Diarrhea may be transitory and pass after a brief acute episode or it may be chronic. In simple acute diarrhea the frequent evacuations gradually change in character from soft to liquid. Intestinal pain and straining to evacuate still further are characteristic; and thirst, abdominal tenderness, and sometimes fever may be present. Frequently some toxic substance or food, such as green fruit, roughage, highly spiced foods, or alcoholic drinks, may be the cause. The diarrhea usually subsides after the elimination of the causative material, although the irritation accompanying it may prolong the condition.

When diarrhea is chronic, medical attention is imperative and failure to treat such a condition can result in serious weakness. The person will lose weight, strength, and appetite, develop anemia, and become prey to various infections. Chronic diarrhea has been classified under eight main headings and forty subheadings, which suggests the variety of disease conditions with which it is associated.

The physician will try to establish the specific cause of the diarrhea and direct the treatment toward elimination of the cause rather than the symptom.

diet, reducing. A regimen of food and drink for the purpose of losing weight. In most cases of overweight or obesity, a reducing diet is the most desirable treatment. In addition to a wish to lose weight, the person should have a knowledge of the nutritional and caloric value of foods. The diet should include sufficient protein to prevent loss of body tissue protein. Carbohydrates should be limited and fat largely eliminated. To insure sufficient vitamin and mineral intake, supplementary multiple vitamin capsules should be taken daily.

After the weight has been reduced to the desired level, it is essential to continue to watch carefully the diet and eating habits. The aim must be to maintain the new weight, and avoid the tendency to regain the pounds lost.

digestion. The complex chemical and physiological process by which food is converted into soluble form for absorption into the tissues and cells of the body.

digestive system. All the parts of the body concerned with intake, digestion, and elimination constitute the digestive system. The digestive tract is really a continuous tube whose parts are the mouth, pharynx, esophagus, stomach, duodenum, small intestine, large intestine, and anus or rectum. The linings of this intricate, convoluted tube perform chemical and mechanical actions on the food and absorb and transmit the resulting substances to the blood and lymph.

digitalis. A powerful stimulant for the heart, and may also be used to provoke the flow of urine in persons afflicted with dropsy or edema.

Digitalis can be dangerous and should never be used except in the dosage prescribed by the doctor. Even a slight excess over an extended period of time may cause the drug to accumulate in the system and act as a poison. The first symptom of poisoning may be palpitation of the heart, since digitalis slows the heartbeat. Often the lips tinge and at the same time the person may find it difficult to breathe. Whenever such an attack occurs, the person should be put to bed at once and a doctor called; sometimes the patient may receive a stimulant such as coffee. If her condition seems critical and the doctor is delayed, she may be given sips of tepid water to encourage vomiting.

dilation. The expansion of an organ, such as the larynx or the cervix, with an instrument to aid in further examination.

disc. A plate of cartilage between the bones of the spine. When one of these discs is broken, the soft material which it contains may protrude in such a manner as to place pressure on the spinal nerves. The person so affected feels as if something has given way in her back, and will complain of a pain which seems to radiate downward along the side on which the break has occurred. This pain, constant and severe, will be intensified when she coughs, bends, or stands erect for a long time. Further symptoms may include muscle spasms, a disposition to protect certain nerve areas, a diminished skin sensitivity in the affected area, and a decrease in tendon reflexes. Sometimes the break is visible under X-rays. *See also* SLIPPED DISC; SPINAL CORD.

diuresis. To release an accumulation of fluids in the blood, a physician may prescribe drugs known as diuretics. The excessive excretion of urine is diuresis. Urine contains both solids and water. Some diuretics increase the discharge of water and others increase the amount of solids released. *See also* KIDNEYS; URINE.

diverticulitis. Pouches, or diverticula, which sometimes develop on the walls of the large intestines of adults, create diverticulosis. Inflammation or infection of these pouches is diverticulitis.

In older people, one of the dangers of diverticulitis is chronic irritation with a possibility of cancer. Treatment of inflamed diverticuli includes rest and enemas to help cleanse the bowels when necessary. Sometimes mineral oil may be used to aid the passage of hardened material. Persistent obstruction or constant inflammation and pain may also necessitate surgical treatment.

Persons with diverticulitis require a soft diet, similar to that for those with ulcer. Irritating spices and sharp foods must be avoided, as well as fibrous foods and those containing seeds or skins.

diverticulum. A small pouch which sometimes develops on the smooth wall of the intestinal tract.

dizziness. Sensation of swimming in the head; one of the commonest symptoms about which people complain. Like a cough, it may be a sign of something seriously wrong that demands prompt attention.

Dizziness follows recovery from all kinds of illnesses. It may result from poisoning by drugs, or sensitivity to certain foods. It is a symptom in high blood pressure, in menopause, migraine headaches, eyestrain, brain injury, punctured eardrum, malformation of the inner ear, syphilis, alcoholism, and many other diseases or disorders.

A common form of dizziness results from inflammation in that portion of the inner ear known as the semicircular canals. Anything that interferes with the delicate mechanism of these canals will produce attacks of dizziness.

dog bites. Because of the possibility of hydrophobia, anyone bitten by a dog should receive the prompt attention of a physician. The wound may be carefully washed with soap and water, a weak solution of iodine applied, and the wound covered with a clean bandage. If possible, the dog should be confined and watched until it is determined whether or not it has rabies. *See also* RABIES.

dorsal. Pertaining to the back.

douche. A jet or current of water applied for cleansing purposes to any part, organ, or cavity of the body.

The danger of germs is always greater when washing an internal portion of the body. Water used for this purpose should, therefore, be boiled, then the temperature brought as close as possible to that of the blood, about 100° F. Cold water must not be used since it is harmful when applied internally.

Certain special equipment is necessary for the administration of a vaginal douche. First is the water container which may be made of tin, glass, rubber, or plastic. A length of rubber or plastic hosing is attached to the container with a vaginal tube of vulcanite or glass at the other end. Glass is more convenient for sterilizing purposes. This equipment must be kept absolutely clean at all times.

The container should be placed two or three feet above the point where the fluid is to emerge, in order that the force of the flow of water be satisfactory. If the container is placed too high, the force might be dangerous, and the liquid could reach unintended areas.

Before the tube is inserted, the fluid should be permitted to run through the entire hose so that all of the air is expelled. Petroleum jelly, if desired, may be smeared on the end of the tube, which should be thrust inward for a distance not exceeding three inches. Afterward the fluid may be ejected into any suitable receptacle. The vaginal douche is useful as an antiseptic, as a means of removing discharge, and also for controlling disagreeable odors. The solution employed will be chosen accordingly. *See also* ENEMA; VAGINA.

Dramamine. The trade name for dimenhydrinate, a compound with antihistaminic properties which has been found to be effective in the prevention and treatment of motion sickness.

dropsy. Accumulation of water in tissues and cavities. A condition rather than a disease. *See* NEPHROSIS.

drowning. Suffocation in water or other liquid. A person removed from the water may be alive, even though she appears to be dead. Without delay her mouth should be cleared of any debris which she may have acquired in the struggle to breathe, and she should be placed on her stomach, the side of her head resting on her forearm. Artificial respiration should be given at once, for at least an hour, until the victim begins to breathe naturally, or the effort is found futile.

drug addiction. The loss of the power of self-control through drug addiction is not only harmful to the person concerned, but also to society. A drug addict has such an overwhelming craving for the drug that she does not count the cost of getting it; crime, violence, and murder have been the price all too often. The addict develops a tolerance to the drug so that increasing doses are necessary in order to produce the desired effect. When not under the influence of the drug the addict tends more and more to manifest typical disturbances of the nervous system. If drugs are withdrawn from the addict, characteristic withdrawal symptoms appear, with acute physical pain in addition to such symptoms as severe cramps in the abdomen and legs, muscular twitching, vomiting, and diarrhea. The addict will be irritable, restless, and unable to relax, and will break out in sweat and "goose pimples." Rest and sleep are difficult or impossible to achieve.

The chief drugs used by addicts are opium and its derivatives, morphine and heroin; cocaine; hashish; and marijuana made from hemp. The widespread use of bromides and barbiturates, sedatives and sleeping pills available to the general public, has also raised problems. The barbiturates fulfill all the requirements of habit-forming drugs. Overdose is often fatal. Therefore, legal control of the sale of the drugs has been tightened.

Information regarding treatment is available from the U.S. Public Health Service in Washington, D.C.

dry labor. Early rupture of the membranes during childbirth. There are few if any ill effects if there is no abnormality present.

d.t.'s. Stands for delirium tremens. *See* DELIRIUM TREMENS.

duodenal ulcer. *See* PEPTIC ULCER.

duodenum. The first portion of the small intestine, leading from the stomach. It contains the openings of the pancreatic and the common bile ducts. *See also* PEPTIC ULCER.

dwarfism. *See* ACHONDROPLASIA.

dysentery. Inflammation of the colon. Its symptoms are pain and severe diarrhea with frequent passage of mucus and blood. *See also* AMEBIC DYSENTERY; BACILLARY DYSENTERY.

dysmenorrhea. Pain at the time of menstruation. Discomfort in the lower abdomen or pains in the thighs or back and a general feeling of pressure may occur. The causes vary from anatomic malformation, such as an undeveloped womb, to disturbances of hormone balance. If pain is constant or severe enough to cause nausea, vomiting, or headache, or to interfere with normal activity, the doctor should be consulted. Mental factors also may be responsible for unusual pain. Often the young girl has been prepared inadequately for womanhood. When the pain is not severe, the use of a mild sedative is helpful.

Strenuous exercise immediately before, during, and after menstruation has been known to produce a period of pain later. Therefore, most physicians believe that violent exercise should be avoided.

While mild non-habit-forming drugs are helpful, the use of habit-forming drugs is dangerous. The relationship between the sex functions and the action of various glands studied by the physician permits him to prescribe endocrine or glandular products which are helpful in controlling dysmenorrhea.

Sometimes called "first-day blues." *See also* MENSTRUATION.

dyspareunia. Pain or difficulty with sexual intercourse.

dyspepsia. *See* INDIGESTION.

dyspnea. The medical term for difficult or labored breathing. This symptom occurs in attacks of asthma, acute laryngitis in children, cancer of the throat, weakness of the heart, and other conditions. *See also* ASPIRATION.

dystocia. Abnormal labor.

dysuria. Severe pain or difficulty in urination. Commonly due to cystitis.

ear. The organ which performs the function of hearing and is involved with the sense of balance.

A number of disorders may affect the ear. Earache is caused by inflammation which, even though slight, should be cared for promptly by a physician, since neglect may lead to serious complications and even mastoiditis. The external ear, because of its position, is susceptible to many kinds of bruises and abrasions, as well as infection and invasion by fungi and insects. Swellings or boils on the external ear should be treated by the doctor. Bony growths on the external ear, known as extosis, are best treated by surgical removal. Congenital malformations are not infrequent and have been effectively treated by plastic surgery.

The eardrum may also be subject to inflammation and is especially liable to puncture or rupture. A sharp instrument should never be used to remove wax or a foreign substance from the ear because of the danger of puncturing. An old saying is, "Never put anything in your ear smaller than your elbow."

In most cases of ear disorder, the minimum amount of manipulation is advisable, since the ear is a delicate and intricate organ through which infections can easily spread. Antibiotics and sulfonamide drugs control ear infection, thus preventing mastoiditis, once a fairly common sequel. *See also* DEAFNESS; MASTOID; OTOSCLEROSIS.

eclampsia. A serious convulsive condition occurring in pregnancy in women of any age. The cause is not definitely known. The prospective mother may suffer convulsions leading to unconsciousness. The first danger signal may be headache or failing vision. The blood pressure may rise sharply and albumin will appear in the urine. These early symptoms are pre-eclamptic. Scientific prenatal care includes constant guarding against this condition. Should any symptoms appear, precautions must be taken at once to prevent eclampsia, which is serious and in the past often resulted in stillbirth.

The woman should be hospitalized promptly. The intake of salt is restricted and a soft diet prescribed. Diuretic agents are given to induce sufficient elimination of urine, since in eclampsia the function of the kidneys is impaired and these organs must be relieved of any extra load. Anticonvulsant drugs are administered to control the tendency to convulsions.

Fortunately the warning symptoms usually develop slowly. However, cases do occur in which serious complications closely follow the first symptoms. Most doctors believe that pregnancy itself is responsible for the development of toxic substances in the body. This toxic reaction may affect certain organs more than others, thus inducing pre-eclampsia or eclampsia itself.

Improved methods of prenatal care in recent years have done much to prevent eclampsia and reduce the mortality rate from that cause. Frequent checking of blood pressure, periodic examination of the urine, and better weight control not only tend to improve the general condition of prospective mothers but make possible recognition of the pre-eclamptic state.

Nevertheless, physicians are always on guard against any eclamptic emergency that may arise. Extreme measures, including the use of oxygen, induction of labor, and even Cesarean section may be necessary in severe eclampsia. Even after a child is born, the mother must be just as carefully watched since pre-eclampsia and eclampsia occasionally occur immediately following childbirth.

ectopic pregnancy. An unusual form of pregnancy in which the fetus develops outside of the normal location, the uterus. It may occur, for instance, in the Fallopian tube. When ectopic gestation takes place the usual signs of pregnancy are present, though they may be overlooked. If a menstrual period is missed and slight bleedings begin to recur from the womb, a physician should be consulted. Prompt operation is the advisable treatment.

Very rarely does an ectopic pregnancy come to term.

eczema. A term which currently refers to a non-contagious skin rash for which a definite cause cannot be cited. Thus, a rash which is produced by a certain type of soap might be described as dermatitis, but not as eczema.

More than two-thirds of all skin diseases are classified as eczema. The symptoms and causes are so complex that successful treatment demands a qualified physician.

edema. Abnormal amounts of fluid in body tissues. *See* NEPHROSIS.

ejaculation. In women, ejection of the secretions of the vaginal glands, especially Bartholin's glands. In the male, ejection of seminal fluids from the urethra.

electrical injuries. Shock or injuries from electricity come from two major sources: accidental contact with electrical current and lightning strokes. In the home, such accidents may result from faulty insulation or careless handling of lighting, heating, or refrigeration equipment.

A person suffering from electric shock must be immediately removed from contact with the source of the electric current. If a live wire must be cut, an axe with a wooden handle is the best tool to use. If the rescuer cannot cut off the current, she must be careful to handle the victim with the aid of some insulating material such as a dry rope, a wooden stick, or a leather belt. She must protect herself from receiving the shock which can be transmitted through the body of the victim. The doctor should be called immediately. If the person is unconscious or breathing has ceased, which is likely if the current has passed through the central nervous system and affected the respiratory center of the brain, artificial respiration should be given at once. Since artificial respiration may have to be continued for several hours, resuscitating equipment should be summoned if possible. The clothing of the victim should be loosened to facilitate breathing and the victim allowed to rest several hours before she is moved to a hospital.

When struck by lightning, the person falls to the ground as if she had received a stunning blow on the head. After the shock, flashes of light seem to pass before her eyes and blindness or deafness can ensue. The nervous system may be dangerously affected with resulting symptoms of paralysis, pains in the limbs, and sometimes hemorrhage.

electric shock treatment. When electric shock therapy is given, two or more electrodes are placed on the sides of the head and a measured electric current is passed through the brain. This type of treatment is used in mental disturbances. The application of electric shock to induce loss of consciousness has resulted in dramatic improvement for some persons, notably for those suffering severe depression, agitation, depression associated with menopause, and catatonic states of schizophrenia.

electrocardiograph. An apparatus or instrument which records the electrical current created by the beating of the heart.

The electrocardiograph is exceedingly useful in diagnosis. It is invaluable in the study of the heart, and in many diseases such as rheumatic fever. It aids in diagnosing suspected cases of coronary thrombosis, a disease caused by clots of blood which block blood vessels leading to the heart and damage the muscle and induce rhythm breaks and other irregularities in the flow of the blood. *See also* CORONARY THROMBOSIS; RHEUMATIC FEVER.

electroencephalography. A method of recording the electrical activity of the brain, especially of the cerebral cortex. Valuable information is gathered by this method in case of tumor, epilepsy, infections, and hemorrhages.

emaciation. Extreme thinness. Emaciation may have many causes, including a psychological basis. For example, a person suffering from depression may refuse to eat and waste away to the point of emaciation. Ordinarily the cause is basically physical, and is usually due to a degenerative disease of the muscles. Emaciation can also result from any degenerative disease of the spinal cord.

Diabetes, syphilis, or a growth in the gullet may cause emaciation. Persistent tuberculosis, in any part of the body, will eventually cause extreme thinness. In addition, emaciation may also be produced by such diseases as cholera, extended diarrhea, disturbances of the thyroid glands, or even by extreme fever.

In the first six months of an infant's life, severe emaciation may seem to develop without any cause.

The term "marasmus" is applied to this condition. Ordinarily the cause will be found in the baby's diet, and a change of diet will bring a cure. *See also* ATROPHY.

embolism. Obstruction of a blood vessel by a blood clot or by any foreign matter floating loose in the bloodstream. An embolus, as the clot or particle is known, is dangerous because it may lodge in an important arterial blood vessel or vein and block the supply of blood to an organ or tissue on which life depends, such as the brain, heart, kidney, or lungs. If an embolus reaches a vital area of the brain, paralysis and even death may follow in a few hours. Embolism in the eye may cause blindness.

embryo. A young organism in the earliest stage of development. In the human being, embryo refers to the organism during its first three months of life in the mother's womb. *See also* FETUS.

emergencies in the home. At least one person in every household should know the basic rules of emergency care.

Falls. Of the millions of serious accidents which occur in the home every day, almost 50 per cent are due to falls. The first rule to observe when a person has fallen is to estimate the extent of his injuries, whether or not he has suffered a broken bone, a hemorrhage, or just a bruise.

Usually, a broken bone can be recognized immediately by failure of the limb to function. A final diagnosis, however, can only be made by a doctor with the help of an X-ray machine. While awaiting the doctor, the injured limb can be placed in a homemade splint if there is someone present able to do it. The splint may be made by wrapping the limb in a large-sized magazine or equivalent which is then tied in place by means of handkerchiefs or strips of material.

A minor hemorrhage can be controlled by placing a piece of gauze against the wound. If the hemorrhage is more severe, pressure against the gauze may be necessary to control the bleeding. A tourniquet should be used with extreme caution. However, if one is absolutely necessary, it is applied in the following manner. A large handkerchief or towel is tied around the arm or leg above the hemorrhage. A small rod of any type, a clothespin or stick for example, is then inserted under the handkerchief. On the other side of the limb the handkerchief is tied in a knot and a larger rod is inserted through this knot in such a way that the tourniquet can be easily tightened, thus closing off the flow of blood.

A bleeding tooth socket can be controlled by filling the socket with antiseptic cotton. Nosebleed may ordinarily be halted by placing the victim face down and then stuffing the nostrils with gauze, or sometimes application of hot and cold packs will bring about the same result. If placing gauze on a scalp wound fails to stop the bleeding, a tight band wound all the way around the head may be successful. A real danger is unexpected hemorrhage of the lung. A doctor should be called and the person placed in bed and kept absolutely quiet.

A bruise is an injury caused by impact in which neither laceration nor external bleeding occurs. The first symptom, pain, is usually followed by redness and swelling. Since blood under the surface has entered the tissue, the skin may become black and blue, and, later, brown and yellow. Though bruises do not ordinarily require treatment, ice packs will often lessen the pain. The pain and discolor of a black eye, which is a type of bruise, will often diminish if iced compresses are applied. Later, when the blackness appears, hot compresses for half-hour intervals are more effective.

Foreign bodies. Foreign bodies accidentally penetrating any orifice of the human body ordinarily should be extracted promptly. This must be done gently, however, since violence might do more harm than good.

An infant who has swallowed a foreign object should be laid face down, or held head down, so that he can cough up the object. If anything is caught in the nostril, blowing the nose or sneezing may help to extract it. Usually, however, the best solution is to call the doctor. When a foreign object lodges in the ear, an insect, for example, it may often be removed by filling the ear with warm oil. The insect cannot live in oil and when it dies it can be floated out with warm water.

Parents are justifiably frightened when a child swallows a broken piece of glass, a pin, or some foreign substance. If small, the object may pass from the body as part of a bowel movement.

A tiny particle in the eye may often be removed with the tip of a clean handkerchief. If it is under the lid, however, the most common method of removal is to turn the eyelid up over a small rod, such as a match.

These suggestions do not apply, however, to a speck which appears on the eyeball itself. When this happens, the wisest course is to place a pad of wet gauze over the entire eye, call a doctor promptly and keep the person quiet until he arrives. Such an accident is often extremely painful.

One should never attempt to pull a fishhook out the way it went in. Rather, it should be pushed all the way through and snipped off at the end. It may then be pulled out without damaging the flesh.

Wounds. A wound is an injury involving a break in the skin. Before caring for a wound, the person in charge should wash his hands thoroughly in soap and water, and perhaps also in alcohol. Any object applied to the wound should also be sterilized and cloth which is used as a bandage ought to be thoroughly boiled. Packages of sterilized bandages may be purchased at a drugstore or other shops.

After the wound has been washed in soap and water, or in some suitable mild solution, it should be covered with a sterile dressing. If any pus appears in the wound, be sure to call a physician. If this is impossible, the pus should be removed before treating the wound, even if it is necessary to open the wound for this purpose.

Burns. Among the possible causes of burns are scalding water, hot irons, electricity and unexpected match blazes. Burns involving more than half the body are usually fatal. Any person who has been burned severely will suffer shock as well as physical damage and requires the immediate attention of a physician. Little can be done by the layman except to make the victim as comfortable as possible.

If a person has suffered lesser burns, however, the injured area may be covered at once with cold water or vinegar. Immersion of the burned part of the body, especially a burned hand, in a bowl full of water and ice cubes will reduce pain and inhibit blisters. The wounds should never be covered with anything since these articles cannot be removed without doing serious damage to the tissues.

Burns caused by nitric or sulfuric acid should be washed at once to remove the acid. This may be done with a solution of bicarbonate of soda. If possible, the wound should then be permitted to soak in the same solution for as long as possible.

Injuries from fireworks, guns, cap pistols and similar toys are no longer as common as they were in the past. Here the greatest danger is the possibility of lockjaw, a disease in which germs, having entered a wound, are sealed in. A doctor is desirable because the wound must be cleansed, after which the victim may possibly need lockjaw antitoxin.

Resuscitation. Asphyxiation, suffocation due to deficiency of oxygen, is often caused by drowning, electric shock or by carbon monoxide gas. When a person has been under water for as long as five minutes, artificial resuscitation is probably the quickest method of attempting to save his life. The most widely accepted method of artificial respiration, or resuscitation, is the direct mouth to mouth breathing, using a special tube if available. This operation may usually be continued for at least an hour, or until the breathing has been restored. The person should be kept under close observation afterward, in case he should again cease to breathe.

If a person has suffered electric shock, the first step is always to remove the victim from the cause. Since every second counts and there is usually no time to turn off the current, the quickest solution is to throw a coat or similar article of clothing around the body of the victim and so pull him away from the current. Artificial respiration should then be administered until the doctor arrives.

Preventive action is the best method of avoiding death by carbon monoxide gas. Windows should always be kept open and an engine should never be permitted to run in a closed garage. Those who are especially sensitive to carbon monoxide gas should avoid any occupation in which such gas is prevalent.

The first symptoms of monoxide poisoning are headache, faintness, nervousness, and irritability. An apparent victim of carbon monoxide poisoning should be removed at once to fresh air and kept quiet and warm. If possible, while awaiting the doctor, the patient should be covered with hot-water bottles or blankets to prevent pneumonia. At the same time, artificial respiration should be administered.

Fainting. If a person has fainted, a physician should be called. While awaiting his arrival, the victim should be placed flat on his back in the coolest location possible. If the face is pale, the head should be brought as low as possible in relation to the rest of the body. If the face is red, however, the head may be moved to a position somewhat higher than that of the rest of the body. Cold water may be applied to the face or chest, and smelling salts or a teaspoonful of aromatic spirits of ammonia in a tumbler of water may be given.

Heat Stroke. Heat stroke may occur, not only in tropical weather, but in any area, a laundry or kitchen, for example, where the heat is intense. Persons working under such conditions should take salt tablets at regular intervals throughout the day.

The signs to watch for in heat stroke are dizziness, drowsiness, and fast breathing. When the attack occurs, it is essential to transfer the victim at once to a cool place and then keep him flat on his back and absolutely quiet. Sponging with cool water will help to control the temperature, and the circulation may be stimulated with coffee or other drugs.

Some authorities advise that the victim of heat stroke be placed on a bed covered with a large rubber sheet, and his entire body then rubbed with ice until the temperature drops to 101. At that point, the cold treatment is terminated and the patient is covered with blankets. If breathing stops, it is necessary to administer artificial respiration at once.

Bite Wounds. If a person has been stung by a bee or similar insect, the sting should be removed at once and a drop or two of diluted ammonia water placed on the wound. When a more serious bite has occurred, however, such as that of a centipede, spider, or scorpion, bleeding should at first be encouraged as a means of removing the poison. Later, iodine may be applied, together with a cold pack to ease the pain. The sting of the black widow spider requires the additional attention of a physician who may employ a local anesthetic and also administer adrenalin to constrict the blood vessels so that the poison will not spread.

The treatment for a dog bite is the same as that which is given for any infected wound. If there is any likelihood of hydrophobia, however, the wound should be cauterized by a doctor and the dog reported to the city authorities at once.

Hiccups. A hiccup is an involuntary spasm of the diaphragm, causing an inhalation which is suddenly stopped by the closing of the glottis. A characteristic sound is involved.

Popular cures for hiccups often involve the use of a ruse which is calculated to distract the victim's attention from his affliction. If the condition persists, a doctor must be consulted.

Migraine or Sick Headache. Migraine may have its source in sensitivity to food, in a disease of the stomach or brain, in hardening of the arteries, in disturbances of vision, in menstruation, or in mental problems. Sometimes the cause cannot be determined.

The headache will either come suddenly or its approach may be heralded by a feeling of depression, perhaps a disinclination to work or to carry on daily activities.

When the migraine headache actually strikes, the victim is usually required to lie down in a darkened room in absolute quiet. Often the patient is so uncomfortable that he rejects any assistance or attention. Drugs provide a satisfying relief for migraine and may become habitual unless their use is carefully supervised by a physician.

Food Poisoning. When a person appears to have eaten poisoned food, an attempt should be made at once to determine the nature of the poison. Evidence may be found in an empty bottle, a cup or spoon, perhaps on the table or floor, or possibly by smelling the patient's breath or inspecting her mouth.

While awaiting the doctor, the white of eggs, milk or strong tea can be given to the patient, all of which are antagonistic to certain poisons. Vomiting can be provoked by means of tickling the back of the throat or by giving the patient a cup of warm water mixed with salt. If there is any possibility that the person has taken an acid poison, vomiting should never be induced.

See ANTIDOTE; BURNS; ELECTRICAL INJURY; EPILEPSY; FAINTING; FOOD POISONING; HEMORRHAGE; MIGRAINE; POISONING; *etc.*

emesis. Vomiting.

emetic. A substance used to induce vomiting for various purposes—for example, to empty the stomach of poison. An emetic should never be used for this purpose if the poison is one which might have a damaging effect on the lining of the stomach, such as an acid.

One of the simplest emetics is a mixture of two tablespoons of salt with the minimum amount of water necessary to produce a liquid solution. Also effective is a mixture of one tablespoon of mustard in half a glass of water, or one tablespoon of alum in the same amount of water.

If an emetic is slow to act, vomiting can often be started by the old method of tickling the back of the throat with the tip of the finger, or with some object of similar shape. When regurgitation has finally begun, the process may be continued if the person drinks a large amount of lukewarm water at frequent intervals. This will also help to cleanse the stomach. *See also* VOMITING.

emphysema. The condition which exists when the normal air spaces in the lungs are dilated and the walls are overdistended. Various types of this disease are related to different causes. An obstruction of the breathing due to asthma or to chronic bronchitis or coughing produced by any one of a number of lung diseases may cause the walls of the small cells in the lungs to stretch and air to accumulate. The stretching occurs chiefly along the margins and upper edges of the lung where the muscular and bony framework of the lung less adequately support it. The stretching tends to destroy the elasticity of the breathing cells and causes distention of the lung.

Among the symptoms of emphysema are breathlessness on exertion and cough. The cough generally is due to chronic inflammation of the bronchial tubes. Cold air, dust, or exercise may start a coughing spell in the irritated tissues. A person with emphysema usually has a large barrel-shaped chest and prominent bones. The disease can be relieved by treatment of the asthma, bronchitis, or other chronic condition that causes it. Medical treatment of the cough which produces the distention is beneficial. Sometimes a properly fitted binder that sustains the chest walls without interfering with the movement of the ribs helps to control emphysema.

Mediastinal emphysema is caused by the introduction of air into the mid-chest region by a blow, strain, or coughing. It may result also from puncture wounds, or from incorrect use of machines for artificial respiration. Symptoms include swelling of the neck and occasionally of the whole face and chest. If the condition interferes with breathing, the air can be withdrawn by an operation. However, if the amount of air in the tissues becomes so great as to interfere with the circulation to the heart and lungs, death may result.

In older people, chronic emphysema may exist because of inelasticity and weakness of the lung tissues. However, the cough generally is not as severe as in the case of younger people suffering from emphysema. A really effective treatment for emphysema associated with old age has not as yet been found.

empyema. A medical term signifying pus in a cavity or organ, especially in the chest cavity, the gall bladder, or in the pericardium which envelops the heart. Usually empyema is associated with infections of the lung and is called suppurative pleurisy.

Pleural empyema affects children more often than adults. Frequently it occurs in connection with pneumonia or influenza, particularly when the influenza virus is accompanied by a secondary infection of streptococci, staphylococci, or other pus-forming germs. Occasionally the tuberculosis germ may be present and fungi of various kinds may also be found. Empyema may also follow an injury or wound to the chest and lung.

encephalitis. Often called "sleeping sickness," an inflammation of the brain which causes drowsiness and slowing down of mental and physical faculties. A number of distinct types of encephalitis are known, most of them caused by viruses. The condition sometimes occurs as a complication of another infectious disease, such as meningitis or measles, or may arise from poisoning or infection of a wound. Virus

encephalitis should not be confused with African sleeping sickness, which is due to a parasite, trypanosoma, carried by the tsetse fly.

Symptoms of encephalitis vary greatly, depending on the severity of the infection and the area of the brain and nervous system affected. The illness may be brief and mild or severe and lengthy. Acute forms usually begin with high fever and headache, dizziness, vomiting, and pain and stiffness of the neck and back. Drowsiness, stupor, and weakness of the eye muscles are common symptoms. In severe cases, delirium, convulsions and insomnia are present.

Damage to the nervous system is the greatest danger in encephalitis. Parkinson's disease (shaking palsy or paralysis agitans) may follow an attack and sometimes a deterioration of mental faculties. Behavior disorders may develop in children who have had encephalitis.

endarteritis. Inflammation of the inner wall of an artery which occurs in certain types of endocarditis. *See also* ARTERIOSCLEROSIS; ENDOCARDITIS.

endocarditis. Inflammation of the lining of the heart. *See also* BACTERIAL ENDOCARDITIS; EMBOLISM; RHEUMATIC FEVER.

endocardium. The thin layer of tissue lining the inside of the heart.

endocrine glands. Any of the ductless glands, such as the adrenals, the thyroid, or the pituitary, whose secretions pass directly into the bloodstream. *See also* GLANDS; HORMONES.

endometriosis. Growth of benign new cells that look like the cells of the endometrium under the microscope but which grow outside the area where such cells normally occur. It is commonest between the ages of thirty-five and forty. The symptoms are pain before, during, and after the menstrual period. There may be low back and abdominal pain. The treatment is surgical.

endometritis. Inflammation of the inner lining of the womb. It may follow normal birth or may occur as a result of abortion or infection. Bad-smelling discharge and fever are the two most common symptoms. This condition demands the attention of a physician. Treatment may require curettage or operation.

endometrium. The membrane lining the inner surface of the uterus.

enema. An injection of liquid into the lower bowel through the rectum. The purpose may be either to cleanse the intestines or to introduce nourishment or drugs into the body.

An ordinary ear syringe, with a rubber tip, may be used to give an enema to an infant. A single bulbful of liquid is the maximum which may be safely introduced into the intestines of a baby at one time. The injection should be performed as slowly as possible.

For enemas of larger quantity, a douche bag with a capacity of at least a pint may be employed. The bag, or can, should be hung not more than two feet above the person's head. Placing it higher gives the stream excessive force. To this bag or can a length of rubber hosing is attached. At one end of the hose is a nozzle, made of bone or vulcanite, or the end of the hose itself, rounded off may be introduced into the rectum. A soft nozzle is preferable, since it is less likely to injure the fragile inner surface of the lower intestine.

To receive the enema, the person may kneel, or she can lie on her left side with her knees pulled up to her stomach. If she lies in bed, the bed should be protected with a rubber sheet. Before the nozzle is inserted into the rectum the fluid should be sent through the entire hose so that all the air is expelled. Petroleum jelly or paraffin should be applied to the nozzle, which may then be inserted for a distance of approximately one inch. Unless the liquid is inserted slowly, it will immediately emerge. If necessary, a folded cloth or towel may be held against the rectum to aid retention.

If the purpose of the enema is to empty the lower part of the bowels rather than to cleanse the intestines, the enema may be given with the patient sitting up instead of lying down, and the liquid, once it has entered, may be permitted to emerge at once. *See also* CONSTIPATION; DOUCHE; SYRINGE.

Enovid. Brand name for an oral contraceptive pill. The hormones that act to prevent ovulation include progesterones. Various pure forms and combinations with estrogens are used.

enteric fever. The technical term for typhoid and paratyphoid fevers. *See* TYPHOID FEVER.

enteritis. The medical term for any acute or chronic inflammation of the intestine due to any one of a variety of causes. Pain and diarrhea are among the symptoms.

enuresis. The scientific name for bed wetting, urinary incontinence in the absence of demonstrable organic causes, at an age when urethral sphincter control is normally expected; a habit disturbance. *See also* BED WETTING; CHILD CARE.

enzyme. A complex chemical substance found largely in the digestive juices of the body which acts as a catalytic agent on other substances and causes them to split up. *See also* DIGESTION.

ephedrine. When injected or taken into the body it causes smooth muscle tissue to go into spasm. In hemorrhage it constricts blood vessels throughout the body, tending to keep the blood pressure normal. As an ingredient of nose drops it shrinks the lining of the nasal passages, permitting more comfortable breathing during colds. It is also useful in asthma, by relaxing the smooth muscle lining of the bronchioles, permitting easier inflow of air into the lungs.

epididymis. That portion of the testicle lying like a hood over the upper end. When it becomes infected as in gonorrhea, the condition is known as gonorrheal epididymitis.

epiglottis. An elastic cartilage resembling a valve or lid, located behind and below the root of the tongue. It covers the glottis, the opening into the windpipe, during swallowing, thus preventing the entrance of food and drink into the voice box.

epilepsy. A disorder of the central nervous system, perhaps among the most misunderstood of all human afflictions. Seizures begin prominently in early childhood and in adolescence, but many persons are subject to them after the age of twenty-one. The number of males and females who suffer from epilepsy is almost equal. The true cause of epilepsy is not as yet known. Epilepsy is known to be related to damaged brain tissue, or to a brain tumor in some cases, but it may be present when such conditions do not exist. Tension, although it does not cause seizures, may precipitate them. A well-adjusted person who is physically and mentally active will have fewer seizures.

Psychologically the illness may have effect. Approximately 80 per cent of all victims of epilepsy are capable of leading normal lives; those persons about them should recognize that epilepsy is not communicable and not a sign of insanity. Unfortunately, through misunderstanding of the disease, a person with epilepsy may find himself shunned by other people and discriminated against in employment. Concealment of the disease may deny many epileptics the advantages of education and marriage. Not only must the public be educated about epilepsy but the epileptic himself must learn to have self-confidence and courage.

epinephrine. One of the chief hormones of the inner portion of the adrenal glands. Its trade name is Adrenalin. *See* ADRENALIN.

epistaxis. The common nosebleed. Nosebleed may be due to many factors. In children, it is usually the result of picking the nose and breaking small blood vessels. In adults with high-blood pressure, nosebleed may occur, which tends to relieve the blood pressure. Nosebleeds may result from frequent blowing of the nose, from a cold, foreign bodies in the nasal passages, or during the menstrual period. Fleshy growths in the nose, such as polyps, vitamin deficiency, food allergy, or even leukemia may all produce a nosebleed.

epithelioma. Any benign cancer or tumor of the skin or other epithelial tissues. *See also* CANCER.

ergot. A fungus that grows on grains and cereals. It is used to aid the uterus to contract after childbirth, to prevent blood loss. It does not affect normal pregnancy.

ergotism. A disease caused by overuse of ergot-containing food or drugs; it is characterized by gangrene of the fingertips and toes.

erysipelas. A skin disease due to streptococcal infection. The inflammation spreads rapidly. The infection appears on the face, but may affect any part of the skin. It usually starts in a wound, fissure, or minute abrasion of the skin.

Erysipelas occurs more often in cold weather when the cracking of the skin due to exposure predisposes persons to its attack. The disease may be fatal, particularly to young children or old and infirm people, and it is essential that a doctor be called at once.

The development of sulfa compounds and antibiotics in recent years has rendered all other forms of treatment of erysipelas obselete.

erythema. A redness of the skin, in uneven patches, caused externally by sunlight, ultraviolet rays, X-rays, heat, cold, friction, or by chemical irritants. Also erythema may result from the action of internal poisons, as in scarlet fever and other infectious diseases.

This condition may be caused by drugs or by poisons generated in the bowels or in other parts of the body. Sometimes it is accompanied by fever, sore throat, and pain in the joints. This type of erythema affects young people, especially girls, and may last for several weeks. *See also* CHAFING; ECZEMA; INTERTRIGO; LUPUS ERYTHEMATOSUS.

erythroblastosis foetalis. When a mother is Rh negative and the embryo is Rh positive, antibodies are developed before birth which may cause the newborn child to suffer from jaundice and anemia. This condition is known, medically, as erythroblastosis foetalis, which means destruction of red cells in the fetus. It is also called hemolytic anemia. *See also* BLOOD TYPES.

erythrocytes. The scientific term for red blood cells. For conditions affecting the red blood cells, *see also* ANEMIA; BLOOD.

essential hypertension. A disease, suspected to be inherited, in which the blood pressure is elevated above normal. The treatment is bed rest, sedation, and hypotensive drugs.

estocia. Normal delivery.

estrogens. The female sex hormones, produced primarily in the ovaries. However, they also occur in the afterbirth, the adrenals, and other glands. Estrogens are responsible for the development of female physical characteristics. They cause the breasts to enlarge, the deposition of fat around the hips, and development of the female reproductive glands. They make the voice high-pitched, the skin soft and delicate, and affect bone growth as well. The female sex hormones cause changes inside the uterus which lead to menstruation. Excessive levels of female hormone may lead to development of fibroid tumors of the uterus, to ovarian cysts, bone defects and possibly to aggravation of tendency to breast cancer or cancer in other areas.

When estrogens cause early puberty, they cause at the same time too early joining of juvenile bones and thus create short stature. Similarly, delayed puberty may cause unusually tall women. The female sex hormones are used medicinally for many conditions—for instance, to help regulate the menstrual periods, to lessen the severity of symptoms of the menopause, and to hasten development of female characteristics. They have been used in men with cancer of the prostate, to lessen the progress of the disease. They should never be employed without the constant supervision of the physician. Production of the female sex hormone ceases at the menopause.

ether. A thin, colorless, volatile, and highly inflammable liquid whose chief use is as an anesthetic in operations and as a solvent.

eunuch. A male deprived of his testicles. *See also* CASTRATION.

excretion. The discharge from the body of waste products, including feces, sweat, and urine. The greater part of this function is performed by the kidneys, which are among the most significant of the excretory organs. *See also* BOWEL; CONSTIPA-TION; DIARRHEA; KIDNEYS; URINATION.

exhaustion. A condition produced by loss of vital power from fatigue or protracted disease. Extreme exhaustion is known as nervous prostration or psychasthenia, sometimes referred to as neurocirculatory asthenia or weakness. The symptoms of exhaustion often include insomnia, loss of memory and appetite, listlessness, palpitations of the heart, and vitamin deficiency. Psychasthenia is rarely fatal, but it may render the person useless to herself, her family, and society. Corrective measures require a thorough examination, both mental and physical, of the person. Ordinarily a complete rest is imperative and possibly a radical revision of diet or even a change of occupation. *See also* ASTHENIA; FATIGUE.

exhibitionism. A variety of sexual disturbance, seen most frequently in men, in which there is a compulsion to display the sexual organs, usually without desire for sexual union. The exhibitionist is typically an immature person, usually beset by feelings of inadequacy. Often he is conscientious in his daily work, and the tendency is not suspected by friends. Exhibitionists act from an uncontrollable inner tension and afterward experience depression and intense remorse. Psychiatrists believe that the disorder is the result of a subdued intense rage of some sort, a feeling of arrogance or hatred toward women, and a desire to shock. Inner feelings of cruelty and sadism exist as well. The exhibitionist usually does not desire to inflict any physical harm. Treatment demands intensive psychiatric study; seldom can the person cure himself.

exophthalmic goiter. Also known as Graves' disease, a disease caused chiefly by overproduction of the thyroid hormone with consequent enlarging of the thyroid gland. It is characterized by goiter, rapid heart action, protruding eyeballs, nervous excitability, fine involuntary tremor, loss of weight, muscular weakness, and a tendency to intense, acute exacerbations called thyroid crises. *See also* GLANDS; GOITER.

exophthalmos. Bulging or forward displacement of the eyes. Usually it is caused by an increase of pressure within the eye or by changes in the muscles of the eye. This condition is seen most often in cases of exophthalmic goiter.

external os. The portion of the cervix of the uterus that opens into the vaginal canal.

eye. The organ of sight.

Nearsightedness, myopia, is the condition in which one is unable to see objects clearly at a distance. It may be hereditary and frequently is not discovered for some time.

Farsightedness, hypermetropia, is the condition in which one sees things at a distance better than things close up because the light is focused at a point beyond the retina.

The eye in its normal functioning has the ability to adapt itself to various conditions of light. Overuse will exhaust this ability, and proper lighting is necessary to prevent the eye from becoming strained or fatigued.

A newborn baby is farsighted and for that reason pays little attention to objects close to her. By two months, she is able to use her eye muscles to bring her eyes into range for what she wishes to see. The baby does not see small objects clearly until she is at least six months old.

As people grow older, their eyes change. The most significant changes are those in which the lens becomes clouded, resulting in cataract. The muscles connected with change of shape of the lens to accommodate seeing at various distances do not respond as well as formerly. People past forty may require glasses when previously they had not needed them. Moreover, all the tissues concerned with the nutrition of the eye change as age increases, and the eye becomes functionally a less competent organ.

Except for time spent in sleeping, the eye is used almost constantly from the moment of birth until death. Overwork of the eyes results in earlier exhaustion, just as with any other organ. Therefore, vision should be facilitated in every possible way. The eye needs regular rest periods. To reduce strain, it is essential that suitable working conditions be given the eye.

The eye may be used for measuring the general state of health. Conversely the body may reflect trouble with the eyes. If the doctor finds the eyes clear and bright he will feel less concern about any immediate danger to general health. When a severe cold, fever or weakness from any cause is present, the eye will reflect this condition by lack of luster, heavy eyelids, and sluggish movement. In jaundice, the white of the eye becomes yellowish.

The eye may also reflect general disturbances of the body, such as hardening of the arteries, anemia, and diseases of the kidney and nervous system. A tumor in the brain is sometimes discovered because of difficulty with eyesight. Frequently double vision, diplopia, is the first symptom of inflammation of the brain. The pupils of the eye may be constantly contracted, dilated, or even unequal in size because of the effects of drugs on the body.

When a child reaches one year of age, parents can, with a simple test, determine whether or not his vision is perfect. A bandage may be tied over one eye. Then a block, a ball, or any toy that the child uses may be placed near him. If the vision of the child is normal, he will pick up the object when either eye is bandaged, indicating that each eye functions properly by itself. If, however, the child is slow to detect the toy or unable to recognize it, an eye specialist should be consulted.

The next significant time for testing vision is when the child begins to read. Difficulties of vision may be present if the child holds the book too close to his eyes, too far away, or at an unusual angle. Such peculiarities call for immediate testing of the child's vision.

Certain other elementary symptoms are quickly apparent. A child with a pronounced degree of astigmatism may frown as he reads; he may have an aversion to reading because he associates it with headaches and discomfort. Sometimes

one eye alone may be farsighted and the child will be able to get along by using just the good eye.

Unfortunately the child who is nearsighted has few readily detected symptoms. He sees things that are close and is not concerned about objects at a distance. The difficulty may first become apparent when the child plays a game, such as baseball or basketball, or is taken to a motion picture.

Any straining of the eye or imbalance of the muscles may result in cross-eyes or squint. Children may be born with one or both eyes crossed. A squint or walleye may develop from excessive strains placed on the external muscle of the eye by the extra effort which is required to see when there is an extreme degree of nearsightedness.

Children rarely outgrow crosseyes. The sight of the crossed eye may never develop and, in many instances, the squint or crossed eye becomes worse. Early diagnosis and treatment are essential for the best results. As soon as one notices that a child is cross-eyed, an eye specialist should be consulted. Frequently good results are obtained merely with proper eyeglasses, which tend to hold the two eyes in position. Children have been found able to tolerate eyeglasses at the age of fifteen months. The earlier glasses are used, the more effective they will be.

The weak eye may be exercised by various training devices to correct the habit of suppressing the image of one eye. In certain disorders, when the deficiency is slight, this orthoptic training is successful.

The most favorable age for such therapy is between three and six years. After the age of seven the results are rarely satisfactory.

The surgical procedure for overcoming cross-eyes is the most certain method of correction. Proper placement of the eye muscles by the surgeon tends to bring the eye back into proper relationship to the other eye and permit binocular vision. The operation is not a guarantee that vision will be improved, but it will prevent the vision from being eventually lost from failure to use the eye successfully. In addition, the correction of cross-eyes is essential in establishing a proper mental attitude in the child. Children with cross-eyes may be so sensitive to ridicule that they become shy, withdrawn, introverted personalities and their lives ruined as a consequence.

Eyestrain is common. Unsuspected eyestrain may be associated with twitching of the eyelids and face. Nausea and vomiting may appear, with headache, loss of appetite, and many other similar conditions. The only conclusive way to determine whether or not eyestrain actually exists is to test the ability of the eyes to see, and then to overcome the condition by rest or with eyeglasses.

Glaucoma causes 15 per cent of all blindness in the United States, and about one-half of the blindness in adults. In this condition, pressure within the eyeball brings about loss of sight. Interference occurs with the circulation of the fluid that comes into the eye. The accumulation of this fluid causes pressure, and as the pressure increases there is pain, the eye becomes hard and reddened and the pupil gray and cloudy. This describes the acute form of glaucoma.

In a second and more serious form of glaucoma, gradual obstruction of the drainage system occurs so that the pressure increases slowly and the loss of sight is gradual.

Older women should be particularly watchful of their eyes, as they are more likely to suffer from glaucoma than men.

Excitement is often a factor in producing glaucoma, because of the increased flow of blood to the eyes during excitement, with consequent rise in pressure. Early symptoms may include headache, blurred vision, eye pain, and nausea. Prompt attention should be paid and an eye doctor consulted.

The most common cancer of the eye, retinoblastoma, is confined to children under ten years of age, and may even occur at birth. Melanoma, perhaps the most fatal and most prevalent form of eye tumor, occurs most commonly in adults, arising inside the eye and spreading throughout the body if not checked in time and removed.

face. The front part of the head, including the eyes, cheeks, chin, forehead, nose, and mouth.

Complexion refers to the color and texture of the facial skin. Many ailments and conditions can affect the complexion. In chloasma, commonly known as liver spots, brown patches appear on the skin. It is often, though not necessarily, associated with pregnancy. Similar patches may occur which are not chloasma. Facial ruddiness has a variety of sources. If permanent it may be a birthmark. It may be associated with fever or with the hot flashes which sometimes accompany menopause. Redness in the vicinity of the nose often accompanies a type of acne, acne rosacea, which is produced by digestive ailments. In alcoholics, the nose may be red and the network of blood vessels chronically swollen. Prolonged exposure to weather can cause the skin to take on a red appearance. A bluish tinge to the facial skin may result from persistent bronchitis or asthma or cyanosis, a heart disease. Anemia may cause the complexion to be pallid. Any of these color tones to the complexion may be perfectly normal. In a healthy person, the gums and inside of the lower eyelid are a rosy color and, as with the skin, a deviation from this may indicate the presence of some undesirable condition. The appearance of the complexion may also be affected by such afflictions as acne, eczema, or impetigo.

A large amount of fat is packed under the facial skin. When this tends to diminish, as in old age or sickness, the skin becomes less elastic and begins to show wrinkles. *See also* ACNE ROSACEA; CHLOASMA; COSMETICS.

fainting. A temporary suspension of consciousness. Originally a depression occurs in the action of the heart. This can be caused by something environmental, such as cold, heat, or hunger, or by mental shock, perhaps from pain or fright. As a consequence, the flow of blood to the brain is interrupted. Dizziness, difficulty in vision, a ringing in the ears, pallor, and an unsteady appearance may follow. The climax is a falling or sinking to the ground, possibly with a long sigh. Momentarily the victim may hardly seem alive. The breathing and pulse beat, for example, are sometimes almost imperceptible. *See also* DIZZINESS.

Fallopian tubes. The two tubes lying close to each of the two ovaries and leading into the womb or uterus. Their function is to transport the egg cell or ovum, liberated each month by one of the ovaries, into the womb and to provide a passage for the spermatozoa from the uterus. The egg cell or ovum may be fertilized if it encounters a spermatozoon within thirty-six hours of coitus.

The patency of the Fallopian tubes is essential to pregnancy. They may, however, like other tissues, become affected by various disorders which interfere with their normal function. Painful twisting and blocking, for instance, may occur and be followed by secondary infection.

Sometimes a fertilized egg cell will begin to develop abnormally in one of the Fallopian tubes rather than in the womb. The condition, tubal or ectopic pregnancy, demands prompt surgery since unchecked growth of the developing embryo within the tube will rupture it, and serious hemorrhage within the abdominal cavity may follow, which may be fatal.

Gonorrhea is the most frequent infection of the Fallopian tubes, accounting, it is estimated, for 70 per cent of Fallopian infections. The symptoms of the acute stage resemble those of acute appendicitis. The temperature rises, the white blood cells increase, and the abdomen is tender to the touch. The infection may become chronic without acute manifestations, causing long-lasting ill health and eventually sterility.

Antibiotic and sulfa drugs are effectively used to treat gonococcal infection of the Fallopian tubes whereas formerly surgery was required. In the most serious cases, however, surgery may still be found necessary.

Tuberculosis or other infectious diseases may also attack the Fallopian tubes. Infection associated with inflammation of the tubes is known as salpingitis. *See also* ECTOPIC PREGNANCY.

farsightedness. *See* EYE; PRESBYOPIA.

fatigue. The cells and tissues of the body have a remarkable power to recover from ordinary fatigue, but excessive, prolonged, and accumulated fatigue is dangerous. Fatigue is a warning that the person is attempting to do too much and if this warning is ignored the fatigue may develop into exhaustion, a condition in which the body is severely depleted. *See also* EXHAUSTION.

febrile. A descriptive term meaning feverish.

feces. The excretion from the bowels. It consists of undigested residue from food, bacteria and substances secreted from the intestinal walls and from the organs connected with the digestive tract.

feeble-mindedness. Mental deficiency or mental defect or mental retardation, a condition in which average intelligence either is not present or fails to develop. It must be clearly distinguished from mental disease, such as neurosis and psychosis, in which functions of a mind of normal capacity become disordered.

Different degrees of mental defect or feeble-mindedness are recognized. A person with an I.Q. below 20, who doesn't advance past a mental age of three, is considered an idiot. Custodial care of idiots is necessary. They usually present no special problem, since only a few live to adulthood and those who do, do not procreate as they are infantile. Imbeciles have I.Q.s below 50. Often they can be taught to do certain tasks, but they may require protective supervision. Morons, who have I.Q.s below 70, generally can be trained to take care of themselves, and may even be able to support themselves. As well as doing domestic tasks, morons have held jobs in factories. Training of the feeble-minded involves sensory stimulation and development of muscular co-ordination. Good physical condition is important to help compensate for the mental limitation.

Symptoms of feeble-mindedness tend to manifest at an early age, although it is essential to have expert opinion regarding each individual case. A baby's failure to be as responsive to sounds and sights as normal, delay in teething and other phases of development may indicate a tendency to feeble-mindedness. However, variations in development are so great that such symptoms are certainly not inevitable indications of mental defect. The condition becomes more apparent as the child grows older and cannot adjust to other children or compete with them in studies or at play. The mentally defective person tends to remain infantile even though he grows physically.

Much can be done to prevent mental defectives from being hopeless and helpless burdens on others. Such capacity as they do have should be developed to the fullest rather than deprecated and neglected. They should be taught physical co-ordination to the greatest possible extent. They should be schooled as far as their capacity permits, but removed from situations in which repeated unsuccessful competition with children may give them acute feelings of inferiority and defeat. Special institutions for training the feeble-minded are available.

Individual attention is essential in caring for the mentally defective. Attempts to apply the same routine to a large group of feeble-minded persons are ineffective, because each one responds quite differently, depending on the extent of his ability.

Feeble-mindedness has a hereditary tendency. Normal people, in no sense mentally defective themselves, may be carriers of mental defect; that is, they are genetically capable of transmitting the defect to offspring. Feeble-minded persons should not marry, and those who have had a feeble-minded ancestor should recognize the potentiality of having a defective child.

Infection of the mother during pregnancy and injury during delivery of the infant have been suggested as possible causes. Parents should not feel themselves to blame when a mentally defective child appears in the family.

feeding, breast. Conflicting ideas about breast feeding a baby—that is, feeding directly from the breast —as opposed to bottle feeding have produced some confusion in the minds of mothers, especially those who are having their first child. The weight of opinion favors feeding at the breast. A formula in the bottle, if the doctor's prescription and the mother's preparation are correct, will provide adequate nourishment, but human milk contains valuable qualities which are not present in other forms of milk. Also, the latest investigations indicate that the breast-fed baby probably has a psychological advantage over the bottle-fed baby; even though the mother who feeds her baby by bottle holds him tenderly and affectionately, the bottle does in some way impede the direct communication between mother and child. However, breast feeding when it is done with a hurried and indifferent attitude can be emotionally unsatisfactory to the child, just as bottle feeding can give the child the feeling of security and love he needs. Above all, the attitude of the mother is important.

During the months of pregnancy much can be done to prepare the prospective mother for the task of breast feeding her baby. The doctor can recommend special care of the breasts, diet, massage, techniques for adjusting the shape of the nipples. A hospital can be selected which offers special facilities for the nursing mother.

The first days of nursing are a time in which the mother and child come to know each other. The child may at first refuse to take the breast, but if the mother is relaxed the child will probably begin to suck as soon as the nipple is introduced into her mouth. The first substance which is received is not milk but a yellowish thick liquid called colostrum. Under the stimulus of the infant's mouth the breasts quickly begin to release a thin blue milk. The nursing mother should keep in touch with her doctor during the first few weeks. The milk may not agree with the child; the child may get too much or too little milk at a feeding; she may eruct part of the intake, get colic pains, or other situations may arise which should be brought to the attention of the doctor. In general, the doctor will want to be sure that the mother is in good health and receiving the proper rest and food, exercise and recreation, and that the infant is progressing normally.

Occasionally breast and bottle feeding may be effectively combined. This may be necessary if the mother is sometimes absent from home during feeding time or if she cannot keep up the necessary supply of milk. Such a combination should be arranged with the help of the doctor. The combination of breast and bottle feeding usually will facilitate weaning.

The mother must decide which method will be used to feed the child. As stated, breast feeding is usually better for the baby, both physically and psychologically. It also eliminates the daily chore of cleaning bottle equipment and preparing the formula. Whatever method the mother decides to follow, the feeding should be administered with love and affection. *See also* CHILD CARE.

feet. Feet are subject to a great variety of ailments. These include sprains, strains, dislocations, fractures, excessive sweating, warts, chilblains, ringworm, hammertoes, painful heels, ingrown toenails, cracked toes, blisters, bruises, circulation disturbances, fallen arches, corns, bunions and calluses, and many others. Some of these are incurred during athletic activities, some are due to faulty footwear, and others are present at birth.

Fallen arches refers to a painful condition affecting the main bone of the foot, the astragalus. This affliction is especially common among people whose work requires many hours of standing or walking. The pain is due to the spasmodic efforts of certain muscles to overcome the strain which is placed on the tissues. Often the person can terminate the pain simply by getting off her feet.

Ordinarily, however, fallen arches require special treatment. Hot applications and massages taken at the end of the day are beneficial. Even more important is the appropriate choice of shoes. Generally shoes should be specially fitted with a medium-width rigid shank which supports the arch.

Among the most common of all foot complaints are calluses, corns, and bunions. When the skin is persistently rubbed, it tends to thicken. Such thickening, callus, develops most frequently on the bottom of the foot, usually at a point where constant pressure is exerted.

A callus on the toes, between the toes, or—especially—on the outer part of the little toes is a corn. The soft corn, produced by a rubbing together of the little toe and the fourth toe, is a frequent point of infection, especially of ringworm. A majority of the numerous commercial cures for corns make use of salicylic acid, a drug which if given sufficient time will cause the corn to fall away. The only cure is an operation, seldom done, which removes not only the corn but also a part of the bone beneath the corn.

A bunion is a swelling produced by the inflammation of a bursa, a fluid-containing sac located between the tendon and a bone which serves to facilitate action. Bunions are found most often on the outer part of the big toe. They may also appear, however, in the middle of the top of the foot, where the person may have laced his shoes too tightly. This type of bunion can be relieved by inserting pads under the laces or by avoiding shoes which lace. Bunions resemble corns in that permanent relief may be found only in surgery. However, surgery for bunions is frequently and successfully done. *See also* ARCHES, FALLEN; ATHLETE'S FOOT; BUNION; CALLUS; FLATFOOT.

felon. An infection at the bottom of a fingernail which may be caused by staphylococcus or another pus-forming germ.

Home remedies are not always effective and the condition may get worse. If the infection penetrates muscular tissue, the bone covering, or the bone, the condition is serious and should be treated promptly by a doctor.

fertility. The power of reproduction has been noted in females as young as eight years and as old as sixty. Among males, the statistics are more difficult to verify.

Fertility varies greatly from one person to another. In many instances, the male may be infertile with one woman but not with another. Similarly the woman may or may not be fertile, depending on the male. Accordingly fertility must be viewed as depending on the reproductive ability of both man and woman and not on one of them alone.

The likelihood of giving birth to more than one child at a time has been estimated as: twins, once in 90 births; triplets, once in 10,000; quadruplets, once in 750,000; quintuplets, once in many million, and the recorded birth of sextuplets includes at least a few instances which are probably authentic.

By the use of X-rays, a multiple birth may be anticipated early enough so that proper preparations can be made for the arrival of the infants. Fecundity, incidentally, and this includes the tendency to multiple birth, is apparently a hereditary characteristic. *See also* BIRTH, MULTIPLE; STERILITY.

fetus. A term designating the unborn child in the mother's womb and applied usually from the end of the third month of pregnancy until birth. The fetal heartbeat of between 120 and 160 beats per minute can be heard as early as the eighteenth week. Movement may be felt from the sixteenth week. *See also* PREGNANCY AND PRENATAL CARE.

fever blisters. *See* HERPES SIMPLEX.

fibrillation. The name of the condition in which a muscle develops a slight shivering or tremor. In certain degenerative diseases, such as amyotrophic lateral sclerosis, muscles fibrillate, but the term is applied particularly to auricular fibrillation in the heart. Instead of having a smooth powerful beat, the heart action and pulse become irregular in relationship to each other. This weakens the force of the pulsation. The condition is treated either with digitalis or with quinidine. If the fibrillation is associated with thyroid disease, surgery of the thyroid may be indicated to effect a cure.

fibrinogen deficiency. Fibrinogen is one of the essential blood proteins manufactured by the liver. In severe liver disturbance this function may be disordered and restrict the clotting ability of the blood.

fibroid tumor. A common benign tumor of the uterus. It does not develop before puberty or after menopause and is more common in Negro than in white women. The symptoms are abdominal enlargement and abnormal bleeding. It is a painless, solid tumor. The treatment may be with hormones, after curettage has ruled out cancer. When treated by surgery, the operation is called a myomectomy.

fibroma. A tumor of fibrous tissue. Most fibromas are benign, as opposed to cancerous tumors which are malignant. However, some tumors have both fibrous and cancerous tissue and are known as mixed tumors.

fibrositis. Inflammation of fibrous or connective tissue of the muscles anywhere in the body outside of the joints. Muscular rheumatism is a form of fibrositis. While rheumatic toxins may be responsible for fibrositis, other toxins, such as those from septic teeth or throat or from some other form of infection may be the underlying cause. *See also* ARTHRITIS; RHEUMATISM.

first-day "blues". *See* DYSMENORRHEA.

fissure. A division or groove between adjoining parts of similar substance. The brain contains many fissures. The term is also properly applied to certain narrow abnormal pathways, such as those which occur in the nipple or anus.

A fissure of the nipple is seen most frequently when the mother is nursing and is commonly due to lack of care, though a certain stiffness of the skin over the nipple may accentuate the breaking of the skin. To avoid this type of fissure, the mother should wash and dry the nipple with care after every feeding. Any rigidity of the skin in this area can be prevented or reduced if an appropriate ointment is applied.

The presence of an anal fissure is usually accompanied by severe pain when making a movement and often reaches down into the thighs. Blood or pus or both may also be seen in the stool. An anal fissure ordinarily occurs at the lower end of the bowel and probably near the rear. A hemorrhoid is often seen where it reaches the anal opening.

The pain of an anal fissure may be somewhat relieved if the person will take laxatives as needed to soften her bowel movement. The surface should then be cleansed with soft paper or cloth, and the anus and adjoining parts should be washed after every movement. After the area is dried, a soothing ointment is beneficial. Most physicians are convinced that surgery is the only successful treatment for anal fissure. *See also* ANUS; HEMORRHOIDS.

fistula. An abnormal narrow passage which leads from some cavity of the body to the outside skin and which may connect one cavity with another.

A fistula present at birth indicates that some passageway, normal while the infant was in the womb, failed to close after birth as it should have done. Sometimes a child is born with an aperture at the navel through which urine escapes. Similarly this opening, normal in the fetus, ordinarily closes after birth.

A fistula may also stem from a wound or abscess which cannot heal because it persistently receives the contents of some body cavity. An anal fistula often originates in this manner. Two types of anal fistulae are the complete, which opens from the rectum and travels outside the bowel to the skin, usually terminating close to the anus; and the incomplete, so-called because it lacks either the surface or the rectal opening.

Another common type of fistula travels from the wall of the stomach to an abscess near the appendix, and still another is the vaginal fistula. If the lining of the vagina has been damaged in childbirth or in gynecological operations such as hysterectomy, this type of fistula may arise between the vagina and bladder or between the vagina and rectum. The symptoms may be constant dribbling of urine. A fistula may also arise from either one of the parotid glands, which are under the ears, and move to a point where it enters the cheek. This is known as a salivary fistula.

If a fistula persists beyond the early stages, surgery is the only cure.

fits. The word fit without a modifier simply means a sudden attack or seizure of any kind. The term is commonly used, however, to designate an attack of convulsions. Fits are associated not only with epilepsy but may also occur in connection with asphyxia, poisoning, lockjaw, hydrophobia, apoplexy, meningitis and in slow-pulse diseases such as anemia of the brain. They may also appear, together with subsequent coma, as a disturbance of late pregnancy. The type of fit known as infantile convulsions may sometimes be a reflex action associated with teething, worms, rickets, fever or diarrhea.

Hysterical fits are of special interest because they do not involve such symptoms as loss of consciousness or incapacity to control the bladder or bowels. Usually they occur to a person in the company of others, which seems to indicate that the victim is subconsciously trying to gain attention. Though hysterical fits are seldom physically dangerous, they do indicate a tense emotional conflict which may require the attention of a psychiatrist. *See* CONVULSION; ECLAMPSIA; EPILEPSY.

flatfoot. A common foot disorder which may be the result of an occupation that requires long periods of standing or walking, overweight, disease, injury, or paralysis. *See also* ARCHES, FALLEN; FEET.

flatulence. An excess of air or gas in the stomach or intestines or in both. Often painful, this accumulation of air may adversely affect breathing, as well as the normal action of the heart. Also called flatus. *See also* INDIGESTION.

flu. *See* INFLUENZA.

fluoridation. The addition of chemical salts, fluorides, to the water supply. It has been carried out in many communities in an effort to reduce dental decay. Fluorine is a chemical element found in the enamel of teeth, bones, and in minute quantities in other body tissues. Experiments with school children, each one receiving a regular intake of one part per million of fluorides in drinking water, have established that there is a definite reduction in dental decay when water is fluorinated.

fluoroscopy. The act of using a fluoroscope; of observing, on a specially coated screen, the shadows of objects which are being X-rayed. This diagnostic technique has the advantage of offering a moving picture rather than a static photograph. The intestines may be examined in action, or the setting of a fractured bone can actually be followed with the eyes. The disadvantage of the fluoroscope is the fact that the image is less precise than that of a photograph. Great skill is therefore essential in the interpretation. *See also* X-RAYS.

fontanelles. The two soft spots in the infant skull.

food allergy. A disturbance affecting people who are sensitive to one or more particular foods. When eaten, such foods cause symptoms of irritation of the stomach and bowels, and often a skin rash such as hives, erythema, eczema, or perhaps asthmatic symptoms.

food fats. As a food, fat is valuable primarily as fuel, a source of energy. The most concentrated food we have, it possesses more than twice the caloric value of carbohydrates. Every ounce of fat has the same value as every other, whether it be an ounce of butter or an ounce of cottonseed oil. One type of fat, however, may be more accessible than another. In the United States, fats are consumed most frequently in the form of eggs, butter, margarine, cream, meat, olive oil, vegetable oil, and nuts. *See also* CHOLESTEROL.

food poisoning. An illness due to disease-causing organisms or harmful foreign substances, such as chemicals, in food. Misconceptions and confusion are common regarding food poisoning. Actually no such illness as "ptomaine poisoning" exists. Ptomaines are products of putrefactive organisms which, because they were toxic to experimental animals when given by injection, were long considered responsible for the effects of food poisoning. Later studies established that ptomaines are destroyed in the human digestive process and almost certainly do not have any connection with the symptoms of food poisoning.

Disease-causing bacteria are the commonest source of food poisoning, the most frequent probably being the staphylococcus. The same type of bacteria is responsible for many local infections of the skin involving abscesses and formation of pus. Perhaps the most severe type of food poisoning from bacteria is botulism, which occurs much less frequently than staphylococcal poisoning. As with botulism, poisoning by staphylococci is actually the effect of a toxin produced by the organisms. Probably everyone is affected by it at some time or other. Possibly what was once called ptomaine poisoning was actually caused by staphylococci. Putrefaction by itself, the process carried on by the organisms which produce ptomaines, is not harmful. *See also* BOTULISM; POISONING.

foot-and-mouth disease. An acute febrile (fever) disease, characterized by an eruption of blisters about either or both the feet and mouth. It affects chiefly cattle and other animals with cloven hoofs. The disease is contagious, involving a virus which may be spread by the infected animal, or, indirectly, through contact with the animal's straw or milk.

freckles. Harmless small brown pigmented spots or blemishes on the skin, caused by exposure to the sun's rays or to ultraviolet light from artificial sources. They are formed by the cells of the skin as a protection against further action of ultraviolet rays. People with red or blond hair and light skin are more prone to freckles than those whose skins bronze under the sun.

Freckles appear about the seventh or eighth year and remain for life, receding in winter and reappearing in spring and summer. If the skin is shaded from the sun their appearance will be retarded.

Ointments for the skin which screen off the ultraviolet rays of the sun and prevent freckles from appearing are available, as are cosmetics that conceal freckles. Freckles may be removed with ointments containing skin-peeling properties. However, these ointments include substances that are poisonous and may cause dangerous irritation to the skin. Such preparations should not be used, especially on children. Freckles may be removed with these preparations, but they cannot be prevented from recurring.

Friedman's test. Also known as the rabbit test, for pregnancy. The urine of a woman suspected of pregnancy is injected into the ear of an unmated female rabbit. The rabbit will show symptoms of pregnancy within two days if the woman is pregnant. A modification is to test a variety of South African toad that will lay large amounts of eggs within twelve hours if injected with the urine of a pregnant woman.

Froehlich's syndrome. Named after the scientist who first described it, a disturbance of the glandular system in which sexual organs remain infantile. The disease is rare.

If the disease occurs in early childhood, it causes dwarfism, but if it appears in children before puberty, the boy or girl will be fat. The victim will be lazy mentally and have a voracious appetite for food. The sexual organs will be undeveloped. Most fat children do not suffer from this condition, and are more likely to be obese because of bad dietary habits.

The adult male becomes effeminate, his skin is soft, and the distribution of flesh around the thighs and breasts has a woman's appearance. Female patients become exceedingly fat, sometimes weighing as much as 300 pounds.

Modern hormone therapy can relieve many of the symptoms if the disease has not progressed beyond control. Treatment includes medical care and administration of hormones, such as pituitary extract. Proper therapy will reduce excessive weight, correct deformity, and restore sexual development.

gall bladder. A baglike, pear-shaped sac lying usually on the underside of the liver. It stores bile which is a primary digestive substance that the liver produces almost continuously. Bile flows to the gall bladder from the liver, and there is condensed by the extraction of water. When food is eaten and digestion occurs, bile enters the duodenum from the gall bladder. Bile is alkaline and neutralizes the acid semi-digested food coming from the stomach.

The gall bladder is susceptible to infection and to obstructions in the tubes carrying bile, particularly by the formation of stones. The probable cause of gallstones is interruption of the bile flow by infections and digestive changes. Gallstones may range in size from that of a poppy seed to that of an egg. The stones will float in water and are soaplike to the touch. They consist largely of cholesterol, a fatlike substance found in the blood and other parts of the body, and of bile pigments. These are derived from the bile itself, but the nucleus around which they coalesce seems to be a foreign substance, such as a small cluster of bacteria or of infected discharge. Approximately 5 to 10 per cent of all adults have gallstones, and they occur in women five times oftener than in men.

Gallstones are not always troublesome, but they may block a gall duct and induce an attack of gallstone or biliary colic without warning. The pit of the stomach is seized with pain which may be agonizing and so severe that the patient collapses. Such attacks are likely to be accompanied by vomiting and fever, and usually end when the stone slips back into the gall bladder or proceeds into the intestine whence it is excreted with the solid wastes. Another attack may not occur for months or years. When the colic symptoms are repeated, the stomach feels full, pains are felt after eating fatty foods, and gas is present.

Removal of the gall bladder is advisable if the person suffers from too frequent attacks of gall bladder colic. Not only is ordinary comfort restored, but certain definite risks are thus avoided. Infection, with dangerous formation of pus, or cancer may develop if stones persist. Some persons, however, cannot undergo the surgical operation and must have continuous medical treatment and care.

Cholecystitis is the serious condition incurred by infection and inflammation when interruption of the flow of bile occurs. Acute pain in the upper right abdomen, abdomen distended by gas, and sometimes jaundice and fever accompany cholecystitis. When such attacks become a major problem, the solution is surgical removal of the gall bladder, preferably not during an acute episode. Nevertheless, if continued vomiting, rapid pulse, and indications of poisoning ensue, it may be necessary to operate immediately.

Chronic infection and inflammation of the gall bladder induce a tendency to formation of stones, and symptoms of chronic indigestion are constantly present. The patient feels too full after eating, especially if she has had fatty foods. Pain on the right side is likely, and may be intensified by stooping or bending. Heartburn often accompanies this condition and medical examination reveals hyperacidity in the stomach.

Many persons live for years with a chronically inflamed gall bladder and without serious consequences. The risk, however, is always present. Surgical removal of the gall bladder obviates these possibilities. The operation is a major one, usually successful. Symptoms promptly disappear, but diet regulation is desirable for a number of months. *See also* CHOLECYSTITIS; GALLSTONES.

gallstones. Small masses of a substance composed most frequently of cholesterol, bile salts, and coloring matter. They often form in the gall bladder or bile ducts, and may cause symptoms varying from mild colicky pain to rupture of the gall bladder and peritonitis or even infection of the pancreas. Gallstones usually occur after the age of forty although younger women may develop them after pregnancy. In general, women are more often affected than men. Gallstones are best seen by X-ray.

Gallstones cause colicky pain as they pass into and along the bile ducts and are often followed by infection in the liver and by jaundice. They may become lodged at the entrance to the duodenum, causing intense jaundice and severe itching.

Mild attacks of gallstone colic are often treated by rest and hot packs on the stomach. However, a severe attack requires the attention of a doctor who may prescribe pain-relieving drugs. Usually the gall bladder and stones are surgically removed; the operation is performed frequently and is rarely complicated. *See also* GALL BLADDER.

gamma globulin. A chemical substance found in the protein globulins of the blood plasma. The blood has the power to develop antibodies to combat disease. The antibodies in gamma globulin have been found useful in developing immunity to measles in children as well as in hepatitis and other infections.

gastric. In medicine many words beginning with "gastro" are used which relate to medical conditions affecting the stomach. Accordingly gastritis is an inflammation of the stomach, gastroenteritis an inflammation of the stomach and intestines, gastrectomy the removal of all or a part of the stomach, gastroscope a device for looking inside the stomach.

gastric ulcer. *See* PEPTIC ULCER.

gastritis. A frequent form of "stomach upset," is inflammation of the stomach wall. When the lining of the stomach is irritated or infected, it becomes red and swollen and in a severe inflammation may even bleed.

Gastritis may be acute or chronic. Acute inflammation is often caused by food poisoning, eating spoiled food, or simply overeating. The lining of the stomach may also become seriously inflamed following the swallowing of irritating substances like lye, acid, or poison, and quick action by a physician to remove the substance is imperative. This must be followed by neutralization of the poison or the stomach wall will be perforated and acute peritonitis will set in. Surgical treatment may also be necessary.

Symptoms of acute gastritis include loss of appetite, a sense of pressure and fullness in the pit of the stomach which is unrelieved by belching, nausea, headache, and a slight rise in temperature. Vomiting then follows, producing a sense of relief. However, the person will feel extremely fatigued afterward. Examination of the material from the stomach enables the doctor to determine the nature and severity of the inflammation. Relief of acute gastritis is usually brought about in a few days by eliminating the irritating substance and being careful of food intake.

Diagnosis and treatment of constant or chronic gastritis are difficult. Many different conditions may produce these repeated irritations of the stomach lining, and treatment requires observation and control by the physician over a long period of time. Certain vitamin deficiencies in the diet produce a tendency to irritation and inflammation. Disorders of the secretion of gastric juice may also be the cause. Gastritis is generally part of the development of an ulcer in the stomach, and a chronic ulcer is likely to produce chronic gastritis. Alcohol taken in excess produces irritation, followed by inflammation.

gastroenteritis. A general term that applies to a variety of gastrointestinal disturbances. In this inflammatory condition of the stomach and intestines nausea, vomiting, and diarrhea occur, generally accompanied by cramps.

Acute gastroenteritis of a nonspecific nature occurs in alcoholism, malaria, acute hepatitis, and as a sensitivity reaction to certain foods. Food poisoning by staphylococci is a form of gastroenteritis. *See also* AMEBIC DYSENTERY; BACILLARY DYSENTERY; DIARRHEA; FOOD POISONING; GASTRITIS.

gastroptosis. Dropping of the stomach, a condition caused by downward displacement of the stomach which may be seen by X-ray.

genes. That part of the chromosome, or male and female germ cells, that is said to account for inherited characteristics. One half of the genes are supposed to represent each parent.

genitalia. The organs of reproduction. The female genitalia are usually divided into internal and external, with the hymen or maidenhead acting as the boundary. The external genitalia in women are the vulva, pudendum, the mons veneris, labia majora and minora, clitoris, the urethral orifice, the glands of Bartholin, and the perineum. The internal genitalia are the ovaries, the Fallopian tubes, the uterus and vagina. None of the internal genitalia possess nerves capable of feeling pain. Injury and infection from childbirth, however, may cause referred pain that may be felt in the skin of the abdomen or in the back or legs.

geriatrics. The science of medical and hygienic care of aged people. It has broadened and expanded in recent years because of the increased number of older people. *See also* SENESCENCE; SENILITY.

German measles. Also known as three-day measles or rubella, a mild but highly infectious virus disease. German measles occurs in epidemics at three- to four-year intervals, often in early spring, together with an outbreak of measles. It affects persons of all ages, though it is uncommon in infants and children under four, and generally occurs most frequently in older children and young adults. German measles during pregnancy may be harmful to the fetus.

German measles, like measles, is transmitted most commonly by droplet infection and direct contact. The incubation period is from four-

teen to seventeen days, occasionally ranging from ten to twenty-one days. The infectious period is generally a day or two before the rash appears.

The first symptoms in younger people are slight, a scant rise in temperature, perhaps a running nose and some soreness of the throat. In older persons, German measles may be accompanied by headache, weakness, slight fever, sore throat, and swelling of the glands at the back of the head and neck, with some tenderness. Usually the rash is the first symptom noted by the patient. It appears after twenty-four to forty-eight hours, first on the face, forehead, scalp, and behind the ears, then spreading over the body. The rash resembles scarlet fever rash more than measles rash. Itching may aggravate the rounded rose-red spots, which are separate at first, then tend to run together. The rash lasts about three days and fades with a fine scaling.

The general treatment is similar to that for measles. The person should remain in bed until the temperature is normal and the rash has disappeared. As in measles, she should be isolated, since she is infectious for about ten days after the appearance of the rash. German measles is not dangerous, but all efforts should be made to avoid secondary infections, since encephalitis is a rare but possible complication. One attack of German measles confers lasting immunity. The patient's bedding and linens and bedclothing should be disinfected and the sickroom thoroughly aired.

If German measles occurs during the first third of pregnancy, the possibility is great that the child may have congenital defects, such as cataracts, heart malformations, deafness, or mental retardation. These serious complications have been known to occur in more than 50 per cent of such cases. Therefore, the obstetrician should be notified immediately. At present, 17 per cent of mothers-to-be have no antibody protection against German measles. Many mothers are now deliberately exposing their young daughters to the infection while it is not serious in order that they will be immune during their fertile years.

germicide. Any substance that kills germs. There is a significant distinction between germicides and antiseptics; antiseptics destroy poisonous material as well as germs and also inhibit and prevent multiplication of germs.

germs. *See* BACTERIA.

giantism. *See* ACROMEGALY.

gingivitis. An inflammation of the gums. Pyorrhea is a form of gingivitis with pus, and the condition called Vincent's disease or trench mouth is also gingivitis. *See also* PYORRHEA; VINCENT'S ANGINA.

glands. Organs of the body which develop a secretion, a substance which performs a specific function, as in digestion. Many of the body's most important processes are effected through the glands and their secretions.

The glands are of external and of internal secretion. The glands of external secretion include the digestive glands and the sweat glands of the skin. Those of internal secretion, also known as the endocrine glands, secrete their products, called hormones, into the blood. These are carried to other parts of the body where they exert specific effects on other glands or organs. Some glands of external secretion also produce substances which penetrate the blood as internal secretions or hormones.

Glands of external secretion include the liver, which produces bile; the stomach, which gives hydrochloric acid and pepsin for digestion; the breasts, which secrete milk; the salivary glands, which produce the saliva that moistens the mouth and contains digestive substances; the pancreas, which produces trypsin used in digestion and also insulin, an internal substance which regulates the use of sugar; and the sex glands.

The glands of internal secretion are more complex in operation and more far-reaching in effect than the glands of external secretion. For example, whereas hydrochloric acid found in the stomach acts directly on food, the products of the endocrine glands function indirectly. Together they form a system which regulates many of the body's most vital processes.

The glands control growth, the body's response to stress of all kinds, and initiate its defenses, and govern the development of sexual maturity. They induce the secondary physical characteristics which distinguish men from women, such as hair on the face and the deeper voice. They regulate the delicately balanced expenditure of energy that persists continuously in the tissues, and are intimately involved in metabolism.

The endocrine glands include the pituitary, sometimes called the "master gland" because it performs a multiplicity of functions and helps regulate other endocrine glands such as the thyroid gland involved in the consumption of oxygen; the adrenal gland, divided into two parts, the medulla and the cortex, which among other functions assist the body in emergencies; the testes and ovaries, male and female sex glands which affect both sexual processes and, even more, general body conditions; the parathyroids which control the calcium and phosphorus content of the blood; and the pineal and thymus glands which are less well understood than the others.

Endocrine disorders may have profound effects. A pituitary gland which is not functioning properly may cause giantism or dwarfism or permanent enlargement of the chin, hands, and feet. A thyroid gland deficient at birth retards the growth of the body and mind, and causes feeble-mindedness. Later thyroid disorder may greatly accelerate or abnormally retard various processes, reacting unfavorably on the heart or other organs. Lack of the hormones of the cortex, which is the outer layer of the adrenal glands, produces death in a few days if they are not replaced. Disturbances of the sex glands and their hormones may cause a woman to assume male attributes or a man to develop feminine attributes. If a duct of a gland is blocked the secretion continues. The accumulation of fluid causes the gland to dilate and form a retention cyst. An adenoma is a tumor with glandular structure.

The normal course of development of a human being comprises the initial period of growth, a plateau through the years of middle life when maturity is reached and then a gradual decline. Many unjustified or actually fraudulent claims are made that the glands promote rejuvenation. None has been substantiated and rejuvenation is as far beyond human reach as ever. *See also* ADRENAL GLANDS; ENDOCRINE GLANDS; HORMONES.

glaucoma. A disease of the eyes in which loss of vision is caused by a pressure inside the eyeball. This pressure occurs when optical fluid tends to accumulate there. In one form of glaucoma, this accumulation is caused by improper circulation. Pain results and soon the eyeball is hard and red, and the pupil itself becomes gray and cloudy. Another form of glaucoma, regarded as more serious, results from the accumulation of fluid caused by failure of the drainage system. The internal pressure and the loss of vision, however, develop more slowly.

In the earlier stages of glaucoma, visual difficulty occurs at both sides of the area of vision, though the person with glaucoma is able to see in front as well as ever. As the disease develops, however, the area of clear frontal vision gradually becomes narrower until finally the person is completely blind.

goiter. Enlargement of the thyroid gland, located in the front of the neck. In exophthalmic goiter the gland becomes overactive and is usually but not always enlarged. Ordinary or simple goiter begins early in adolescence and is directly associated with an inadequate supply of iodine in the diet. Goiter is most common in inland and mountainous areas away from the sea where there is a deficiency of iodine in the soil and water. Simple goiter occurs infrequently in coastal areas, and is five times more common in women than men. A goiter during pregnancy may sometimes cause cretinism in the fetus.

As a preventive measure against goiter, small amounts of iodine are sometimes given to young people, particularly those who live in areas where the water and soil are low in iodine. Iodine is also administered to pregnant mothers to prevent undesirable changes in the thyroid gland of the developing embryo. Iodine is often added to table salt, "iodized" salt, and can be added to drinking water. Iodine-containing tablets are also available.

In cases in which the thyroid gland becomes so large as to be a deformity and a discomfort to the person, it is ordinarily removed by surgery. However, this condition is rare today.

Exophthalmic goiter is usually more serious than simple goiter. A typical symptom of the condition is bulging eyes, the derivation of the term "exophthalmic." The disorder occurs most frequently in young adults, especially young women, in urban areas, and is apparently associated with stresses on the nervous system. The overactivity of the thyroid gland causes the basic chemical changes throughout the body to accelerate abnormally; the basal metabolism rate rises; the heart beats faster. The person tires easily, her appetite increases, she feels warm, is more nervous than usual and inclined to excitability, she begins to lose weight, her hands may tremble, and she often engages in excessive activity. Substantially these same symptoms can be produced by ingestion of too much extract of the thyroid gland.

For permanent relief part of the thyroid gland is removed surgically. Enough of the gland is left to perform its normal functions and provide the necessary thyroxin. The amount of the gland to be removed is established by the surgeon at the time of the operation. Sometimes supplemental thyroid material must be given for a time after surgery until the gland and body adjust properly to the loss of part of the thyroid gland.

Recently other means have been found for controlling excessive thyroid activity, such as radioactive iodine. Radiation from the iodine directly affects the cells of the gland and permanently lowers its activity.

Hyperthyroidism may also result from the growth of a tumor in the gland which may in turn have developed from a simple goiter. Because of the possibility of cancer as well as hyperthyroidism, these tumors are often removed surgically. *See also* EXOPHTHALMIC GOITER.

gonorrhea. A contagious venereal disease, characterized by inflammation of the genital mucous membranes and caused by a micro-organism, known as the gonococcus germ. Gonorrhea is the most common venereal disease and occurs throughout the world. Adults are almost always infected by sexual contact with an infected person. An epidemic form occurs in young girls which is spread through nonsexual objects, such as clothing or toys.

Symptoms of infection appear in about three days, although they can take as long as three weeks, after exposure.

In women, gonorrhea affects the urinary passage and may extend to the bladder and kidneys. The symptoms include malaise, raised pulse and temperature, vaginal discharge, pain in the abdomen, lower back, cervix, or urethra. It should always be treated promptly. Gonorrhea has far-reaching effects and is a common cause of many of the inflammatory conditions found in gynecology. In the past, treatment of the infection in women was much more difficult than in men, because the organs are less accessible. Formerly a person infected with gonorrhea was incapacitated for weeks or even years, but new methods of treatment with penicillin and other antibiotics, under direction of a physician, can bring about a cure in one or two days, provided the infection is brought to the attention of a physician in time.

In the male the first symptoms are usually a slight feeling of irritation or burning sensation when urinating because of the inflammation of the urethra. If not treated, a large amount of pus is produced and an increased amount of discharge may be noticed. Complications can ensue which cause damage to other areas of the sex organs, such as the sex glands, and to other parts of the body, such as bones, eyes, joints, kidneys, and heart.

Gonorrheal infection of the eyes, although it does occur in adults, is more frequent in newborn infants, who become infected as they pass through the birth canal. Doctors may administer dilute silver nitrate solution or penicillin into the eyes of newborn infants to prevent this infection.

In treating gonorrhea with penicillin, the physician must be particularly careful, since the patient may seem to be cured but still be able to transmit the disease, and penicillin, although it may cure the gonorrhea, may cover up, but not cure, an unsuspected case of syphilis, also present. Syphilis requires larger doses of penicillin. Therefore, if syphilis is also suspected, the physician may use a sulfonamide drug, which will not cover up a developing syphilitic condition.

gout. A disease in which the primary symptom is a painful inflammation of the joints of the hands or feet, and especially of the big toe. This inflammation arises when uric acid in the blood increases, is not destroyed by the body, and accumulates in the blood, where it combines with sodium to create sodium urate. The sodium urate may eventually be deposited in the cartilage and other tissues. It is not as yet known why the excess of uric acid appears in the blood, why the excess is not destroyed, or why urates are deposited in the tissue.

Gout usually begins with pain in the big toe, occasionally in the ankle, heel, or even instep, and is ordinarily accompanied by chills and fever. The pain resembles that of a violent dislocation. The affected joint becomes so sensitive that any pressure, even that of bedclothes, is unendurable. This disease attacks men, and occasionally women, in their middle thirties as well as in their sixties or later, contrary to popular belief that it is a condition resulting from a diet of rich foods in advanced years. Gout finally becomes chronic.

Among the drugs used in the treatment of gout are salicylic acid, cortisone, ACTH, Butazolidin, Benemid, anturan, and colchicine, a drug used to treat gout since the fifth century. These drugs should be taken only under supervision of a physician, since they can be toxic with many side effects if improperly used. Gout is also relieved by application of heat to the painful joint and by protecting it from disturbing external contacts.

Graafian follicles. A follicle means a little bag. The Graafian follicles are in the ovaries and are responsible for the whole female physiology, including puberty, ovulation, menstruation and reproduction. At birth there are between 100,000 and 400,000 immature follicles. At puberty one of these becomes mature and ruptures to allow the ovum to escape in the process known as ovulation. Some 450 follicles are utilized during childbearing years.

granulocytopenia. *See* AGRANULOCYTOSIS.

granuloma inguinale. A disease usu-ally regarded as venereal although no evidence exists that it is transmitted by sexual contact. Its main symptom is deep ulcerations on and around the genitals and is thought to be caused by a micro-organism. There are approximately five to ten thousand cases of granuloma inguinale in the United States and it is associated with uncleanliness.

Following exposure, the disease becomes noticeable one to four weeks later. The first symptom is swelling, usually in the groin, and this swollen area then ruptures and ulcers form. As the ulcers heal, new ulcers continue to appear, and the disease may eventually cover the reproductive organs, lower abdomen, and buttocks. These lesions have an unpleasant odor. A person with granuloma inguinale apparently develops little immunity and may have the condition for many years. Streptomycin and Terramycin have both proved successful in treatment of the disease.

Graves' disease. Another name for exophthalmic goiter. *See* EXOPHTHALMIC GOITER.

grippe. *See* INFLUENZA.

gynecology. The medical science concerned with the diseases of women, particularly those of the organs related to childbirth. A gynecologist is a specialist in these diseases.

gynecomastia. Derived from two words meaning women and breasts, a condition of enlargement of the breasts which affects males only. It is usually related to some glandular disturbance. Excessive enlargement may be surgically treated.

hair, excess. Expert opinion inclines to the view that the endocrine glands, or glands of internal secretion, have a definite relationship to excessive growth of hair, particularly on the upper lip and chin of women. Certain forms of overgrowth of glands may be associated with excessive growth of hair. In women excessive growth of hair is more likely to occur after they have passed the menopause. If a young girl has a fine mustache, the matter can be lightly regarded unless the mustache is too dark in color.

For removal of superfluous hair three different methods are known. The safest and the only one generally recommended is the use of the electric needle. This requires patience and endurance both on the part of the woman undergoing the treatment and the doctor. In this process a needle or wire carrying the current is inserted into the hair follicle and a weak current turned on for a brief time. Only from ten to fifteen hairs may be removed in a single session. Since there may be 1200 to 1500 hairs on the upper lip, the time involved is a major consideration. Even with the best operators, from 10 to 50 per cent of the hairs that are removed recur, depending on the efficacy of the electric current in destroying the hair follicles.

Most experts warn against removal of superfluous hair by X-ray. The results are so uncertain and the possibilities of harm so great that this method should not be used except in extreme cases. A dosage of X-ray sufficient to cause the hair to fall out is likely also to produce permanent damage to the skin.

Temporary measures for relief from excess hair are shaving, rubbing with pumice stone, application of depilatory waxes, which harden and are pulled off, taking the hair with them, and other methods. Hydrogen peroxide is sometimes used to bleach the hair so that it is not so visible. *See also* BALDNESS.

halitosis. The scientific name for bad breath. The cause may be tooth decay; or an infection of tissue in the mouth, tonsils, or nose; or chronic intestinal disturbances. Certain foods and seasonings, such as garlic, leave a temporary smell on the breath.

hallucination. An impression, involving any of the five senses of sight, smell, taste, touch, or hearing, without actual basis in fact. Hallucinations occur frequently in alcoholic delirium, when the victim thinks he sees, for example, rats or snakes. Victims of paranoia often claim to hear voices.

Hand-Schuller-Christian disease. A rare disease which occurs chiefly in children and young adults. Deposits of cholesterol appear in the bones and subcutaneous tissues with consequent disturbance of the metabolism. Growth and development are retarded and other symptoms usually appear, such as bulging of the eyes, a tendency to develop diabetes insipidus, and defects in the formation of the skull.

hardening of the arteries. *See* ARTERIOSCLEROSIS.

harelip. A cleft or clefts in the upper lip, so-called because of its resemblance to a hare's lip. *See also* CLEFT PALATE; LIPS.

hay fever. A common allergic disorder, involving the nose and eyes. The symptoms are sneezing, watery discharge from the eyes and nose, itching, swelling, burning sensations, and general discomfort. In chronic cases, the sinuses also may become infected.

headache. A pain or ache across the forehead or within the head; it is not a disease but a symptom. It may be the result of profoundly complex and obscure conditions, little understood until recent years.

One theory establishes three basic types of processes underlying headaches: mechanical, such as blockage of the sinuses by infection; toxic, resulting from too much alcohol or ingestion of a poison; and functional, in which the parts and phenomena of the body involved do not manifest any detectable disease. Under these three classifications are placed altogether 203 separate causes of headaches.

A common mechanical cause of headaches is dilatation of the blood vessels of the head by a temporarily excessive blood supply under too great pressure. The dilatation, in turn, may arise from different sources, such as high blood pressure or the effect of an infectious disease which evokes outpouring of fluid in the body. Thus, many infections seem to begin with a headache.

One of the most frequent sources of headache is tenseness in the muscles of the head and neck, sometimes because of local injury or a nervous disturbance, sometimes because of emotional tension. Such headaches, usually felt at the rear of the head and down into the neck, tend to respond well to heat and massage.

Persons who have headaches only occasionally may find them closely related to some experience that is also only occasional, such as excessive drinking, eating, or smoking, or exposure to toxic gases or other substances. The actual source of pain is often a change in pressure within the head due to the toxic materials.

Inflammation of internal structure of the head which characterizes severe infections, such as encephalitis or meningitis, incurs acute headache, and inflammation following brain hemorrhage has the same effect.

A seemingly general headache may actually come from a disorder in a small isolated part of the head, especially from the eyes. Excessive use of the eyes, particularly in reading or working under glaring light, will induce headache. Strain and failure to correct defects of vision also bring the same discomfort. Correction of the causative factor generally eliminates the distress.

Migraine, often called sick headache, designates a particular kind of disorder marked by its intensity, its association with vomiting and nausea, and its tendency to recur. Migraine is believed to be a response by the body to some protein to which it is especially sensitive which induces fluid and swelling within the head. However, this kind of headache varies considerably from person to person and from time to time in the same person. Mental factors are closely related to the degree of acuteness experienced in a migraine attack, as are other physical conditions in the body.

In the functional headache, physical cause is not detectable, nor is tissue change discernible even to the closest examination. Frequently, however, it can be correlated to a mental or emotional disturbance. This kind of headache produces as much acute pain as if it had a clearly defined physical origin. The study and treatment of such ailments are in the field of psychosomatic medicine, which examines the interaction of the mind and body.

Frequently headache is the most acute symptom of some minor underlying condition, such as constipation, indigestion, fatigue, or menstruation.

Headache remedies are as varied as the causes, and some are dangerous for a number of reasons. The simplest and most basic remedy should be tried first: elimination of excesses in the use of alcohol and tobacco and food, adequate rest, and establishment of good hygiene relative to excretion of body wastes. A large measure of relief may thus be effected without resort to drugs.

Although the majority of commercial headache remedies are mild analgesics or pain relievers, this is not true of all. Some should be approached with great caution or not at all. Aspirin is the least injurious.

A physician should be consulted when recurrent headache is a new experience. Medical advice is also essential when attacks are of unusual severity or persistence. Sedatives and pain-relieving drugs merely mask symptoms. Expert diagnosis and detection of the real cause usually brings relief. *See also* MIGRAINE.

head banging, head rolling. Toward the end of the first year an otherwise normal, healthy baby may roll his head from side to side at bedtime and also bang his head up and down or against his crib. Sometimes this banging will be so violent as to cause bruises on the head, or so prolonged as to rub the hair away from the scalp.

While parents are understandably disturbed by such behavior, they need not be alarmed. Head banging is not a vicious habit or a mental or emotional disturbance. Neither is it associated with any organic disease. It seems to occur at the period when the baby begins to crave some rhythmic activity; occasionally it seems to be more than enjoyment and an expression of development.

A relationship has been noted between head banging and an obstruction in breathing, such as may be caused by adenoids. Removal of adenoids is advisable and successful in many cases. Nevertheless, head banging may continue if chronic congestion of the nasal passages results from other causes.

Sedatives, which induce sleep quickly, have been found useful in correcting this condition, especially if the child has a tendency to be tense before going to sleep. Head banging, under such circumstances, is similar to thumb sucking, a means of relieving tenseness. If parents or those who attend the baby are themselves tense, this may reflect on the child. Definite or specific suggestions to cure these habits have not as yet been developed. However, babies outgrow the tendency to head banging and rolling. Cuddling and rocking a child to relax it (and the parent) is helpful and this custom is no longer disapproved of. The bottom and sides of the crib may be lined with quilting for protection. In any case, head banging need not cause great concern.

heart. The organ whose function is to keep up the circulation of the blood. At birth the heart beats about 130 times a minute, gradually diminishing to 100 at 6 years, 90 at 10 years, 85 at 15 years, and, among adults, anywhere from 60 to 80. Sixty to 65 beats per minute is exceedingly slow but has been noted, particularly in long-distance runners. The heart beats more than two billion times during a lifetime and pumps millions of gallons of fluid. The heart lies inside a sac, called the pericardium, a little to the left of the breastbone, at about the fifth rib. It is essentially a muscle about as big as a fist. It beats from before birth until death and seldom rests, even by diminishing its rate. It is an involuntary muscle that responds to excitement, effort, and other activities by beating fast.

You can give it rest by lying down so as to slow the beat a little and decrease its force.

Coronary Arteries. The heart gets its own nourishment from small blood vessels that pass into its muscle tissue from the large blood vessels that carry the blood away from the heart. Blocking of these coronary arteries is called coronary thrombosis; the symptoms that follow such blocking are known as coronary disease. In hardening of the arteries, blocking of the coronary blood vessels is more frequent than otherwise. Associated with temporary spasms of these vessels or temporary lack of blood supply to the heart is angina pectoris.

Heart Failure. Failure of the heart to carry on its work is serious because the whole body depends on the blood. Failure may be due to inability of the muscle to pump, inability of the pump to force out enough blood at one time, or failure of the pump to force the blood all the way around and back again. If any of these failures occurs, fluid collects in the feet and in the abdomen; the brain gets insufficient nourishment; occasionally the heart muscle will enlarge in an attempt to do what it cannot. Signs of heart failure are shortness of breath, and a blue tinge to the skin resulting from lack of oxygen in the blood.

Heart Disease. Heart disease is not a single illness but may be one of several, such as that resulting from rheumatic fever, one of the foremost foes of health in children, which is related frequently to streptococcus infections of the throat. People of advanced years sometimes suffer breakdown of the heart; death may be prevented by seeing to it that the victim avoids stress and strain.

Coronary Thrombosis. Coronary thrombosis is the forming of a clot or clots in the coronary arteries. The moment an attack occurs, the victim should be put immediately at complete rest in bed. Then, by careful study involving the use of the electrocardiograph, the doctor will determine the nature and scope of the condition and take the necessary measures to relieve pain and, if possible, bring about improvement. Any attack of acute indigestion in a person past forty-five years may actually be the beginning of coronary thrombosis and should not be regarded lightly.

When the heart is damaged by disease so that the connections between the upper and lower portions of the heart are interrupted, these portions will beat independently of each other. The condition is called heart block. Any interference with the rhythmical, steady beat of the heart demands careful investigation. (See also ANGINA PECTORIS; BLOOD PRESSURE; BLOOD PRESSURE, HIGH; BLOOD PRESSURE, LOW; CORONARY THROMBOSIS; PERICARDITIS.

height. A person's height is determined by the span of the vertebral trunk and the length of the bones of the lower limbs.

Children's growth in height is influenced by climate, including weather and sunlight, by diet, exercise, and posture, and particularly by glandular action. The growth hormone, secreted by the pituitary gland, stimulates the growth mechanism of the body for the first ten or fifteen years of life. Then the same gland begins to function in such a way as to affect the reproductive glands of both males and females. When a balance of secre-

tion is reached, about the time of adolescence, the growth mechanism generally stops and adult growth is achieved.

Overactivity of the pituitary gland produces acromegaly or giantism. Underactivity of the same gland results in achondroplasia or dwarfism.

The injection of growth hormones in children whose rate of growth is such as to indicate that they will be abnormally short in stature has been helpful. The results have been more effective when the injections are given before adolescence, because of the relationship between the pituitary and sex glands. See also ACHONDROPLASIA; ACROMEGALY; GLANDS; PITUITARY.

hematoma, of the vulva. A distention and purplish swelling caused by a direct injury such as a fall or a kick. It sometimes occurs after an operation or because of the rupture of varicose veins during pregnancy or after childbirth. The treatment is bed rest with cold compresses and, occasionally, surgery.

hematuria. Blood in the urine. This condition is abnormal and requires immediate medical attention.

A number of possible causes of hematuria, all related to the urinary system, are known. This disease may result from severe infection or inflammation of the kidneys, or when a tumor of the kidneys breaks through a blood vessel. In addition, various chemicals and drugs, such as the sulfa group, may act on the tissues of the kidney to cause bleeding. A kidney stone, rupture of the kidney, bladder, or other portion of the urinary tract may induce hematuria. Blood in the urine may also be an indication of cancer of the kidney or bladder.

A person with hematuria should be put to bed and the doctor promptly consulted. Uncontrolled or continuous bleeding may be critical if not apprehended and treated immediately and properly.

hemoglobin. The red coloring matter in blood cells, is a protein consisting of hematin and globin. It takes oxygen from the air into the lungs and transports the oxygen to the cells of the body through the arteries. Hemoglobin also combines with carbon dioxide, carrying it from the cells through the veins. Hemoglobin contains iron, which when absent from the diet causes anemia. *See also* ANEMIA; BLOOD.

hemolytic anemia. *See* ANEMIA; BLOOD TYPES.

hemophilia. A hereditary blood condition in which clotting is delayed or does not occur, perpetually threatening the sufferer with death from hemorrhage. In normal persons, when the surface of the body is injured and blood escapes, the blood coagulates into a solid mass within five or six minutes, and in this way seals the wound. In hemophilia, the blood does not clot properly and the person may lose quantities of blood from even a trivial wound. The inability of the blood to clot is apparently involved with a relative deficiency of specific factors in the blood. Estimates indicate that in the United States between 20,000 and 40,000 persons are affected.

It is a hereditary disease which does not affect women, but is transmitted from the mother to her chil-

dren. Such women, called carriers or conductors, do not themselves have any of the symptoms of the disease. If the gene is transmitted to a son, he may suffer from hemophilia, and be able to pass on the gene to his offspring. If the gene is transmitted to a daughter, she in turn becomes a carrier, without having any symptoms of the ailment. Though it is believed that the daughter of two parents who each carry the gene of hemophilia might show the symptoms of hemophilia, a case of a woman with the symptoms of hemophilia has never been reported.

Queen Victoria, whose ancestors left no record of the disease, transmitted hemophilia to one daughter, a granddaughter, great-grandson, the czar of Russia, and to another daughter, who brought it into the royal house of Spain.

The first severe bleeding in hemophilia may be controlled, but subsequent hemorrhage may prove more serious. Persons with this tendency should always report the fact before having a tooth extracted, or undergoing the most minor surgical procedures, so that transfusions of the proper blood type can be available.

Any person who has hemophilia must avoid activity which might result in injury. When hemorrhage is not severe, it may be controlled by cold compresses, by judicious pressure, or by local application of thrombin, a basic blood factor, and Oxycel, a commercially prepared agent. Transfusions of fresh blood or preserved plasma can shorten the clotting time to nearly normal.

hemorrhage. A flow of blood, such as might result from a ruptured blood vessel. Uncontrollable bleeding indicates that the blood of the patient, because of some deficiency, will not easily clot. The supply of blood platelets may be less than adequate.

In adult women, other than menstrual bleeding, the commonest causes are abortion or ectopic pregnancy. The flow is irregular and does not resemble menstruation.

hemorrhoids. Piles, swellings that appear at the lower end of the bowel on the margin of the anus. These are actually varicose veins and are classified as either external or internal, depending on their location inside or outside the anal sphincter, the muscle that closes the lower end of the bowel.

Hemorrhoids result from interference with the flow of blood in the vessels of this area. A number of factors may be responsible, such as extremely sedentary habits, overweight, constipation, or the excess use of cathartics. Pregnancy, too, may cause this condition, as may also congestion or cirrhosis of the liver.

External hemorrhoids may apppear as little folds of brownish skin protruding from the anus, and may produce little more than itching or a feeling of tightness during a bowel movement. Internal hemorrhoids sometimes become infected and inflamed with consequent clotting or thrombosis. These may also protrude, and if scratched or broken bleed until the blood clots.

Treatment of hemorrhoids ranges from preventive measures to erase the cause to surgery for hemorrhoids that have become intolerable. People who lead sedentary lives must exercise. Poor circulation must be improved. Overweight must be corrected by reducing. Foods that may irritate and increase congestion in the blood vessels should be avoided or their use curtailed. Vinegar, spices, and coffee in excess are often harmful. Much can be done to regulate the movement of the bowels and a little mineral oil will help to soften the stool.

Hemorrhoids may be treated by the application of various ointments, suppositories, and hot wet packs, but such methods are only temporary and not curative. Surgery to remove piles is a radical but effective method. Electrical coagulation is effective, and injections of compounds similar to those used to treat varicose veins in other parts of the body are also means of controlling and curing hemorrhoids.

hepatitis. An acute or chronic infectious disease of the liver, caused by a filtrable virus. An acute form of the disease with similar symptoms may appear after injection of serum, as was seen during yellow fever vaccinations given in the army, and also following transfusion of blood or plasma. In these cases, a serum was given containing a virus of which no one was aware. The disease may appear after an incubation period that varies from forty to sixty days to as much as a year, and has also become an occupational hazard for hospital workers.

In ordinary hepatitis, which develops without any previous injection, the spread of the virus may be traced to water or food that has been contaminated. Here the latent period, before the appearance of the disease, is much shorter.

Infectious hepatitis of the ordinary type may be mild, with jaundice as the most noticeable symptom. Other symptoms preceding the jaundice may include loss of appetite, fever with or without accompanying chills, aching of the back, joints, or eyes. Sometimes the gastrointestinal tract is affected, with heartburn, nausea, vomiting, and diarrhea as possible symptoms. The jaundice may last for weeks or months and disappear slowly or rapidly.

Treatment includes bed rest during the period of most severe jaundice, with a curtailment of activity for the duration of the disease. The diet must be controlled carefully and the invalid should be encouraged to eat since starvation is a special hazard to people with hepatitis. A high-protein, high-carbohydrate diet with few fats is a requisite.

While a few people develop chronic low-grade liver insufficiency as a result of hepatitis, the majority are completely cured in time and the liver returns to its normal functioning. *See also* JAUNDICE.

heredity. The congenital transmission of characteristics and tendencies of parents to their offspring.

Certain physical traits are inherited, such as hair color and type, pigmentation of the skin, and color of the eyes. Tendencies to tallness or shortness are transmitted; tall parents generally have tall children and short parents have short children. Heredity is also accumulative; that is, many generations may contribute characteristics as well as the immediate parents.

A tendency to allergies and sensitivity to various protein substances may be hereditary. Hemophilia, the tendency to abnormal bleeding, is transmitted through the female to the male progeny, although the female does not suffer from the disease. It has occurred notably in some of the royal families of Europe. Diseases themselves are not inherited, but possibly a tendency or susceptibility to certain diseases can be transmitted. Superstitions and popular notions about the effect of a prospective mother's thoughts and experiences on her child do not have any foundation in fact.

A child does not inherit fixed traits or characteristics. Rather, she is born with genes from both parents which interact to produce characteristics. The possibilities for interaction of genes are so numerous that several children in one family may display widely different traits.

Mental instability may be manifested through heredity by inheritance of defects in the brain structure, and many states have laws controlling propagation among insane or mentally defective people. By the same token, superior qualities in brain tissue may be transmitted. *See also* HEMOPHILIA.

hermaphroditism. A person with both an ovary and a testicle is called a true hermaphrodite. More common is the male pseudo-hermaphrodite who may have undescended testicles and an underdeveloped penis. Nevertheless, at puberty the voice may deepen and sexual feelings may be those of a male. A female pseudo-hermaphrodite may have ovaries but external genitals resembling those of a male. At puberty breasts may develop. Female contours and hair distribution and in some cases menstruation leave no doubt that the person is really a woman. Skin biopsy for chromosome study can determine the true sex when there is doubt about any person. *See also* ANDROGYNY.

hernia. Rupture, a protrusion of a part of the contents of the abdomen through a weak spot in the abdominal wall, or any protrusion of a loop or part of an organ or tissue through an abnormal opening.

Certain parts of the muscular wall of the body are less well reinforced than others. One weak point is in the groin along the lowest point of the abdomen; another is at the navel, and a third is in the area of the sex organs. When the muscle at one of these points separates sufficiently to permit part of the contents of the abdomen to bulge through, a hernia occurs. A hernia may result from any of many possible causes. A muscular weakness may be present at birth; a hernia may develop in infancy from straining—for example, in whooping cough; it may result from lifting a heavy object or other overstraining, or during childbirth, or because tissues have not healed adequately after a surgical operation.

herpes simplex. An acute virus disorder, commonly called "cold sores" or "fever blisters," characterized by blisters or sores which appear in clusters of small painful swellings about the lips. They frequently follow severe colds, pneumonia, malaria, or other acute conditions with fever. Although usually confined to the lips, herpes simplex may occur on the conjunctivas, corneas, or on the genitals. The swellings develop into watery blisters which break, form a crust, and eventually heal.

herpes zoster. Also known as shingles, a fairly common virus disease found most frequently in adults. It usually occurs during the spring and autumn. The word zoster is derived from the Greek, meaning girdle. The condition is characterized by the appearance of clusters of large painful blisters running in a bandlike pattern on patches of reddened skin. The rash follows the course of one or more of the cutaneous nerves that transmit sensation to the skin. Generally only one side of the body is involved, though it may affect nerves leading to the eyes or other vital structures. When the eye is affected, blisters form not only on the forehead and eyelids but sometimes even on the eyeball itself. This condition requires expert attention.

Shingles (derived from *cingulum*, meaning belt) is most apt to occur when body resistance is low. It is usually preceded by severe smarting pain in the involved area and a general feeling of indisposition, with perhaps some respiratory or digestive disturbances for three to four days before the rash appears. The patches of blisters may persist for a week or two, then dry up and be covered with shinglelike scabs.

The same virus that causes herpes zoster may also be responsible for chickenpox.

In treating herpes zoster, efforts are made to relieve pain and prevent any secondary infection of the blisters.

high blood pressure. *See* BLOOD PRESSURE, HIGH.

histoplasmosis. A disease closely resembling coccidioidomycosis, histoplasmosis is probably the second most significant systemic fungus disease. The fungus histoplasma capsulatum grows chiefly in moist soil and the disease is acquired by inhaling the airborne spores of the fungus. Men are more often affected than women, and children of both sexes seem to be more susceptible to this mold than to any other mycotic infection.

At one time, histoplasmosis was considered to be rare and usually fatal. During the past two decades, however, it has become evident that the mold is also responsible for a milder form of the disease which has affected many thousands of people living in the central portions of this country, principally around the valleys of the Mississippi, Missouri, and Ohio rivers. At times the disease has reached almost epidemic proportions.

hives. Urticaria, a condition in which whitish elevated areas, painfully itching, appear on the surface of the skin.

These eruptions may follow the eating of certain foods, or exposure to particular atmospheric conditions. Theoretically these or other physical influences can alter the chemistry of the skin so that the absorption of certain substances will produce the rash. Psychological factors, however, may also cause the appearance of hives.

Hives often appear and disappear within the space of hours, but may persist for longer periods, become chronic, or recur persistently. Most frequently they will disappear after several days unless the person irritates or infects them—for example, by scratching.

The obvious first step in the treatment of this annoying malady is to locate the specific source. If this can be done, and if the cause, perhaps a type of food, can be eliminated, control of the disease should not be difficult. The person is advised to avoid chocolate, cocoa, nuts, peanut butter, shellfish, fish, tomatoes, fresh pork, fresh fruits, and spices.

Frequently a person may be desensitized to the food which makes him susceptible to hives. For example, the extract of shellfish can be administered in increasing amounts until the patient is able to eat this food without ill effect. Antihistamines have also been used to control the susceptibility to hives. In acute urticaria, the condition usually can be promptly controlled by injection of epinephrine hydrochloride. Severe cases also respond to treatment with ACTH, cortisone, or Meticorten.

Hodgkin's disease. An ailment which involves the lymph glands. The disease is fairly widespread throughout America and Europe and is believed to be increasing. It is most common in men between the ages of twenty and forty, although it has been reported in older people.

As the disease develops, the spleen and sometimes the liver are often enlarged, and frequently the bone marrow is affected, causing secondary anemia. When the process reaches the vertebrae and spinal cord, a paralysis of the lower part of the body results. These symptoms are accompanied by a loss of weight and the patient appears to be in extreme ill health and wasting away, a condition called cachexia. As other glands in the body become enlarged, they press in on neighboring organs. Coughing and chest pains are caused by compression in the chest, and pressure on the trachea or surrounding structures makes breathing and swallowing painful and difficult. The condition gradually becomes generalized.

Treatment consists of X-ray for the localized enlargements. When the swellings are widespread, nitrogen mustard is used in addition to the radiation of selected areas. Cortisone and ACTH have been effective in temporarily reducing the size of the spleen and lymph nodes. The periods of relief vary and are unpredictable.

Known treatment, however, can provide temporary relief, but does not effectively halt the progress of the disease.

homosexuality. Sexual attraction toward persons of one's own sex rather than the opposite sex. In females it is called lesbianism. In psychoanalysis the term can also include sexual interest which does not receive genital expression.

The causes of homosexuality are extremely complex and difficult to ascertain, and science or psychiatry have only partial answers to the treatment of the problem. This deviation from normal heterosexuality may develop at puberty. A lack of hormones, or such emotional factors as a father complex in the female adolescent, or a similar identification toward the mother in the male adolescent, may be the basis of homosexuality.

hookworm. *See* WORMS.

hormones. A hormone is a substance produced by one of the internal secretion or endocrine glands which exerts a specific effect elsewhere in the body on some other gland or organ. Other glands also secrete special substances, such as the sweat of the sweat glands, the milk of the mammary glands or breasts, and the saliva of the salivary glands. The products of these glands of external secretion, however, as contrasted with those of internal secretion, do not have regulatory effects on other organs.

The pituitary gland produces several of the most important hormones. It secretes a growth hormone which produces human growth, a hormone stimulating the development of the sexual organs, hormones regulating the thyroid gland, the adrenal cortex, and other important internal secretions.

Some glandular parts of the body produce both external secretions and hormones. The pancreas, for instance, provides the body with both insulin, an internal secretion or hormone regulating the body's use of sugar, and trypsin, an external secretion involved in the digestion of protein foods.

Hormones and the glands in which

they originate constitute an organized system for regulating many fundamental bodily processes in a co-ordinated way, including growth, reproduction, mobilization of defenses against stress and many forms of disease, and also basic aspects of metabolism, such as the use of oxygen and sugar.

In recent years, ACTH and other hormones of the cortical group have been produced from animal pituitaries and made available to the medical profession for therapeutic use in a wider variety of diseases. *See also* GLANDS; PITUITARY.

housemaid's knee. *See* KNEE.

hydatidiform mole. A disease of the chorion, the outer membranes of the uterus. A mass of cysts develops and the uterine cavity becomes distended. The symptoms are bleeding, excessive vomiting (hyperemesis), general malaise, and local pain. The treatment is usually surgical.

hydramnios. A disease of the late stages of pregnancy characterized by an abnormal amount of amniotic fluid. It is most common with diabetes but is a rare condition, occurring about once in 10,000 pregnancies. The patient is anxious, breathless, and the skin becomes slightly blue. The treatment is complete bed rest.

hydrocephalus. Commonly called water on the brain, a condition in which large amounts of cerebrospinal fluid are around or within the brain. Normally this fluid flows through the ventricles of the skull and is drained off by the venous sinuses. An excess of the fluid or inefficient drainage, which may be caused by blocking of the drainage canal by inflammation or by a tumor, will produce hydrocephalus. Obstructions may also exist at birth due to malformation of the internal portions of the skull concerned with proper drainage.

hydrocortisone. *See* CORTISONE.

hydrophobia. *See* RABIES.

hymen. Maidenhead, the membrane found at the opening of the vagina, partially blocking the entrance to the female sex organs. Although its presence is usually considered a sign of virginity, occasionally it may be entirely lacking or it may be ruptured by strain, such as occurs during horseback riding.

hyperacidity. Excessive secretion of gastric juice, which may appear in a temporary disturbance of the digestion or be present in chronic gastritis or in gastric or duodenal ulcers.

hyperemesis gravidarum. Neurotic or toxic vomiting during pregnancy. It begins as morning sickness and meticulous care should be taken to prevent its getting worse. (Gravidarum means starving.) The treatment is with diet, hormones, and drugs.

hyperhydrosis. The scientific name for excessive sweating. *See* PERSPIRATION.

hypertension. *See* BLOOD PRESSURE, HIGH.

hypertrophy. Disproportionate growth of any organ or tissue of the body. Vigorous exercise of the muscles can cause enlargement and bulging. Certain conditions in the heart may cause enlargement or hypertrophy, as when an improperly functioning valve impedes the outflow of blood from the chambers of the heart. Enlargement of the breasts is a common form of hypertrophy and may occur in both males and females, young or old. A compensatory hypertrophy may occur, as in the case of the loss of a kidney; then the other kidney tends to grow larger to make up for the one that is lost and even to take up some of its functions.

hypnosis. A state of sleep or trance induced in a person by means of verbal suggestion by a hypnotist or by concentration on some object.

In hypnoanalysis, hypnosis is employed by the psychoanalyst to uncover the unconscious drives and mechanisms of the personality of the patient in an effort to analyze the causes of her emotional conflicts in the conscious state. The person may seem to be asleep after the hypnotist has induced the trancelike state and in this state she remains responsive to ideas suggested by the hypnotist. The unconscious mind is then exposed, repressed ideas or experiences recalled which have a bearing on the person's emotional disturbance, and a relationship later established to the conscious personality.

Narcosynthesis is a technique based on the same principle, but drugs are used rather than hypnosis. Here the hypnotic drug is introduced intravenously to induce the state which will reveal the underlying emotional conflict. This state is then followed by discussion. This form of psychoanalysis has particularly been used to treat neuroses resulting from war experiences.

Hypnosis is sometimes useful in dealing with drug addiction, dipsomania, or other injurious habits or impulses. Disorders such as insomnia, diarrhea, or constipation, due to nervous influences, have responded to this form of treatment. Certain menstrual irregularities related to a disturbed emotional state have also been treated by hypnoanalysis.

Hypnosis should be practiced only by those who are skilled and under medical supervision.

hypochondriasis. A person who is constantly concerned with her health or believes she is suffering from a serious disease, without factual basis, is known as a hypochondriac. The condition of morbid fear is called hypochondriasis.

In true hypochondriasis, the person's fears are related to the functioning of one particular organ of the body—the lungs, kidneys, heart, eyes, or digestive tract. Some women constantly develop imaginary symptoms concerning the organs of childbirth. A hypochondriac can mistake the slightest cough for a sign of tuberculosis. If the gastrointestinal tract is the center of anxiety, the interrelationship of the mind and the functions of the organs is such that certain symptoms can actually develop as a result. Loss of appetite, nausea, vomiting, fullness of stomach, and belching after meals are a few of such symptoms which may develop without physical cause.

The hypochondriac may be so beset with fears and symptoms that frequently the cure demands much time and patience. Persuasion that her fears are groundless is not sufficient to convince such a person. Psychotherapy is helpful, but again such treatment is slow. Persons suffering from hypochondriasis to a lesser degree have been helped sometimes by turning attention from the subject of health to new interests. Older people have most frequently responded to this type of treatment.

hypomenorrhea. Scanty or deficient menstrual flow.

hypoplasia. Abnormality of the genitalia. Absence of the ovaries, the Fallopian tubes, the uterus, the vagina, or the vulva may be seen in all degrees from mild to severe. The condition is not uncommon but complete absence occurs only in monsters.

hypotension. *See* BLOOD PRESSURE, LOW.

hypothyroidism. Any condition characterized by deficient activity of the thyroid gland and its secretion, thyroxin.

When such a condition occurs in a child before it is born, the infant will be retarded in both physical and mental development, and will grow to be a dwarf of low mental capacity, termed a cretin. The same deficiency may arise spontaneously in later life, leading then to what is called myxedema. Abnormal tissue develops beneath the skin of the face, arms, and legs, giving a puffy appearance. The person becomes lethargic, mentally as well as physically. Sometimes this condition develops after surgical or other treatment for hyperthyroidism, when the remaining amount of thyroid tissue is insufficient for the body.

Treatment of all these conditions is by administration of thyroid substances, such as thyroid extracts, and thyroxin, which are taken daily by mouth. Only the physician should prescribe such treatment and determine the amounts to be taken, because of the dangers involved. *See also* CRETINISM; GOITER; MYXEDEMA.

hysterectomy. Medical term for removal of the womb or uterus. The presence of a tumor or any of a variety of other conditions determines the desirability of a hysterectomy. Whether or not one or both of the ovaries, the female sex glands, or the Fallopian tubes, which transport the egg cell from the ovary to the womb each month, should be removed at the same time depends on whether or not those organs are disordered in such a way as to require it.

The ovaries, especially through their internal secretions or hormones, are fundamental to a woman's health. Removal of the ovaries induces menopause or change of life, a serious development which may require administration of the missing hormones for a long time until the patient's body adjusts. Accordingly, if the ovaries are healthy, the doctor will not include them in a hysterectomy without compelling reasons. Among the most common of such reasons is the existence of cysts, encapsulated collections of fluid glandular material, which sometimes grow to unwieldy size and cause great discomfort. The ovaries may also be affected by tumors and infections in such a way as to make removal necessary. Since the ovaries supply the female body with the vital female sex gland secretions or hormones, elimination of the uterus alone will not disturb the regular onset of menopause. The womb is simply an organ to cradle the developing embryo and child until birth; it does not by itself secrete hormones. Removal of the womb does, however, permanently stop menstruation.

Hysterectomy, which is undergone by thousands of women every year in the United States, is definitely a major operation, requiring anesthesia, a stay in the hospital, and a period of careful convalescence to permit the tissues affected to mend adequately. Heavy exercise and lifting are not advisable and ample rest is necessary. The choice of the two surgical methods used will depend on the condition of the individual patient and the judgment of the gynecologist. Alternative routes, either of which may be used, are through the lower opening of the body, the vagina, or through the abdomen.

A common question of women who must undergo hysterectomy is whether or not the operation will disturb or stop regular marital relations. The answer is a definite negative. Once the postoperative repair has begun and healing is complete, marital relationship continues undisturbed.

hysteria. A psychoneurotic disorder, involving intense emotionalism with various psychic and physical disturbances. It often results from repressed conflicts within the person, and occurs most frequently in young women. Most people think of a hysteric as a person alternately

crying and laughing in an excited and distracted manner. The concept of hysteria was not understood, however, until the introduction of the psychoanalytic approach by Freud. There are many varieties of hysteria. In the ordinary course of experience, the tantrum type of hysteria may be encountered, in which the person may cry, shout, walk about aimlessly, or even attack a friend. In another, more serious type, the person may not talk or move or hear what is said to him. First-aid measures, such as slapping the victim or throwing water into her face may be effective; but if symptoms are severe, relief of hysteria requires expert medical advice.

Another dramatic manifestation of hysteria is the falling fit, which may resemble an attack of epilepsy. However, certain signs will indicate real hysteria: the person usually does not hurt herself in falling, and does not bite her tongue or have other symptoms of epilepsy; a certain degree of consciousness of action is present in the hysteric. Strange behavior may be manifested in hysteria, relating to such activities of everyday existence as eating, sleeping, working, memory, and conversation. The hysteric, being extremely impressionable, may also imitate symptoms of many diseases.

The development of hysterical paralysis may involve a single limb or perhaps half of the body, a condition known as hemiplegia. Certain signs aid the experienced observer to distinguish between paralysis due to a definite organic cause such as apoplexy and a hysterical semi-paralysis.

In all types of hysteria in which real organic damage is not present, definite psychological causes are the source and are known as conversion reactions. Whatever the manifestation, the development indicates that the person to some degree has lost a sense of her own identity, and is seeking refuge in hysterical symptoms as a device to obtain attention or sympathy. Disappointment in love or some other deep frustration are examples of emotional upset which may stimulate a hysterical attack.

Shell shock or even blindness are forms of hysteria manifested in soldiers who may be seeking to escape an intolerable situation.

In the treatment of hysteria the diagnosis must be certain. Failure to detect and distinguish between a real physical cause and one of hysterical origin may be extremely serious.

Sometimes a person who for years has been blind or deaf may suddenly recover the lost sense in what is apparently a miraculous cure. Similarly people confined to bed for months because they are unable to walk or stand may unexpectedly leap from the bed if shocked by a startling alarm.

A hysterical person is unduly open to suggestion and just as she may simulate symptoms that are prompted by well-meaning but injudicious friends, so her craving for sympathy will make her respond to friendly psychotherapy, which is the most effective form of treatment. When the victim of hysteria

is made to understand the basis of her disturbance, the cure of the symptoms may be as sudden as the onset. The deeper attitudes and motivations of the person must be understood to effect a real cure of hysteria.

ichthyosis. A disorder of the skin characterized by dryness and extreme scaliness, which gives it the common name of "fish skin disease." It is a congenital disease; babies are born with scaly skin or it appears in the early months of life.

icterus. *See* JAUNDICE.

iliac glands. Carriers of lymphatic material in the genital area.

ileitis. Chronic inflammation in that portion of the small intestine known as the ileum may produce a partial obstruction which grows progressively worse. This comes from scar tissue formation such as may be caused by tuberculosis and other causes.

The symptoms include cramps or colicky pain following meals. Fever and diarrhea often accompany this condition, and there is weakness and general signs of debility. Anemia may also accompany this disease.

The condition can be managed by careful attention to diet, medical treatment, and a sympathetic approach where the emotional state of the patient is a complicating factor. The disease may progress to a point where surgery is required to resolve the condition. Postoperatively patients may continue to have occasional diarrhea, but other symptoms clear up completely and in dramatic fashion.

immunity. The state of being temporarily or permanently able to resist an infection. Immunity to a disease exists when the antibodies, substances which combat invading micro-organisms and their toxic effects, against that particular disease are present in the body. The antibodies may be present for several reasons: (1) the person has had the disease once and developed the antibodies; (2) the antibodies have been artificially provided by inducing the body to produce them; (3) the antibodies have been introduced into the body from an external source. Sometimes a natural immunity exists, such as the immunity which human beings have against many animal diseases and vice versa. Depletion of the body through deprivation may render the system susceptible to an infection to which ordinarily it would be immune.

immunization. Immunity, freedom from or resistance to disease, either temporarily or permanently. The body itself may produce immunity, as in the case of most infectious diseases, or it may be induced artificially. Great progress has been made in artificial immunization against disease, the Salk immunization against poliomyelitis being the outstanding recent example.

The body has the power to develop antibodies which act directly against disease-producing germs, or antitoxins which act against the toxins produced by micro-organisms. In many instances, the body can develop the disease-fighting antibodies against killed bacteria or viruses as readily as against live micro-organisms, with the advantage that

risk of disease is eliminated. For example, the Salk vaccine is based on killed viruses, and a similar method is used against typhoid fever when killed bacilli of typhoid are injected to render the body immune to typhoid fever for a period of years.

Immunity against diphtheria is established by injecting a substance to produce antitoxin which combats the poison produced by the diphtheria germ. For smallpox, the virus of cowpox is injected which produces a mild case of the disease at the region of injection.

Schedules for active immunizations to common infectious diseases have been standardized and are followed by most physicians and clinics for diphtheria, tetanus, smallpox, whooping cough, and poliomyelitis. Whooping cough, especially dangerous to babies, and diphtheria immunizations are usually given at the same time, at four to six months of age. The primary smallpox vaccination may be given at any time, generally when the child is about a year old, and should be repeated about four or five years later.

Immunity against plague, yellow fever, typhus, cholera, and Rocky Mountain spotted fever can be obtained by people traveling to regions where these diseases are apt to be present, and in epidemic areas. Immunization against rabies, hydrophobia, is given after a person has been bitten by an animal suspected of having rabies, or after the presence of rabies has been definitely established.

Scarlet fever immunization is

available, but is not usually given except to children living in institutions or sanatoriums or in the event of an epidemic.

The value of immunization has been proved over and over again, and death rates in such diseases as diphtheria and smallpox have been reduced to relative insignificance through immunization. *See also* IMMUNITY; VACCINATION.

impetigo. An infection, most frequently affecting children, in which the skin is covered with pus-filled eruptions. Although impetigo occurs most often on the face, other parts of the body, especially the hands, may be involved.

Impetigo is transmitted either directly from one person to another or by contact with articles used in common. If the infection is promptly treated, a cure can often be achieved in a week or two. Otherwise the problem becomes more difficult and may continue for a long time. Another complication which arises if the disease is permitted to linger is that the infected areas become susceptible to germs other than those of impetigo and thus prolong the treatment. Impetigo may occur simultaneously with infestation by lice or mites, with one condition tending to enhance the other.

Impetigo is now successfully treated not only with antiseptic ointments such as ammoniated mercury but also with preparations which contain sulfa, penicillin, and other antibiotic drugs such as bacitracin, neomycin, and polymixin.

A school child with this disease should remain at home until he has recovered completely.

impotence. Lack of power in a male to have or maintain an erection of the penis, and consequent inability to perform or complete the sexual act. Impotence must be contrasted with infertility or sterility in a male, which denotes inability to propagate offspring.

The cause of impotence may be a small or deformed penis which may be corrected by surgery, or it may be the result of some disease such as gonorrhea, diabetes, Bright's disease, or a disorder of the spinal cord. Medical treatment is necessary.

A common cause of impotence is emotional disturbance. This may occur temporarily in the early months of marriage due to self-doubts and usually disappears during the adjustment period natural to this stage of life. Impotence, unfortunately, often results from incompatibility which develops later in a marriage relationship. In such cases, psychotherapy may be the only way to resolve these marital conflicts.

Age is often a factor in impotence. Men over fifty-five sometimes begin to lose their capacity for erection and their interest in sex. Many men, however, retain their powers for years beyond this age.

indigestion. Dyspepsia (a term now considered a misnomer and seldom used), denotes discomfort that accompanies or follows the intake of food. It is usually associated with difficult or painful digestion and may be related to actual failure of some phase of the digestive process.

infantilism. A condition in which

growth is retarded or inhibited because of malfunctioning of certain glands or other causes. When the pituitary gland is affected and there is a lack of growth, hormones, teeth, bones, and the sex glands will be involved and the result is an underdeveloped body, a dwarf, seldom over three to four feet in height. Mental retardation will take place and childish characteristics will persist into adult life. Overactivity of the same gland will produce giantism with the mental and sexual retardation characteristic of dwarfism.

Infantilism may also be the result of certain congenital defects, thyroid deficiency, or other diseases. In one type, characteristics of senility such as baldness and hardening of the arteries may develop along with dwarfism. Thyroid cases respond sometimes amazingly well to injections of thyroid extract, while many of the other types have no known cure. Another form of infantilism is brought about by early kidney disease which results in death.

infections. An infection is the condition which occurs when the body or a part of the body is invaded by disease-causing germs or organisms. One or more organs or parts sustain at least temporary damage and impairment. The body as a whole reacts protectively, in most cases, with general symptoms such as fever. An infection restricted to one fairly sharply defined area, such as a tooth or a finger, and not serious enough to provoke general symptoms, is called a local infection, as distinct from a general infection.

In women, conditions are much more favorable for infection after childbirth or abortion.

infertility. Relative sterility. The term means that pregnancy is possible if certain unfavorable conditions are overcome. The commonest causes of infertility in women are sexual incompatibility, menstrual irregularity, certain occupations which involve chemicals, and past operations or illnesses. The physician requires a full investigation to discover the cause or causes of infertility.

inflammation. A reaction of the tissues to injury, characterized by redness, heat, swelling, and pain, regardless of the cause. (The inflammation may be a symptom of a disease or ailment, but this discussion concerns itself with the actual condition of the inflamed tissue.) The redness and heat are due to an influx of blood to the affected area; the swelling and pain are also due to blood but even more to the inflow of watery fluid or lymph which distends the tissue, compresses the nerve endings, and causes pain. The white cells of the blood accumulate at the affected area and attempt to kill the invading micro-organisms. If they do not and too many white cells are destroyed, an abscess forms. Inflammation is usually due to micro-organisms, but may also result from severe irritation of the skin, as from rubbing, chemical action, or heat.

influenza. Commonly known as the flu or grippe, a highly contagious disease caused by a filtrable virus, one capable of passing through a Berkefeld clay filter. It usually appears in the winter in epidemic form throughout the world and spreads with amazing rapidity during these outbreaks. Generally influenza is self-limited; that is, it runs a definite course within a specific period of time and is of short duration. While rarely serious in itself, influenza tends to predispose to secondary infections of the lungs, which may become serious.

During pregnancy, special precautions must be taken to prevent miscarriage or fatal results.

inguinal glands. The glands that carry lymph secretions in the groin and also have direct communication with the lymph glands around the clitoris.

injection. Certain drugs and remedies are best introduced directly into the tissues rather than by mouth because the digestive juices react chemically upon them and nullify their effectiveness.

inoculation. The introduction of a disease agent, serum, infective material, or micro-organism into the tissues through the skin or mucous membrane. The purpose may be to immunize, as in smallpox vaccination, or to increase resistance to certain diseases by introducing controlled quantities of dead germs or their poisons into the body where antibodies will develop to combat future invasion of the same micro-organism. *See also* IMMUNIZATION; VACCINATION.

insanity. The legal term for a mental disorder.

insomnia. Any degree of sleeplessness during the time when most people ordinarily sleep. Aside from being incidental to a number of illnesses, including fevers, heart trou-

ble, and certain brain disorders, insomnia may be due to a variety of causes.

insulin. The hormone produced in the part of the pancreas known as the Islets of Langerhans. It is significant in regulating the sugar level in the blood and in the burning of sugar to produce heat and energy. Persons who suffer from diabetes mellitus have a deficiency of insulin.

Insulin is not a cure for diabetes, but it supplements a deficiency. Care must be taken in using it. Patients who take too much insulin may have an insulin shock which involves a reduction in the blood-sugar requiring immediate attention to avoid serious consequences. Common symptoms of insulin shock are agitation, weakness, trembling, sweating, pallor, listlessness, speech difficulty, nervousness, and unconsciousness. If the victim of insulin shock is still conscious, sugar in some form, such as fruit juice or candy, is given to him. If he is unconscious, Adrenalin may be injected to revive him and then the sugar given to him. In some cases of unconsciousness, glucose must be administered intravenously. *See also* DIABETES; INSULIN SHOCK THERAPY.

insulin shock therapy. Insulin shock treatment or therapy for schizophrenia and other mental disorders is used in mental hospitals. By injection of insulin, the patient is put into a state of coma for a given period of time and then brought out of the coma by the administration of sugar. By this treatment, the patient during the coma period is in a condition in which psychotherapy can be more effectively used.

intermittent claudication. *See* LIMPING, INTERMITTENT.

intertrigo. An irritation of the skin caused by friction between two moist adjacent skin surfaces. The most common locations for this condition are the folds of the groin, the inner surface of the thighs, between the buttocks, under the arms, under the neck, and behind the ears. In obese women it may occur between the breasts. In infants, intertrigo is caused by the rubbing of a diaper and is known as diaper rash.

To treat intertrigo, the opposing surfaces should be dusted thoroughly with talcum powder containing zinc oxide and then separated by a piece of lint. If the skin is macerated from the effects of perspiration, the skin should be thoroughly cleansed and dried before the powder is applied. Such care will help to avoid inflammation and infection of the skin surface. *See also* DIAPER RASH.

intervertebral disc. A circular plate or pad of fibrous cartilage located between the vertebrae of the spine. The disc allows movement of the vertebrae and acts as a buffer against shocks to the spinal column. Its action is that of a cushion, the disc flattening under pressure, with the ability also to shift its position to accommodate the motions of the spinal vertebrae. Sudden strains or movements may damage the disc. "Slipped disc" is a fairly common occurrence, and refers to the vertebrae of the lumbar and sacrum. The term intervertebral disc syndrome is applied to the low back pain which results from compression or protrusion from falls, jumps, or strains in the bent-over position. A protruded disc may complicate a case of slipped vertebrae.

The intervertebral disc is also subject to degenerative changes, fracture, and calcification, or may be destroyed by tuberculosis of the spine. Rarely is it attacked by cancer. *See also* SLIPPED DISC.

introitus vagina. The entrance to the vaginal canal, partially closed in virgins by the hymen. It is a highly variable structure and rupture or even non-rupture is not of the slightest value as proof that coitus has or has not occurred.

intussusception. An obstruction in the intestine, brought about when one part of the intestine passes or is drawn into another part. It occurs most frequently at the ileocecal valve, located at the opening from the small intestine into the large intestine. It may be due to a tumor, to the presence of hardened and impacted indigestible material, or it may be caused by a rupture into which a portion of the bowel is pushed.

Acute intussusception is most common in young children, usually during the first year. It is usually caused by straining, and is characterized by severe pain and vomiting. The straining ordinarily results only in the evacuation of blood-stained mucus. Only a surgical operation will correct this condition.

Chronic intussusception occurs usually in adults and is not too serious unless the obstruction becomes acute or results in acute peritonitis, at which point an operation is also imperative.

inversion of the uterus. A condition in which part of the uterus protrudes through the cervix or even the vaginal introitus. It may occur after birth when the placenta emerges too abruptly. It may also occur as a result of a tumor.

involutional melancholia. A mental disturbance characterized by mental depression. Ordinarily this disease occurs during middle age or later. The person realizes at this time that life's long and ambitious dreams will probably never be wholly fulfilled. Moreover, as contemporaries begin to die, and as the burden of family worries and responsibilities increase, the person becomes less capable of facing and overcoming his problems. Delusions of a serious nature are sometimes experienced. Women are more particularly the victims of this affliction, perhaps because a sense of uselessness and isolation comes to them with special abruptness.

In treating involutional melancholia, the physician stresses the importance of a nourishing diet, adequate sleep, a healthful and pleasant environment, proper exercise, and absorbing avocations. Glandular drugs have also been used with success. Another source of help is undoubtedly found in psychotherapy.

iritis. An inflammation of the iris, the circular disc of the eye, and sometimes also the ciliary or eyelash region of the eye. *See also* EYE.

iron. A constituent of hemoglobin, the red coloring matter of the red blood cells, and the carrier of oxygen from the lungs to all parts of the body. Iron as a vital part of hemoglobin not only assists the hemoglobin in the disposition of waste products and carbon dioxide from the kidneys, lungs, skin, and large intestine but is essential in the manufacture of hemoglobin itself within the body. When the body is deficient in hemoglobin, and therefore iron, the body tissues fail to receive their quota of oxygen. A large number of red blood cells are destroyed each day and must be replaced.

At birth, most babies are oversupplied with hemoglobin, the mothers having generously supplied them with a store of iron-rich blood from their own reservoir.

Iron deficiency and its symptoms can be due to blood loss—such as injury or bleeding peptic ulcer—diet deficiency, and defective absorption of iron in the body. The high incidence of anemia in women may generally be attributed to increased demands of menstruation and pregnancy. *See also* ANEMIA; BLOOD; HEMOGLOBIN.

itch. *See* SCABIES.

itching. Or pruritis as it is scientifically known, an irritation of the fine terminations of the sensory nerves at the skin. It may be due to a variety of causes.

Itching occurs in many different diseases of the skin; it may be a result of an eruption from sensitivity to certain foods, drugs, chemicals, material, or dusts; or it may be produced by invasion of the skin by parasites, such as the louse or itch mite, or a fungus infection, such as ringworm. Abnormal states of the blood, present in diseases like diabetes, gout, jaundice, and in various digestive disturbances, may produce itching. Nervous disorders, either of a mental or physiological type, may also cause itching. Itching often follows recovery from a case of dermatitis.

Itching may be general and nonspecific, or it may be located in one part of the body. Scratching the area may give temporary relief, but it also may lead to damage to the skin and intensify the discomfort.

Control of itching depends on locating the cause and eliminating it. For example, treatment of an allergy or sensitivity will remove the cause and cure the itching. Itching due to a lack of moisture in the skin may be helped by repeated applications of bland lubricating ointments to relieve dryness and provide flexibility.

jaundice. Or icterus, is a symptom rather than a disease and is characterized by yellowness of the skin and of the whites of the eyes. The color of the skin may range from bright lemon yellow to dark olive green. Itching is often associated with jaundice, especially in cases of long duration.

Causes of jaundice are varied. An excess of bile from the liver or any damage to the liver which affects the normal excretion of bile pigments may be responsible. Obstruction of the bile passages through which the pigment is normally excreted into the intestinal tract from the liver may result from gallstones, tumors, or parasitic invasion of the ducts. In obstructive jaundice, the feces are clay-colored and the urine

may vary in color from light yellow to brownish green. The liver enlarges and its function gradually deteriorates unless an operation is performed to remove the cause of the obstruction.

Infectious diseases such as malaria and pneumonia may damage the blood, causing excessive destruction of the blood cells and ensuing jaundice. Chemical poisoning, resulting from absorption or inhalation of toxic substances like arsenic or phosphorus which affect the liver, or other poisons or infections which affect the rate of destruction of blood cells may also cause jaundice.

Catarrhal jaundice, the most common type, is caused by an infection with a specific virus and is fairly common among young people. The acute form of jaundice is the disease hepatitis.

The poisons of eclampsia may affect the liver and cause jaundice. Jaundice in newborn babies is usually due to excessive destruction of the red blood cells that may result from septic infection of the umbilical cord, or from other infections associated with childbirth.

Ordinarily jaundice is a symptom of damage to the liver or bile ducts. Treatment depends on the nature of the causes, but in general includes the injection of glucose to prevent further damage to the liver. Any severe case of jaundice, whatever the cause, requires bed rest and careful diagnosis by a physician who can make the necessary tests and prescribe the proper treatment. *See also* BILE; HEPATITIS; LIVER.

jejunal ulcer. An ulcer located in the

jejunum, the portion of the small intestine between the duodenum and ileum. The jejunum is about eight feet long.

joints and joint disorders. A common disturbance is water in a joint such as the knee. This results from the flow of serous fluid into the joint following an injury. When the condition appears without apparent cause and disappears within a few days, it is called intermittent hydrarthrosis, accumulation of fluid in a joint.

Following an injury, blood may flow into the joints of some people who bleed easily. This condition is hemarthrosis, passing of blood from its proper place into a joint.

As a result of violence applied to a joint, the joint may become sprained. In sprains, parts of the ligaments may be torn or stretched, and the bones partially or completely displaced from contact, as in dislocations. In the knee, for example, such an injury may result in displacement, bruising, or fracture of a semi-lunar cartilage, which will get caught between the bones and result in locking of the knee joint. Such injury frequently occurs to basketball and tennis players. The condition can be relieved by extending the leg and turning it inward. When locking occurs too frequently, a surgical operation may be indicated to relieve the condition.

Another frequent joint injury is the pulling away of the ligament which extends from the kneecap to the large bone of the lower leg.

Some forms of sprains are treated by cold applications, followed by strapping or by applying an elastic bandage. Healing of a severe sprain can occasionally be hastened by bathing the affected joint in hot water or by applying heat in some other manner. Light massage, followed by more intense rubbing, helps restore circulation and motion.

Inflammation of a joint may be limited to the synovial membrane, called synovitis, inflammation of the lining of the membrane, or it may involve the entire structure, as in arthritis. Acute synovitis may develop as a result of any of these forms of injury, or it may be due to some other disorder, such as rheumatism or gout. The symptoms are almost the same as in sprain, and the treatment too is similar to that for sprain. Pain and swelling of the joint occur; and following injury, there is discoloration from blood effusing into the joint. The best treatment is an elastic bandage and promotion of circulation by moving about until gradually the amount of fluid diminishes and finally disappears.

Acute synovitis may be followed by stiffness and adhesions, which should be overcome by movements of the affected parts as soon as possible in the course of the disorder. There is always a possibility of ankylosis, or permanent fixation, to some degree, which can be avoided by careful treatment.

Acute synovitis may become chronic, with not much pain but with weakening of the joint, thickening of the membrane, and the presence of fluid. The movements of the joint are interfered with, and there may be a sense of grating or rubbing present when the joint is moved. Diathermy or hot baths may help, but in severe cases an operation may be indicated.

A dislocation of a joint is promptly followed by swelling to a disproportionate size and impairment of the ability to move the particular limb or part. Once the doctor is called, he will make every effort to reduce the degree of dislocation in order to avoid pseudoarthrosis, the process whereby the displaced bone makes a fresh socket.

Kahn test. A procedure for detection of syphilis. It has largely superseded the Wassermann test. *See also* WASSERMANN TEST.

keloids. Overgrown scars which usually develop after surgery but which may occur following any break in the skin, such as a pinprick, pimple, or insect bite. Actually a keloid is a benign tumor of fibrous tissue growing in a scar. Keloids occur most frequently in young adults, and are most common among Negroes. Their exact cause is unknown.

kidneys. Bean-shaped organs located high on the rear wall of the abdominal cavity. Their chief function is elimination of waste substances from the blood through the formation of urine.

The kidneys are the channels through which approximately 40 to 60 per cent of the water which is discarded passes out of the body. (The rest is eliminated largely by evaporation from the breath and in sweat.) These organs separate and incorporate into the urine the digested products of protein, substances in the blood which are formed continuously as a result of the normal constructive activity of the body. The kidneys also help to keep the fine balance between acid and alkaline conditions in the tissues by removing excess acid. The preservation of alkalinity in the tissues and blood is essential to life. They also maintain the necessary relation between salt and water in the body; a disturbance of this balance leads to overretention of moisture, as in dropsy, or to insufficiency of water, which may cause acidosis, dehydration, or reduce the necessary chemical changes.

Various disorders may involve the kidneys. Fortunately, however, one kidney is sufficient to perform all the functions of both, in the event that one is incapacitated or must be removed.

Kidney stones are small, hard masses in the organ. Often they pass into the bladder, causing acute pain and kidney stone colic, with nausea, vomiting, and sometimes collapse. These stones may cause an obstruction of normal flow of fluid within the kidney, with various adverse effects including local infection. Frequently the stones, or occasionally the entire kidney, must be removed surgically. Internal obstruction in the kidney may also cause hydronephrosis, a condition in which urine collects and cannot escape. Here, too, surgical treatment may be required.

Other disorders of the kidney include nephritis, inflammation of the tissues; pyelitis, infection of the pelvis of the kidney; pyelonephritis, which affects both pelvis and the rest of the tissues. Such infections may result when organisms infecting some other part of the body travel to the kidney in the bloodstream. High fever, tenderness in the loin, and a high white blood cell count are characteristic. Most organisms causing kidney infections are controlled by the antibiotics, such as penicillin or Aureomycin, but frequently sulfonamide drugs, mandelic acid, or furacin derivatives are more effective. Tuberculosis of the kidney may arise, although the disease may not be present in any other part of the body. New drugs provide efficient means of treating this disease. If the condition is far advanced and affects only one kidney, surgical removal often results in elimination of the condition.

Bright's disease is a term commonly used to designate chronic inflammation of the kidney. The presence of albumin in the urine (albuminuria) is a symptom of any of a whole group of disorders, just as fever is a symptom of infection by any of innumerable organisms.

Thus Bright's disease may designate a bacterial invasion of the kidneys, poisoning by toxins from invasive organisms or from those which originate in other infected tissues, poisoning by artificial poisons, disturbance of the kidneys caused by obstruction of the normal passage of urine, tumors or other abnormal growths, and the effects of interference with the kidneys' blood supply because of a disorder in the blood vessels themselves.

Kidney disturbances may produce symptoms ranging from those which are scarcely noticeable to those which are severe.

A slight elevation of blood pressure, listlessness, undue fatigue, headaches, and failing appetite may also be noticed. As the disease progresses, however, regardless of the specific cause, symptoms develop such as spots in front of the eyes, dryness of the mouth and constant drinking of water, loss of weight or, conversely, gain in weight due to excessive holding of liquid within the tissues, and sometimes fever. Dizziness, nausea, vomiting, and other more acute symptoms will be noticed as the disease progresses.

Treatment of kidney ailments is directed not only to removing the cause of the trouble but also, and of special significance, to resting the kidneys themselves. Bed rest will relieve the kidneys of much of the work they ordinarily must perform. Fewer waste products will form, and thus there will be less to be rejected. Additional strain may be taken from the kidneys by encouraging the elimination of wastes through the bowels and perspiration. Diet control also can exclude substances which require work on the part of the kidney.

Uremia occurs when both kidneys are removed or their functions totally blocked. The retention of the poisons in the body brings death in a short time. The chief characteristic of uremia is drowsiness, sometimes interrupted by convulsions. Occasionally it appears without any warning.

Structural abnormalities may be present in the kidneys at birth. For example, they may be joined at one end and form a "horseshoe kidney," which does not have any notable consequences. Or the two kidneys may be fused to form one large one. Occasionally, especially in women, the kidneys change position, which is usually without significance except when twisting occurs which blocks the flow of urine. Pain and vomiting may result, but are relieved when the kidney again moves into another position. Recurrence may be prevented by wearing a suitable padded support, or by surgery.

Cysts and tumors also occur in the kidneys, blood in the urine being the most common symptom. Such symptoms should be promptly reported to a physician. *See also* AL-BUMINURIA; HEMATURIA; NEPHRITIS; NEPHROSIS; URINATION; URINE; WILM'S TUMOR.

knee. Inflammation of the knee joint can cause pain, swelling, and limited movement. The ligaments may become weakened and to some degree affect the stability of the knee in walking or even standing. In such cases, a support of some kind may be required for the knee. When inflammation of the knee is severe enough to require the person to remain in bed, proper splints are essential to prevent ultimate displacement of the tibia head.

The knee, more than other joints, is liable to effusions of fluid by the synovial membrane of the capsule. This may follow any strain, twist, fall, or blow severe enough to damage a significant part of the joint. It may also be caused by infection or accompany rheumatoid arthritis.

The whole joint will swell, obscuring the outline of the kneecap which is raised by the swelling and "floats." An effusion will generally subside of itself, but rest is essential.

Housemaid's knee results from bursitis or from accumulation of fluid in the patellar bursa. This bursa is a sac in the kneecap which lies between the tendon, the anterior surface of the kneecap, and the skin. The condition occurs when a person kneels frequently. The fluid collects in front of the kneecap; whereas in water on the knee, the kneecap floats in the fluid which is behind it.

If the condition remains untreated, the fluid accumulates until a sizable swelling forms over the kneecap, and bending the knee or kneeling becomes painful. If infection reaches the fluid through a scratch or break in the skin, an abscess may form inside the bursa, and the knee becomes more painful and extremely tender. The fluid, once it forms, can be drawn out of the bursa with a syringe and hollow needle, under local anesthetic. If an abscess develops, it must be opened and drained. Often it is desirable to remove the entire bursa to avoid chronic recurrence of the condition.

To prevent housemaid's knee, always kneel on a soft pad.

In knock-knee, the knee is bent inward, the foot carried outward, and the toes turned out abnormally. Both legs are usually affected. In early childhood, knock-knee usually results from rickets, but may also affect a child with weak ligaments. In the earlier stages, only the soft parts of the joint are involved and the condition may be corrected by manipulation and a correct alignment, preserved by splints or braces. When the knock-knee condition is of long standing, certain stages take place in the body structure which can be corrected only by an operation, which includes breaking through the lower part of the femur.

kraurosis. A dryness and atrophy of the skin or mucous membrane, particularly of the vulva, characterized by severe itching.

labia majora. Part of the vulva. These are the skin folds on either side of the vagina. Their outer surface is covered with hair and the inner surfaces with smooth, shiny soft skin, many secreting glands, and a rich vein complex.

labia minora. Two thin skin folds next to the labia majora. They are without hair but well supplied with blood vessels and erectile tissue.

labor. The process whereby the pregnant woman expels the products of gestation from the uterus, via the birth canal, into the outside world.

laceration. A wound made by a tear through the tissues. The damage is usually greater than when the wound is clean cut, and danger of infection is also increased.

Laceration sometimes occurs during childbirth or illegal abortion. The treatment is ligation, or sewing up.

Lacerations may be caused by a blow from a blunt instrument, from machinery, or from a fall against angular surfaces. Dirt or debris may be ground into the wounded tissues. An extensive or extremely dirty wound should be covered by sterile gauze as a first-aid measure, and then be cleansed and dressed by a doctor. A small laceration can be cleaned with soap and water, treated with mild antiseptic, and bandaged.

laparotomy. Abdominal incision for an operation on the internal organs.

laryngitis. Inflammation of the mucous membrane of the larynx. In acute laryngitis, the usual symptoms are hoarseness and dryness of the throat, difficult and painful swallowing, coughing, discomfort and pain in speaking, and even partial or complete loss of voice. Acute laryngitis may occur in certain eruptions of the skin and mucous membranes, from swelling in certain gastrointestinal disorders, or as a secondary complication of such infectious diseases as scarlet fever, measles, and chickenpox. It often is associated with the common cold.

Adults should rest in bed and refrain from using their voice. Cold, moist compresses and ice packs, in other cases warmth, may be beneficial. Inhaling steam, to which aromatic oils may be added, is also helpful. In serious cases, particularly when infection is present, the doctor may prescribe drugs and soothing sprays to aid in alleviating soreness in the larynx.

Chronic laryngitis is characterized chiefly by a change in the voice, hoarseness, and often a persistent cough and need to "clear the throat." It may follow a single attack or series of recurring attacks of laryngitis, a misuse or overuse of the voice, and is also associated with chronic irritation of the nose and throat. Excessive drinking and smoking predispose to chronic laryngitis.

Any persistent hoarseness may also be symptomatic of early cancer of the larynx, of laryngeal tuberculosis, and of paralysis of the vocal cords, and medical attention should be sought as soon as possible. Treatment of chronic laryngitis always includes rest of the voice, sprays and other remedies directed toward relieving the condition. *See also* LARYNX.

larynx. Or voice box, a cavity at the upper end of the windpipe which contains the vocal cords and serves as the organ for the voice.

The larynx is subject to nervous and physical disorders. Laryngitis is acute or chronic inflammation of the mucous membrane of the larynx. Paralysis of the laryngeal muscles may be due to nervous causes, to a tumor in the chest, or result from syphilis. Laryngeal tuberculosis is generally secondary to pulmonary tuberculosis. Tumors are fairly common and are generally benign; they can be removed by surgery. Cancer of the larynx may originate in the larynx or develop from adjoining areas of the body, and surgery to remove all or part of the larynx is generally indicated.

Foreign objects drawn into the larynx may cause spasm and produce an urgent danger of suffocation. First-aid measures, such as slapping the victim on the back, may help remove the object; and if breathing has stopped, artificial respiration is necessary. If the object does not cause unusual pain

and removal does not seem urgent, a doctor should remove it, since unskilled efforts can cause damage. *See also* LARYNGITIS.

laxative. *See* CATHARTICS.

left-handedness. When the left hand is stronger or more expert or used in preference to the right hand, the person is said to be left-handed. Left-handedness may or may not be inherited. Attempts to direct a normally left-handed child to use her right hand will only confuse her and has been associated with the development of stuttering and awkwardness. True left-handed people are likely to favor using the left eye, left ear, and left foot, just as right-handed people prefer the right eye, ear, and foot. Beyond this type of preference, differences between right-handed and left-handed persons are not apparent. *See also* STUTTERING AND STAMMERING.

leg. The part of the lower limb between the knee and the ankle; the upper part of the limb is the thigh.

Varicose veins, which are quite common, may lead to secondary disorders such as eczema, ulceration, and discoloration. Frequent exposure to intense heat may also lead to a brownish discoloration of the legs. Eczema on the shins, apart from that caused by varicose veins, is not unusual. Dropsy or edema also affects the legs early in their development. In infantile paralysis the muscles waste away, and in another form of muscular paralysis known as pseudo-hypertrophic muscular paralysis the muscles develop unduly. *See also* ANKLE; FEET; KNEE; VARICOSE VEINS.

lesbian. A woman who desires sexually only members of her own sex.

leucorrhea. Any whitish discharge from the vagina and uterine tract. Popularly such discharge is called "the whites." Leucorrhea may be indicative of an abnormality. The mucous glands of the vagina and cervix normally secrete small amounts of whitish material which moistens the tissues. Minor inflammation and congestion may similarly cause discharge, and premenstrual conditions sometimes stimulate activity of the mucous glands. However, inflammation of the Fallopian tubes, which can be due to gonorrhea, tuberculosis, or some other infection, can produce an abnormal discharge. Cancer of the uterus may also be the cause. Therefore, any abnormality in quantity, color, or odor of the discharge from the vaginal tract should be referred to a physician.

leukemia. A disease of the blood in which the production of white blood cells or leukocytes increases tremendously without apparent reason. In the normal person there are about 7500 white blood cells in every cubic millimeter of blood. In leukemia the number may increase to from 100,000 to one million white blood cells in every cubic millimeter of blood.

Leukemia is generally classified as acute or chronic although several different types of leukemia are recognized. Chronic leukemia generally attacks persons over thirty-five years of age. Frequently the first sign of acute leukemia is prolonged bleeding after a minor operation or tooth extraction. Other early signs are anemia, fever, pain in the bones and joints, and, in some cases, a swollen mouth and thickened gums. Chronic leukemia is also characterized by anemia and bleeding. In addition, the lymph nodes and spleen are noticeably enlarged. Small lumps, composed of the infiltrating white blood cells, may appear under the skin. Chronic leukemia may also be accompanied by loss of weight, nervousness, shortness of breath, and abnormal night sweats.

Treatment of leukemia depends on careful diagnosis to determine the exact type and extent of the disease. Blood transfusions may be required during the procedure to control anemia, to keep the red blood cells at a proper level, and to prevent purpura which is characteristic in some forms of leukemia. Antibiotics may also be used to prevent secondary infection.

leukocytes. The colorless blood cells, generally called white blood cells or corpuscles. The blood contains several varieties of leukocytes which can be differentiated and counted by staining and other techniques, including observation under the microscope.

The number of leukocytes in a person's body varies over a lifetime and during the course of a single day. More leukocytes are present in childhood and in pregnancy. After meals an increase of leukocytes occurs, due to an increase in the number of lymphocytes from the lymph glands. Any increase in the number of leukocytes is known as leukocytosis.

In certain diseases, such as granulocytosis, leukocytes are almost totally absent from the blood. Sensitivity to certain toxic drugs may cause complete absence of leukocytes; and, since these cells are essential to resist infection, their absence may be fatal. In typhoid fever and certain other diseases, the number of leukocytes may fall below normal, a condition known as leukopenia. In cases in which it is desirable to increase the number of leukocytes, certain drugs and serums may be injected. *See also* BLOOD; LEUKEMIA.

leukoplakia. A disease affecting middle-aged or elderly persons, in which white patches develop on the tongue and on the inside of the cheeks and the gums. The exact cause of leukoplakia is unknown, but the condition has been associated with excessive smoking and was once known as "smoker's patch." Leukoplakia has also been related to drinking and, in some instances, syphilis.

In time the patches become painful, especially in swallowing and talking. Continuous irritation is sometimes followed by cancer. Smoking and liquor, condiments and hot food must be avoided. Treatment by X-rays or radium and the application of antiseptics have been beneficial.

libido. Sexual desire; the term also refers to the energy derived from the primitive impulses. In psychoanalysis, libido refers to the motivating drive of the sex life. In Freudian psychology, it denotes psychic energy in general.

ligaments. Tough fibrous bands of tissue connecting bones at the joints and holding them in place.

Ligaments can be torn from the bones at the points where they are attached, or otherwise damaged. They may heal of themselves if the part that has been injured is immobilized. In some cases surgery may be imperative to bring together torn ends of ligaments. Plastic surgery is also employed to restore motion in cases of paralysis by transferring ligaments from one part of the body to another. *See also* JOINTS AND JOINT DISORDERS; SPRAINS.

ligation. Tying off of a blood vessel to constrict it, or the application of any type of ligature, either cord or thread. Ligation is often indicated in surgery and may be required in cases of accidental bleeding.

Ligation of the Fallopian tubes prevents passage of the ovum into the uterus and thus prevents pregnancy.

limping, intermittent. Intermittent limping is a particular symptom of Buerger's disease. Other disorders associated with limping are dislocation of the hip, breakdown of the arch, various nervous and muscular disorders, and even ill-fitting shoes. All require diagnosis and treatment by a specialist in orthopedics. Color of the skin is associated with circulation, and a test is made by raising the leg and flexing the foot toward the knee; if circulation is adequate, the color will return when the leg is lowered to a normal position.

lipoma. A fatty tumor or a tumor made of fatty cells. Although lipomas are painless and not malignant, they are unsightly and may become the seat of gangrene or fat necrosis. If infected or annoying, they should be removed by surgery.

lips. Harelip, a congenital malformation, results from failure of the lips to grow together properly and is a serious and often unsightly handicap. Plastic surgery is most effective in correcting it. Another condition of the lips which is successfully treated by surgery is overgrowth of the glandular tissue, which ordinarily results in enlargement of the upper lip.

Chapping or inflammation of the lips is often due to exposure to sun, wind and cold. Sensitivity to chemical ingredients of lipstick may also produce similar conditions. Cracking of the lips may follow. A protective ointment helps give relief.

A deficiency of riboflavin provokes cracking and blistering in the corners of the mouth. Supplementary vitamins together with careful hygiene and protective ointments usually cure the condition.

More serious are carbuncles and abscess of the upper lip. Because of the presence of large blood vessels in this area, care must be taken to prevent spread of infection to vital parts of the body. Use of sulfa drugs and antibiotics has greatly reduced the danger of this condition, which was formerly fatal in some cases.

Also serious is cancer of the lip which may be induced by chronic irritation. Early detection and treatment by surgery is imperative; treatment by irradiation or electric coagulation or a combination of both has proved effective.

In the common cold and in fever, blisters known as herpes frequently form on the margins of the lips. Nervousness in menstruation and sensitivity to certain foods may also induce blisters. *See also* HARELIP; HERPES SIMPLEX; HERPES ZOSTER.

lithotomy. An incision into the bladder for removing a stone.

liver. The largest gland, and one of the largest organs in the human body; it is located in the upper right abdomen, immediately under the diaphragm and attached to it by ligaments.

The liver is involved in many significant body processes, such as affording protection from disease, supplying sugar to meet the needs of muscle tissues, and regulating clotting of the blood.

Another vital biochemical activity of the liver is the formation of many antibodies, the substances developed by the body to counteract invasive organisms and their toxins. The liver synthesizes proteins, stores copper and iron, and produces both vitamin A and one of the ingredients essential to the creation of the red blood cells.

A serious condition results when the liver becomes infected, inflamed, or otherwise disordered. One significant factor is the effect of the liver on the body's sugar supply. Liver cells respond to major damage by discharging their glycogen. Injection of glucose may then be indicated to supply the required sugar. This in turn may demand the injection of insulin to assist the body in taking care of the replenishment of sugar. Unusual fatigue, listlessness, drowsiness, and confusion are symptoms of a relative lack of sugar or, often, a relative excess of insulin. The same circumstance may arise from sources other than liver damage, and the cause can be established when the quantity of sugar in the blood is checked.

Among the serious diseases of the liver are cirrhosis, or hardening; atrophy, or wasting; overgrowth; and bacterial or parasitic infection, which cause abscesses. Recent research indicates that the liver is vulnerable to dietary deficiencies, especially those of vitamins. Vitamin deficiencies may be associated with hardening of the liver.

Acute hepatitis is a form of liver disease caused by a viral infection, and the proper diagnosis is urgent, since the symptoms often resemble other disorders. Fatal complications may ensue with little or no warning.

Abscesses in the liver may originate from infection by amebae, as in amebiasis, or from a general infection of the blood, as in pyemia. Abscesses caused by amebae are more serious, since they tend to be single rather than multiple, and thus to concentrate their virulence in one spot in the liver. Frequently, though not invariably, the history of the patient reveals previous dysenteric infection. Usually a liver abscess must be treated surgically. It must be exposed and cleansed or it is likely to rupture and empty its contents into the abdominal cavity and result in peritonitis which might be fatal. Sometimes an operation is advisable to establish the actual existence of an abscess. Operative treatment is accompanied by injection of amebicidal drugs.

The proportion of fat in the liver is increased by its reaction to various poisons, to a high-fat diet, sometimes to general obesity or chronic alcoholism. In reacting to poisons, the liver replaces functioning cells with fat. Storage of fat in the liver occurs with an overfatty diet. Carbon tetrachloride, a common drycleaning substance, phosphorus, arsenic, and chloroform are all particularly damaging to the liver. *See also* ALCOHOLISM; BILE; CIRRHOSIS; HEPATITIS; JAUNDICE.

liver spots. Or chloasma, yellow and brownish spots and discolorations in patches on the skin. They may occur in pregnancy, tuberculosis, and digestive disturbances. They may also follow exposure to sun or heat and may appear in areas where pressure from a pad or belt has been exerted on the skin.

Pigmentation has been successfully treated with an ointment containing benoquin, a drug derived from an Egyptian plant, ammi majus. In certain instances, peeling techniques have also been used successfully.

lochia. The vaginal discharge that occurs in the early weeks after childbirth. It resembles normal menstruation.

lockjaw. *See* TETANUS.

longevity. Long life or the condition or quality of being long-lived. It is an inherited tendency, but a higher standard of living, better nutrition, and advances in medicine have in recent years increased the life span.

Statistics indicate that women in the United States generally live longer than men. In 1965 men had a life expectancy of about seventy years, women about seventy-five.

lordosis. Or sway back, a condition caused by an increase in the forward curvature of the lower spinal column or small of the back. It comes from an effort to improve the body's balance, as in the later stages of pregnancy.

Lordosis is also associated with hip-joint diseases and other disorders. In a person with a large, heavy abdomen, a strain is placed on the muscles and ligaments which can produce pain and an increase in curvature of the lower spine. *See also* SPINAL CORD; SPINAL CURVATURE.

low back pain. One of the commonest complaints brought to the attention of doctors. A symptom rather than a disease, low back pain may be caused by a great variety of conditions which are classed as congenital, mechanical, produced by disease, or the result of injury or strain.

Some of the mechanical causes are poor posture, overweight, or occupational strain. Injuries to or strains of the vertebrae, their ligaments, muscles, or nerves can cause low back pain. Such diseases as lumbago, rheumatoid arthritis, tuberculosis, syphilis, osteomyelitis, and degenerative arthritis of the sacroiliac joint produce low back pain.

Low back pain can originate in a number of areas of the spinal cord and may result from disorder of the sciatic nerve, which passes through the thighs, legs, and feet from the back. The sacroiliac joint may also be the seat of low back pain, as the result of strain, injury, or disease.

Early treatment is essential in order to avoid development of chronic conditions or complications such as arthritis. A physician should be consulted at the first sign of pain in the lower back. In most cases treatment is non-surgical, and, if the diagnosis is correct, largely effective in at least 90 per cent of the cases. Treatment includes rest, physical therapy such as heat, baths, and radiant light; strapping; drugs; and mechanical aids such as splints, belts, and braces.

Most therapy can be carried out at home, although more prompt and efficient treatment can be administered in a hospital. *See also* BACKACHE; LUMBAGO; NEURITIS; SACROILIAC; SCIATIC NEURITIS; SLIPPED DISC.

low blood pressure. *See* BLOOD PRESSURE, LOW.

lumbago. An acute attack of pain and stiffness in the lower back region which may appear without warning and without a sign or symptom of general illness. It may occur after ordinary housework or gardening, exposure to cold or wet weather, or sitting for a period of time in a draught of cold air blowing on the lower back region. It is usually characterized by a twinge of pain on moving.

Lumbago can generally be helped by heat from a hot-water bottle, heating pad, infrared ray, or with diathermy. Drugs such as aspirin may be taken or the doctor may inject a local anesthetic to be followed by limited movement and rest periods. Repeated attacks of lumbago may be due to an infection elsewhere in the body which the doctor will try to locate. *See also* LOW BACK PAIN.

lumbar. Describes anything pertaining to the loins. A lumbar puncture is made to remove spinal fluid for diagnosis or for the injection of an anesthetic.

lungs. The respiratory organs. The lungs lie on either side of the chest and occupy a large part of the chest cavity.

Tuberculosis and pneumonia are among the most serious diseases infecting the lungs. Other infections may cause bronchitis and bronchiectasis. The lungs may be affected by various viruses, by parasites and fungi, and by different poisons and dusts found in industry. Certain other disorders like abscess and emphysema or dilation of the air cells may invade one or both lungs.

During the last twenty-five years, cancer of the lung has considerably increased in incidence, and is now the most common form of internal cancer among men, in whom it is more likely to occur than in women.

Removal of the lung is usually the preferred treatment for patients with cancer of the lung. Unfortunately, however, detection in a large percentage of cases is too late for this means of control of lung cancer.

Advances in surgical techniques, in anesthetics, and in the use of antibiotics have made surgery on the lungs more possible and successful than it once was, and the death rate has now been decreased. *See also* ASPIRATION; ASTHMA; BRONCHITIS; BRONCHOPNEUMONIA; CHEST; EMPHYSEMA; PLEURISY; PNEUMONIA; TUBERCULOSIS.

lupus erythematosus. Usually a chronic, but sometimes severe acute disease, marked by the appearance of red scaly patches of various sizes on the skin.

The disease may seriously affect the internal organs. Infusion into the joints may occur, and the toxic effects may be extreme, sometimes fatal. This acute form of erythema requires drastic treatment. The use of ACTH and cortisone, and the injection of gold salts have been found effective in many cases. *See also* ERYTHEMA.

lymphatic system. An interconnected series of spaces, ducts, and glands within the body which carry lymph, a fluid which is constantly being circulated throughout the body.

Certain disorders may affect the lymphatic system—for example, infectious mononucleosis and glandular fever in which the lymph nodes become swollen and tender. In agranulocytosis, the production of white blood cells stops. The lymph vessels and glands may become inflamed. Septic sores on toes and fingers may result in acute inflammation of glands in other parts of the body through spread of the infection. Tuberculosis frequently causes inflammation of the lymph glands. Malignant and benign tumors may occur in the lymph glands or the glands may enlarge as a result of malignant growths carried to them from other parts of the body. Cysts often form in the glands when the lymphatic vessels are dilated.

Any disturbance of the lymphatic system must be taken care of by a physician. Proper treatment of the causes of the infection will usually relieve the symptoms affecting the lymph glands. *See also* HODGKIN'S DISEASE; LEUKEMIA.

lymphogranuloma venereum. Known popularly as bubo, a world-wide virus-produced disease usually spread by sexual contact.

The chief symptom is swelling of the lymph glands following infection. Five to fourteen days after the disease is contracted, a small ulcer, or papule, appears on the sex organs. This may heal within a few days, but frequently a secondary infection results in a larger sore. The infection spreads along the lymphatic ducts and in a short time reaches one of the large lymph glands.

In the early stages, fever, inflammation of the joints, skin rashes, and infection of the brain and dura may be present. Other symptoms are stiffness and aching in the groin, followed by swelling. These swellings, hard and about the size of a walnut, are known as buboes. They may break down and leave a draining abscess but this is rare. Elephantiasis in which the whole vulva may swell sometimes occurs in women, and in more severe cases the whole body may be affected.

After healing, men are generally considered incapable of transmitting the disease, but women may be carriers for years. Although rarely, the disease may be transmitted other than through sexual contact, by way of the mouth, nose, and eyes.

The duration of the disease can be controlled successfully by vaccines, made from material taken from infected glands. Sulfa drugs, penicillin, and other antibiotics including Terramycin and Aureomycin are used; lymphogranuloma is one of the few virus diseases that yields to such treatment. *See also* BUBO.

mammary. Having to do with the breast. The two mammary glands secrete milk after childbirth.

mammography. X-ray of the breast for diagnosis of tumors.

manic-depressive psychosis. Manic-depressive psychosis is a form of mental disturbance, almost as common as schizophrenia, the most frequent mental disorder. About one-third of all the patients in mental institutions belong to this group. Manic-depressive psychosis may attack at any age, but is more prevalent in the age group between twenty and sixty. Women are more subject than men, comprising about two-thirds of all cases.

Manic-depressive psychosis has been called cyclical insanity, because it is characterized by periodic and alternating cycles of mania and depression. In the manic phase, the person may manifest overabundant energy, incessant activity, and exaggerated well-being. Impulsiveness and motor excitement will be pronounced, and her ideas lofty and unmistakably pleasurable, expressed in incessant talk. Her judgment will seem disordered and her ability to make decisions weak. The mood may suddenly change to extreme irritability, temper, and anger, and then she may give advice and criticism to others in an attempt to show her superiority.

As in other psychoses, the afflicted person is apt to have lofty goals. The manic-depressive psychotic imagines that she is an exalted and powerful personality, perhaps a great scientist, actress, queen, or savior of mankind. She will aggressively demand attention to her claims, which she may express without cessation. During the manic phase, she may completely change her former moral and ethical standards. In most instances, pronounced eroticism and sometimes alcoholism and drug addiction occur.

Hypomania or lesser mania is a milder form of mania. Here, too, an overabundant energy and quest for incessant activity appear. The person's humor and talk will be boisterous or childish and giggling. While delusions of grandeur are absent, the hypomaniac still manifests an irritating and overdone self-esteem. Outbreaks of anger and irritability are frequent.

The manic phase alternates in manic-depressive psychosis with a painful emotional condition in which the person is dangerously depressed and miserable. In this state she will be self-derogatory, driven to deep despondency by some sense of guilt about often illusory misdeeds and sins. She may contemplate suicide, considering herself unworthy to live. Delusions and hallucinations are habitual, and symptoms such as sluggishness, inability to make decisions, and lack of power of concentration are pronounced. This depressive stage of manic-depressive psychosis may be accompanied by physical symptoms such as constipation, coated tongue, sleeplessness, loss of weight, and many others. Intellectual activity is suppressed while the person is deeply involved in her harrowing delusions, and stupor is not uncommon. Women become antagonistic to sex and men.

Manic-depressive attacks, which may occur originally from great emotional tension, may be short or last for many months. If they are isolated and infrequent, chance for recovery is possible; however, full and complete recovery is rare.

marasmus. A word derived from the Greek *marasmos* or decay, is a disease characterized by progressive wasting of body tissue of infants. It also denotes severe malnutrition due to poor diet or protracted intestinal disorders that prevent proper utilization of food. Only rarely is the underlying cause of marasmus a constitutional disease.

The symptoms of marasmus are similar to those of gradual starvation. The infant has a low temperature, loose skin in folds, wasted limbs, large sunken eyes, and a general appearance of old age. Marasmus occurs most frequently in bottle-fed babies, in slum and unsanitary conditions, and in institutions.

Treatment, if in time, may restore the health of some infants, especially those older than six months. Large quantities of mother's milk must be given; if necessary it can be procured from a mother's milk bank. If human milk is not available, powder or evaporated milk may be substituted. Vitamins A and B complex, massages, and an abundance of fresh air have been found helpful.

marijuana. Also known as hashish in the Orient, a habit-forming drug. It is the dried leaves and flowers of the Indian hemp plant, usually smoked in cigarettes. Addiction to marijuana is as widespread in the United States as in other countries. Every country in Asia has a centuries-long history of marijuana drug addiction.

Marijuana or hashish affects its users in many ways, since it stimulates the nervous, respiratory, circulatory, digestive, excretory, and genital systems. The drug clouds the mind and reduces self-control; the person becomes restless and talkative, relaxed and exhilarated with a sense of well-being, followed by drowsiness. Generally difficulty in focusing and sustaining mental attention is noted.

marriage. The physical, personal, and legal union between a man and woman for the establishment of a family. The beginning of marriage is a new experience for both partners. Sexual adjustment must be made and techniques adapted to the needs and preferences of the husband and wife. Although sex is the biological foundation of marriage, many adults are misinformed or confused about it.

Differences exist between men and women which affect the degree of sexual gratification, and for women especially the success of the sexual life depends in large measure upon the degree of emotional accord enjoyed with her husband. Sex is not all of a marriage; but if this area is a source of satisfaction to the husband and wife, success in the other areas will be more easily assured. *See also* CONCEPTION; CONTRACEPTION; IMPOTENCE; ORGASM; STERILITY.

masochism. A psychopathic condition which demands the stimulation of pain, or abuse, before the subject can respond to sexual stimulus.

mastectomy. Surgical removal of the breast, usually for cancer. In recent years many measures have been taken that enable the patient to lead an almost entirely normal life after recovery.

mastitis. Inflammation of the breast; it occurs in various forms and degrees of severity. An injury to the mammary glands can produce an infection by staphylococci or streptococci. The breast becomes swollen, reddened, knotty, and tender to the touch. Pain may be severe and fever high.

The acute form, puerperal (pertaining to childbirth) mastitis, is frequent among nursing mothers, occurring a few days or weeks after delivery. A so-called "caked breast," the result of excessive milk secretion with retention, may precede it. In some instances, chronic mastitis follows the acute form. However, it may be the outgrowth of an injury to the tissues of the breast or due to menstrual disorders, miscarriage, or abortion. Women during menopause are frequently affected. Young girls may suffer a painful swelling and hardening of the breast during puberty. Mastitis at puberty is rarely a serious inflammation and in most cases quickly subsides.

Mastitis must always be diagnosed and treated by a physician. Treatment may involve surgical emptying of abscesses and extraction of milk with a pump. Drugs, such as the sulfonamides and antibiotics, are prescribed to act specifically against the germs. *See also* BREAST.

mastoid. The mastoid (breast-shaped) bone is a part of the skull just behind the ear. This spongy network of bone connects with the middle ear. Disorders of the middle ear, nose, throat, or upper part of the breathing system may cause infection to spread into the mastoid. When this occurs with inflammation of the bone, the condition, mastoiditis, is dangerous, not only because it may cause permanent damage to the inner ear but because the close proximity of the mastoid tissues to the brain may lead to meningitis, the spread of infection into the membranes around the brain.

Symptoms of mastoid infection include high temperature, pain, and redness behind the ear, and occasionally a stiff neck. Often earache, sore throat, or a cold have preceded the symptoms. Infection of the mastoid may follow measles, scarlet fever, or diphtheria.

Prompt treatment of infections of the nose, throat, tonsils, and ear with antibiotics has made mastoid infections rare; twenty years ago the condition was common. Treatment of severe mastoid infection may include surgery in which the diseased inner contents of the mastoid bone are removed.

masturbation. Self-production of a sexual orgasm. Any harmful effect is due more to a sense of guilt and secrecy than any physical result that may occur.

measles. An acute, highly communicable disease, common throughout the world. The characteristic symptoms resemble those of the common cold with fever and the early appearance of a rash on the mucous membranes of the cheeks and lips and later over the entire body. Epidemics usually occur in late winter, at two-year intervals in large communities and four- to five-year intervals in smaller communities. Everyone is susceptible to measles and the transmission of the disease takes only an infinitesimal dose of the virus. Most of the cases occur among children, adults usually having had it in childhood. However, older people have been known to contract measles in areas where an epidemic appears after a long absence. Measles during pregnancy is apt to cause miscarriage; it has been observed in newborn infants when the mother has had it simultaneously.

In recent years a successful living attenuated virus vaccine has been developed that gives immunity to measles.

Measles is transmitted through secretions from the eyes, nose, and throat by direct contact or droplet infection and is spread through the air by coughing, sneezing, or talking. It may be transmitted from seven to eleven days after a person has contracted it. Transmission is at its highest peak just before the rash appears. Complications that may follow measles do not spread the disease, though they may transmit the secondary infection.

The first symptoms generally resemble a cold, with running nose, sneezing, an irregular fever and chills, pains in the head and back, and watering eyes. There may also be inflammation of the upper respiratory passages and congestion of the mucous membranes of the nose and mouth. A day or two later, bluish white specks, called Koplik's spots, appear opposite the first molar teeth and inside the lower lip. They are pinpoint in size and surrounded by a bright red area. At first there are only a few, but soon the spots increase and run together. Koplik's spots may be seen two or three days before the rash appears. As soon as these spots appear, the person should be isolated, not only to avoid spreading the disease but also to aid his own recovery. Fever will be fairly steady, gradually rising to its height when the rash appears.

The rash, which usually appears over the body about fourteen days after exposure and about three or four days after the fever begins, seldom lasts longer than four or five days. It first appears in the hairline, behind the ears, on the neck and over the forehead, then extends downward, gradually covering the entire body. These tiny red pimples become larger and redder and tend to increase and group together, giving the skin a blotchy appearance. Temperature often ranges between 104° to 105°, the skin itches and burns, the face is puffy, the eyes red and swollen and sensitive to strong light. A discharge from the nose ensues, as well as a hoarse cough without discharge, and the patient generally feels miserable. When the rash has reached its peak, the fever drops rapidly, the symptoms disappear, the cough lessens, and the patient begins to improve rapidly. As the rash fades and dries, the skin sheds gritty brownish scales.

Uncomplicated measles is not a particularly severe disease, but, like many of the virus infections, it tends to reduce the normal resistance of the body so that the patient becomes susceptible to secondary infections, which may involve the upper respiratory tract, the ears, nose, sinuses, larynx, and lungs. The most serious complication is bronchopneumonia or conjunctivitis which may damage the eyes. At one time tuberculosis was a frequent aftermath of measles, particularly in cases in which prolonged signs of lung involvement and persistent low-grade fever were present. In addition to these secondary invasions by bacteria, another serious complication due to the virus of measles itself is inflammation of the brain or encephalitis. Fortunately this is rare.

Of utmost consideration are all measures which will prevent development or spread of measles. Children who have been exposed to it should be isolated for fourteen days after their first known contact. If globulin has been given to modify the disease, the child should be isolated for a minimum of eighteen days following the last exposure. Unnecessary exposure should always be avoided, particularly of older infants, preschool-age children, and pregnant women. This is important not only as a preventive of transmitting the disease but also to minimize the incidence of secondary infection.

While a specific drug for treatment of measles is not yet known, the improved methods and drugs used to treat the complications have materially reduced the already low death rate as well as the effects of secondary complications.

meatus. An opening or passage. The term is applied to various orifices or openings of the body, such as the auditory or external ear, the meatus of the nose which connects the pharynx and the nasal passage, and the urethral meatus through which urine is discharged.

medicine chest. Every household should have an orderly, adequately stocked medicine chest—that is, a cabinet or container in which medicines, drugs, bandages, and other related supplies are kept. Too often the family medicine chest is a catch-all, and the medicines and drugs it does contain are old or unlabeled or their original purpose forgotten. Drugs wrongly used can do infinite harm, and all old medicines for illnesses since cured should be thrown out. Not only can random taking of medicine be harmful, but many drugs deteriorate and are not safe after a certain time. Every item in the medicine chest should be labeled and, if necessary, dated. It may be a wise idea to keep the cabinet or container locked if there are children in the household, since even a seemingly mild medicine can have fatal results. The key should be kept in a safe place

where it can be found promptly. Following are items which most families will want to keep in their medicine cabinets.

Laxatives and cathartics. A wide variety of substances are used as laxatives. Castor oil and Epsom salts are not generally advisable, since they are irritants and may drastically disrupt the normal pattern of bowel movement. Mineral oil, a mechanical lubricant, is somewhat less potent; however, if used over a period of time, it may interfere with the absorption of vitamins A and D. Perhaps the safest laxatives are the so-called bulk laxatives. Some persons, however, are sensitive to the natural type, and synthetic bulk producers are more consistent in their action, non-allergenic, and do not swell until they reach the intestine. Other common popular preparations include phenolphthalein, Seidlitz powder, sodium phosphate, milk of magnesia, aromatic cascara, and mineral oils mixed with sugars. A laxative or cathartic should never be taken when the abdomen is painful, since it may cause serious harm—for example, in the case of appendicitis. Persistent use of laxatives will eventually chronically interfere with the normal bowel movements, and is a habit to be avoided.

Pain relievers. Most pain relievers are used for headache, although they are sometimes taken for neuritis, neuralgia, toothache, colds, and pains of unknown origin. Most headache powders purchased commercially contain phenacetin or acetanilid in varying doses. The most common general pain reliever is acetylsalicylic acid, commonly called aspirin, which is usually sold in 5-grain tablets. If kept in a tightly-capped bottle, aspirin will keep indefinitely, except in the tropics. Aspirin does not cure, but will relieve certain types of pain. It acts as both an antipyretic (antifever) drug, and an analgesic (antipain) drug. Various combinations of aspirin are available—for example, with phenacetin and caffein. Although it is one of the safest drugs, serious and even fatal effects from aspirin poisoning point up that no drug is always safe.

Aspirin is available for children in smaller tablets, which are sometimes flavored. This has proved to be a mixed blessing, since children may confuse the aspirin with candy and consume large quantities of it. An editorial in the *Journal of the American Medical Association* has advised against the use of sweetened aspirin and aspirin chewing gum. Hundreds of cases of aspirin poisoning occur each year and usually because through negligence the bottle of aspirin has been left in a place accessible to children.

Most cases of aspirin sensitivity are not serious, but two or three persons out of a hundred have reactions, usually nausea or stomach upset. This is especially likely in those who have allergies or asthmatic conditions, and such persons should be especially cautious in using aspirin.

Sleep-producing drugs. Most of the sleep-producing drugs are chiefly derivatives of barbituric acid—for example, Seconal, Amytal, Veronal, Trional, and combinations of barbituric acid with other drugs. These drugs should be used only under medical care, and then extreme caution should be taken to keep them out of the reach of children, and to have the bottle clearly identified.

Narcotics. Among the strongest of medicinal preparations are the narcotics and anesthetics, which should never be used by anyone without a doctor's prescription. A drug that must be administered with a hypodermic syringe should not be kept in the family medicine cabinet. Some persons with diabetes have been taught by their doctor to inject themselves with insulin, and they usually keep the syringe outfit in a special separate place.

Antibiotics. Formerly antibiotics could be obtained only by prescription, but now, in some states and in certain dosages, they can be purchased at a drug store without a prescription. Antibiotic lozenges for mouth infections or sore throats, and bandages medicated with antibiotics are now available.

Any antibiotic preparation should be used with discretion. Locally they can produce definite sensitizing effects and result in irritations far more serious than the one the drug was purchased to cure. Also, taken orally, antibiotics, such as Aureomycin, Terramycin, penicillin, are known at times to produce serious side effects. Any antibiotics that are left over from a prescription should be destroyed; and if, for any reason, old antibiotic preparations are taken and signs of nausea, vomiting, or other unusual symptoms appear, the doctor should be contacted at once.

Antiseptics. Many different antiseptics are available for use on the skin, for cleansing parts of the body, or as a gargle. Iodine, Metaphen, Mercurochrome, Zephiran, and similar preparations are often used.

First aid. Among the materials needed for first aid are adhesive tape of various widths, sterile cotton, sterile gauze bandages, sterile gauze pads, petroleum jelly, zinc oxide ointment, and scissors, which should be kept in the medicine chest exclusively for such purposes. Other first-aid items which may be included are ready-made sterilized bandages to cover small wounds, which can be purchased in a waterproof type and premedicated, and milk of magnesia and sodium bicarbonate (baking soda) which are frequently recommended by doctors as alkalies.

Poisons should never be kept in the family medicine chest, or any chemicals used around the household for bleaching, killing insects and rodents, dry cleaning, and similar purposes. Even when children have been cautioned again and again to stay away from such chemicals, accidental poisonings do occur; the rate of accidental poisoning in children under five is 2.6 per 100,000 children. Too often the labels on, for example, cleaning fluid bottles, do not tell of potential dangers or the precautions which should be taken when the solution is used. Many such solutions contain carbon tetrachloride, a toxic chemical. Inhalation of a small amount can poison a child, and be dangerous for an adult.

In addition to first-aid materials, most families will find it desirable and convenient to have a bedpan, glass drinking tube, syringe for giving an enema, atomizer, hot-water bottle, electric pad, ice bag, and sometimes a special device for creating steam, to be medicated with small amounts of tincture of benzoin or other drugs for relief in various types of throat conditions.

The family medicine cabinet should be checked at least four times a year, and all unnecessary items thrown away, such as old razor blades, which should be kept in a special container and then discarded.

Following are several rules to be observed.

1. Do not save poisonous preparations of any kind, unless absolutely necessary. Keep them separate from medicines, and label plainly.

2. Every drug should be clearly labeled, and the correct dose plainly marked.

3. Keep bottles tightly closed; drugs may concentrate and become dangerous, or evaporate and become useless.

4. Do not keep samples of any patent medicine whose composition is not known.

5. Never keep any opium or morphine preparations in the family medicine chest.

6. Discard all prepared prescriptions when the special purpose for which they were prescribed is past.

7. Read labels carefully, especially

again before giving any drug or medicine.

melancholia. *See* INVOLUTIONAL MELANCHOLIA.

melanosis. The condition which exists when abnormal deposits of melanin are formed in the blood or placed in organs or surfaces. Melanins are metabolic, dark brownish, granular pigments which are produced by the activity of cells. As a normal pigmentary matter, melanins occur in hair, skin, or muscles. Pigmentation of the skin or some internal organs is not always associated with a medical disorder. Tanning or freckling results from exposure of the skin to the ultraviolet rays of the sun, or from radium therapy. Prolonged treatment with certain chemicals—such as arsenic, for example—will also result in skin pigmentation. The nipples of the breast and other parts of the body may be pigmented during pregnancy.

Melanosis, however, is sometimes related to serious ailments. In Addison's disease, some skin disorders, and ochronosis, a discoloration of cartilage and allied tissues, melanosis is a symptom. It also occurs in pellagra and other disorders resulting from vitamin deficiencies.

Tumors containing melanins, the so-called malignant melanomas or melanocancers are especially serious. They originate in discolored flattened moles and spread, adding pigmentation to other parts of the body. In such cases, melanuria is pronounced. Since pigments may be involved in all sorts of tissues, the prefix "melano" may also refer to the pigment in sweat (melanidro-

sis), to the pigment in the menstrual flow (melanorrhagia), to the pigments in the mucous membranes of the mouth (melanoplakia), and to the black fungus growths (melanomyces). *See also* FRECKLES.

melanuria. The condition in which urine takes on a brownish black color because large quantities of pigments are present.

Ménière's disease. A chronic ailment in which the major symptoms are dizziness, deafness, and noises in one or both ears. It is usually due to an interference with the function of the inner ear or labyrinth, and is frequently accompanied by nausea and vomiting. It begins in late life and affects both sexes.

The disease begins with mild deafness and head noises, called tinnitus, which are high-pitched and hissing, roaring, or ringing. The noises are generally heard on one side of the head only, and vary in intensity from day to day. The vertigo, which is a strong feeling of swaying, rocking, or turning, begins abruptly, and may last from a few minutes to several hours, and is generally associated with nausea and vomiting. It recurs at long, irregular intervals. Complete rest helps to lessen the severity of the attacks. Impairment of hearing is progressive, and on rare occasions, during an acute attack of dizziness, there may be a rolling of the eyes from side to side, known as nystagmus.

meningitis. An inflammation of the meninges, the membranes covering the brain and spinal cord, caused by infection of the cerebrospinal fluid by various micro-organisms.

The term is, however, usually applied to an epidemic form, caused by the meningococcus.

The doctor diagnoses meningitis not only from the history of the patient, which may indicate that he has been in contact with the infection, and from the symptoms, but also by obtaining specimens of the spinal fluid which are studied for the presence of germs and for other changes which indicate infection and inflammation.

The symptoms of meningitis arise from the changes that the germs and their poisons produce in the tissues of the nervous system. During the period of invasion, sore throat, dullness, fever, chills, rapid pulse, and a general soreness of the body indicate that an infection is present. Then a rash of pinpoint-sized red spots or even large spots appears over the body. In the stage when the infection has spread to the nervous system, severe pain is felt, with intolerable headaches, vomiting, and even delirium and convulsions.

The conquest of meningitis is one of the great triumphs of medicine. Before the discovery of a serum which could be used against meningitis, the death rate used to be 80 or 90 out of every 100 cases. Sulfa drugs, antibiotics, and other advances in treatment have reversed the situation so that today recovery is the rule and death the exception, even in the most stubborn form of the disease, tuberculous meningitis, a variety caused by the tuberculosis germ. Medicine may well be within sight of a meningitis recovery rate of 100 per cent. Because of the many possible complications, hospital care is necessary for persons with meningitis. *See also* CEREBRO-SPINAL MENINGITIS.

menopause. Or more popularly, change of life, the characteristic physical changes which most women undergo between the ages of forty-five and fifty, though sometimes earlier or later. Early onset of menstruation is usually associated with late appearance of the change of life.

The basis of the retrogression is the gradual cessation of the secretion of certain major endocrine glands. The most noticeable aspect is the gradual or abrupt disappearance of menstruation. Loss of sexual desire and sexual activity are rarely involved. There are a number of physical changes in the genitalia that occur at this time. They reverse the procedure occurring during puberty. Not only do the ovaries, the female sex glands, become relatively inactive, but other changes take place in the body. The spleen, the lymphatic system, and the intestines are affected, at least slightly.

The manner in which the changes of menopause take place is subject to tremendous variation among women. With some it occurs quickly and with only minor disturbances. With others, however, the change of life lasts three or four years, accompanied by much difficulty. The most troublesome factors sometimes associated with the menopause are mental depression, heightened irritability, and excitability. Unless these are extreme, however, little medical treatment is necessary. Nevertheless, mental difficulties may develop at this time and then medical advice is desirable.

The most common physical symptom is the hot flush, which sweeps the entire body with sudden warmth and perspiration, then leaves it chilly. Flushes occur without perceptible reason or often in association with excitement. Itching skin and constipation of the bowels may be noticed but are readily controlled, and heart palpitations, headache, dizziness, and insomnia are not unusual.

Most of the unpleasant developments of menopause are of minor consequence, and these, and others of a more serious nature, can usually be controlled with hormones. Because of the complications which may be involved and the long duration of change, medical supervision is helpful. The same symptoms may characterize other developments within the body and demand prompt medical attention when they occur. Artificial menopause may also result from the surgical removal of the ovaries or from their destruction by X-rays or radium. Men often experience many of the unpleasant symptoms of menopause, related to retrogression of the sex glands. *See also* MENSTRUATION.

menorrhagia. The loss of an exceptional amount of blood at the monthly menstrual periods, in contrast to metrorrhagia in which an excessive flow of blood occurs between menstrual periods. Several possible causes have been found for this uterine bleeding, including poor functioning of hormones involved in the menstrual cycle, poor blood clotting, an unusual condition of the blood, or some emotional or psychological factor. It has been frequently noticed when women move from a cold climate to a hot one. It is also a symptom of a considerable number of diseases.

A physician must be consulted to diagnose the cause. Among successful therapeutic measures employed are complete bed rest and drugs to relieve anxiety and to bring about contractions of the womb. Hormones, such as estrogen, progesterone, and androgen, have also been used successfully.

menorrhalgia. Painful menstruation. *See* DYSMENORRHEA.

menorrhea. Normal menstruation.

menostaxis. Prolonged menstruation.

menstruation. The periodic flow of blood experienced by women in the years of sexual maturity and the associated changes that occur in the body at this time.

When the discharge ceases, the lining of the uterus or womb begins to thicken and continues the process for a week or longer. In the next stage, lasting about two weeks, the lining of the womb becomes engorged, in readiness to receive a fertilized egg. Approximately two weeks before the regular menstrual flow begins the ovary releases an egg. If the egg is not fertilized and pregnancy has not taken place, by the end of the cycle the womb lining, called the endometrium, breaks down, alterations in the blood vessels occur, and the menstrual flow washes away the residue.

Characteristics peculiar to this cycle vary greatly in different women. Although the average period is exactly four weeks or twenty-eight days, some women complete the cycle in three weeks and some take as long as five. In others, irregularity may be usual. Although the age of sexual maturity is usually between the twelfth and the sixteenth years, development earlier or later is not abnormal.

Slight variations in the individual cycle are not significant, but sudden major changes, such as complete cessation of menstruation in the absence of pregnancy, should receive prompt medical attention. Suspension of the menstrual period may be caused by a variety of factors. Undernourishment and associated disturbances such as anemia, or severe infections like tuberculosis, rheumatic or typhoid fever may be responsible. Disorders of the pituitary gland or thyroid gland or the ovaries themselves may be involved. Two ovarian secretions or hormones, estradiol and progesterone, are the chief regulators of the menstrual cycle, and the ovaries in turn are controlled to some extent by the pituitary.

Conspicuous delay in the onset of menstruation in a young woman should be investigated by a physician. Although nothing more serious than personal variation may be involved, other difficulties may be responsible. Delayed development, if it persists, may eventually lead to psychological changes, rendering normal childbirth impossible.

Menstrual pain may be caused by such factors as a narrow cervix, the passageway from the womb, by fibroid tumors in the uterus, by cysts, or by variations in the position of the uterus. Most of these conditions can be remedied by a physician. Pain and discomfort which sometimes accompany menstruation may often be relieved by simple measures such as mild sedatives, application of heat, and plenty of rest and sleep. Nevertheless, a physician should be consulted if these remedies are not effective. Glandular substances, to modify the behavior of the mechanisms involved, or the use of more potent pain-relieving drugs may be necessary. Some drugs are harmful if not employed under medical supervision and milder ones may become habit-forming if care is not exercised.

Menstruation is a normal physiological function, and is not concerned, as some suppose, with ridding the body of "poisons." Unless special factors are involved that prompt medical advice to the contrary, young women need vary only slightly their ordinary routines. Violent and competitive athletics are not advisable or should be closely controlled because of the general stress they impose on the body, and bathing need not be interrupted. Swimming may cause extra blood to be lost, but there is rarely any risk of infection from the water itself. *See also* AMENORRHEA; DYSMENORRHEA; MENORRHAGIA; MENOPAUSE; METRORRHAGIA.

menstruation anovular. Menstruation without ovarian secretion, particularly common during the first few years after puberty and at the menopause.

metabolism. *See* BASAL METABOLISM.

metastasis. A process in which primary agents or cells, through blood vessels or lymph channels, transfer the seat of a disease from one part of the body to another. For example, tumors of one organ may spread to the brain, especially from a focus in the lungs and breasts. Cancer in any part of the body may metastasize—that is, transfer—from the kidney, uterus, prostate, or breast and become secondary cancer in another part of the body. The condition is dangerous since it can become widespread before any symptoms are apparent.

Another example of metastasis is the wandering course of acute rheumatism, which has the tendency to involve the lining of the heart and the pericardium, the membranous sac which envelops it. In mumps, the testicles of males or ovaries of females may be involved, as a result of metastasis.

Meticorten. *See* CORTISONE.

metritis. In medicine, diseases of the uterus are referred to by the prefix "metro," denoting relation to the womb. Metritis is an infection and inflammation of the uterus. A metroscope is an instrument used for examination of the uterus.

metrorrhagia. A hemorrhage from the uterus between menstrual periods; it may be a sign of a serious disorder. Full examination and treatment by a physician is desirable. The excessive flow of blood between menstrual periods is often related to disorders in the womb and pelvis, and sometimes to acute fevers and glandular conditions. *See also* MENSTRUATION.

micturate. To urinate. The need to urinate increases greatly in frequency between the fourth and the twelfth weeks of pregnancy.

migraine. Commonly called "sick headache," has an age-old history dating back to the ancient Greeks. The name is believed to be derived from the Greek word *emikrania*, meaning half head, which became *mikrania* and eventually migraine. The complaint is widespread, usually beginning some time around puberty and lessening in late middle age. Migraine is more common in women, and often more than one member of a family suffers from it.

Certain features distinguish migraine from other types of headache. It is limited to one side of the head, recurs periodically, and for each person follows a rather consistent pattern, so that it can often be predicted where the headache will begin, how severe it will be, and how long it will last. The headache is described as a throbbing, aching pain, limited to the forehead, temple, or back of the head. In some cases it seems to arise from the back of the upper teeth and strikes the face and the area below the eye, or it may spread behind the angle of the jaw, reaching down the neck and into the shoulders. This pattern of pain is often accompanied by an unusual throbbing in the neck. In some instances the first symptoms are not confined to the head, but instead the person will suffer pain in the abdomen, chest, or arm, or an attack of vomiting or diarrhea, or a passing fever. A frequent accompaniment to the migraine headache is a disturbance in vision, which may take the form of temporary blindness, blinding flashes of light, or a general blurring of vision. These symptoms disappear as the headache abates.

Migraine, primarily a tension headache, is believed to result from continued muscle contraction which causes distention of the blood vessels in the brain. The general tightening of the body associated with anxiety and emotional tension contributes in most cases to the preliminary symptoms—the tingling sensations in the hands and feet, the impairment of vision, and noises in the ears or mental depression.

In the treatment of migraine, much emphasis is now placed on prevention of the attack. At the first indication of its approach, steps are taken to avert the headache or reduce its severity. Complete quiet, a dark room, hot or cold applications to the head and a hot-water bottle at the feet are often helpful. Aspirin and ordinary analgesics give little or no relief once the headache has begun. Histamine and intramuscular injections of ergotamine tartrate, administered by a physician, have been effective.

The psychological factor is of primary significance in treatment of migraine. The patient must feel that he is receiving the best possible care and that his physician has a thorough understanding of those emotional factors in his background and environment which may be at the root of his condition. Patients with migraine headaches almost invariably fit into a common pattern. They are tense, driving, rigid in their standards, conscientious, and constantly striving for perfection. The treatment of migraine must include and evaluate all the factors that may give rise to the disorder. The patient must be made to understand the nature of his drives and how these create frustration and anxiety. Psychotherapy, a long-term project in these cases, has yielded fruitful results and promises to be even more successful in the future.

milk. The whitish liquid secreted from the mammary glands of all mammals; it is the only natural food, intended for the very young, which comes straight from the living body. Nature provides it in abundance, and more than eighty different animal sources have been classified.

Milk has always been highly esteemed and from time immemorial many nourishing, healing, and spiritual qualities were attributed to it. Mother's milk was long considered the only suitable food for an infant, and children were breast fed for three years or longer before animals were domesticated and the milk of cows, goats, camels, and sheep able to be substituted for that of the mother.

Milk is often called a food of near perfection. It furnishes proteins to replace and repair body tissues, it supplies minerals such as calcium to build sound bones and teeth and to perform other functions, it is a good source of natural sugar and of vitamins A, C, D, B_1, and B_2, and it is abundant in fats which are more easily digested than any other edible fat.

miscarriage. *See* ABORTION.

mongolism. A type of idiocy, with some similarities to myxedema and cretinism. Also called Down's disease. The name apparently derives from the slightly oriental look, due to the obliquity of the eye slit mongoloids have. However, mongoloids occur throughout the world. Three mongoloids are born in every thousand births. They are small, rarely reaching the height of a normal twelve-year-old child. They have broad faces with flat or stubby noses, and an open, apparently undeveloped mouth with large protruding lips. Their legs and arms are abnormally short, the hands thick and the muscles flabby. In most instances the senses are deficient, with weak eyesight, impaired hearing, and an undeveloped sense of smell. Mongoloids have speech difficulties and very limited vocabularies and usually are only able to utter unintelligible sounds. They reach puberty exceedingly late and may learn to walk as late as the age of eleven or twelve. Frequently mongoloids show little or no interest in their environment, live in a stupor, and seem unable to perform even simple tasks or to take care of themselves. Thus their retardation is pronounced enough for them to be considered true idiots.

Often organic defects are present. Mongoloids may have a faulty circulatory system, or underdeveloped brain, liver, and kidney. Physical weakness and a susceptibility to lung and intestinal infections have always been high contributing factors to the high death rate among mongoloids before the age of maturity. However, antibiotics and other drugs have increased their life span considerably.

The cause of mongolism is not known. The condition has been related to the splitting of a chromosome. Since mongoloids are prenatal casualties, they can be considered as part of the broader problem of congenital anomalies.

A specific cure for mongolism is not known. Even under the most ideal circumstances, mongoloids will only become about 30 per cent normal. Dr. Thomas Benda, an authority on this subject and author of *Mongolism and Cretinism*, reports that mongoloids can learn to do simple manual chores such as household or farm work. He points out that they learn by imitating others. *See also* CRETINISM; FEEBLE-MINDEDNESS; MYXEDEMA.

moniliasis. A disease caused by a yeastlike fungus, *Candida albicans*, and occurring throughout the world, among all races and ages, and in both sexes.

The fungus causes a wide range of infections, from mild disorders of the skin and mucous membranes of the mouth or vagina, to invasion of the deeper tissues, particularly the bronchi, lungs, or meninges. The fungus is widespread in nature, and has been found in the normal mouth, throat, and gastrointestinal tract, as well as in patients with long-standing diseases, in which the wasted tissues offer a good medium for the growth of this organism.

The most common infection, oral thrush, is an acute inflammation of the mouth, tongue, gums, or pharynx, often found in undernourished children and during the first few weeks in infant life. It is highly contagious. Another variety is vaginal moniliasis, which often occurs during pregnancy and in diabetics. Monilia infection of the skin of the hands often develops in bakers, waiters, bartenders, housewives, and others whose hands are softened from continual soaking in water.

The symptoms vary with the location and the intensity of the infection, from creamy whitish patches in the mucous membranes to fever, cough, abscess formation, and meningitis.

The infection generally responds to treatment. Alkaline mouthwashes or irrigations with dilute solutions of gentian violet clear up infections of the mouth. Skin infections have been controlled by potassium permanganate soaking, and daily application of an ammoniated mercury ointment. Mystatin (Mycostatin), a new antibiotic which is the first of these drugs to be effective against this fungus infection without causing undesirable reactions, has brought encouraging results.

mononucleosis, infectious. A virus infection which causes a swelling of the lymph glands and changes in the white blood cells. The condition occurs in epidemic form as well as in scattered cases, most commonly in people between the ages of ten and thirty-five. Recent research has demonstrated passage of the virus in saliva during kissing.

Some five to fifteen days after exposure to the disease, there may be a flulike feeling of malaise, fatigue, and headache. Fever develops and the lymph glands, especially those of the neck, become enlarged, giving the condition its common name, glandular fever. Sore throat is generally present.

The condition develops in many different ways. Sometimes skin eruptions with discolored rashes are perceptible; the liver may be affected, causing a jaundiced appearance of the skin; and occasionally the heart, lungs, and central nervous system are involved. The spleen is also frequently enlarged. In still other cases, all the symptoms may pass unnoticed. Infectious mononucleosis is manifested by characteristic changes in the blood, an increase in the white blood cells and some changes in their structure.

Infectious mononucleosis usually runs its course within three to six weeks, and recovery is generally uncomplicated and complete. Occasionally the spleen and the lymph nodes may remain enlarged for some time after the other symptoms have disappeared.

Bed rest and limitation of activities are considered essential and in severe cases may have to be prolonged, even after all fever or acute symptoms have subsided. Hot salt gargles or throat irrigations are often given to relieve sore throat. Special diets are usually prescribed when jaundice develops. Aureomycin and chloramphenicol have recently been used, and may be effective in controlling the condition.

mons veneris. Or pubis. The slightly fatty pad over the female genitalia, covered with short, wavy hair.

morning sickness. The nausea and

vomiting that sometimes affects women during the first few months of pregnancy. Taking a deep breath on rising may compensate. Eating a dry biscuit before getting up is also recommended.

morphine. Of the approximately twenty alkaloids in opium, morphine is the chief one and largely responsible for the effects of opium. As morphine acts reliably and quickly and is especially suited for hypodermic use, medicine employs it widely as a pain reliever. Morphine can be habit-forming. *See also* DRUG ADDICTION.

motion sickness. A condition produced in some persons when they are in a moving boat, car, bus, airplane, elevator, swing, or other conveyance. Characteristic symptoms are nausea, headache, dizziness, and vomiting.

Certain conditions aggravate the tendency to motion sickness—for example, a stuffy unventilated enclosure, unpleasant odors, or irritating or loud noises. More people become sick during the day than the night, some persons are sick when they ride backward but not when they ride forward, and reading or other close use of the eyes will sometimes be contributory. Persons with chronic infections of the sinuses and of the ears are more likely to suffer from airsickness than others.

The best and most effective drugs now available for prevention or treatment of motion sickness are Marezine, Bonamine, and Dramamine. Marezine does not bring on as much drowsiness as the other drugs and its effect is almost immediate. It lasts about four hours and should be taken fifteen minutes before departure. Bonamine lasts an entire day, but, like Dramamine, is apt to cause drowsiness. Dramamine is excellent for quieting the nerves and therefore of benefit to nervous travelers and persons with organic conditions in whom vomiting might be injurious. For severe cases of vomiting, the doctor may prescribe a combination of Dramamine and Marezine, which is administered in the form of rectal suppositories.

Several measures can be taken to help prevent motion sickness. When riding in smaller vehicles, sitting low near the center of gravity subjects the person to as little motion as possible. Children may sit on the floor of a car. In an airplane, a left-hand window should be avoided, since most turns and banks are made to the left. Rich, heavy, and gas-forming foods should not be eaten before beginning a trip. It is a good idea to eat moderately and not overload the stomach, and keep alcoholic beverages at a minimum. If symptoms of motion sickness appear during flight, the person should slide down the seat as far as possible with her head and neck supported. In severe cases of motion sickness, ample bed rest is advisable, and a plentiful intake of fluids, intravenously if necessary. The person susceptible to motion sickness should be kept warm, but make sure she gets plenty of fresh air at all times. Adequate sleep before and during the trip will also help stave off motion sickness.

mucous membranes. The lining of

passages and cavities that lead from the interior of the body and come in contact with air. They secrete a viscous fluid called mucus. The color of the mucous membranes and the amount of their moisture are valuable in diagnosis.

Müllerian ducts. Organs formed early in the female embryo that later become the Fallopian tubes, uterus, and vagina. The failure of the ducts to develop may cause a number of abnormalities, many of which are symptom-free.

multipara. A woman who has delivered two or more children.

multiple sclerosis. One of the commonest disorders of the nervous system. This disease is marked by interference with muscular movements which are finally lost. Degeneration and scarring of the nervous tissue develop slowly, and outward symptoms of multiple sclerosis appear only gradually over the years. Symptoms depend on how and where the nervous system is damaged. Frequently the first symptom is a gradual failure of the leg muscles. Leg movements become jerky and spastic and eventually paralysis occurs. Another common symptom is the slowing down of speech. The person talks in a monotone, and each syllable is uttered with great effort and difficulty. The hands tremble, especially when a purposeful movement is attempted. Sometimes, too, the head tends to shake. Those suffering with multiple sclerosis generally maintain a good frame of mind, even when the disease reaches an advanced state. Occasionally they become depressed and emotionally and mentally disturbed, but this is not characteristic.

The rate of development varies in all cases. However, eventually the basic functions, such as sight, hearing, and digestion, are involved, and constant nursing becomes a necessity. Sometimes this point is not reached for many years.

The adequacy of the care given can make a real difference. General and medical care must be properly given in order to secure any relief. Also, the patient can be protected from those conditions which are especially threatening to her condition.

Medical researchers are still working to determine whether or not a virus infection or inflammation coming from some toxin is responsible for multiple sclerosis. No organism has yet been found to which it can be attributed. There are instances in which the disease makes its appearance after childbirth or a major operation, but apparently this is a matter of coincidence. No special hereditary factor seems to be involved. It generally appears before the age of forty. Based on the concept that the cause may be autosensitization, treatments of injections of cortisone into the spinal fluid are tried.

mumps. An acute contagious disease of early winter and spring. It is more dangerous to adults than to children. Mumps usually attacks children between five and fifteen years of age and is rare among infants of less than ten months of age. While complications are serious, they occur in only about one out of a hundred cases. The commonest complications, according to a report of the U. S. Public Health Service, are "inflammation of the sex glands, sometimes causing sterility in men, and inflammation of the brain. Mumps may also lead to deafness, inflammation of other glands or kidney disease." However, mumps is usually such a mild disease that approximately a third of those who contract it recover without having definitely known that they have had it.

Mumps is caused by a tiny virus, the smallest form of infective organism.

Mumps is a communicable disease, though not as contagious as measles and chickenpox. The mumps virus is found in discharges of the nose and mouth, most frequently in the saliva, and is spread to others by personal contact or contaminated objects. Usually a person has mumps only once in a lifetime, since the first attack gives the body protective substances against subsequent attacks. Cases are known, however, in which the disease has occurred two or even three times.

The first symptoms of mumps appear from twelve to twenty-six, but usually eighteen, days after exposure. Usually pain under the ear is preceded by chills, fever, headache, and loss of appetite. Vomiting and nosebleeding may occur, with gradual swelling of the gland in front of and below the ear and along the angle of the jaw. The parotid gland of the cheek is the most commonly affected, and the technical term for mumps is parotitis. The face of the patient becomes puffy, and usually the swelling is confined to first one side of the face for a few days and later both sides. The pain increases when food is swallowed. The temperature may reach 101° to 104° during the second or third day. Fever and swelling will subside within a week or ten days.

While treatment of mumps is not specific, it is simple. The patient should be kept in bed. Her mouth must be kept clean, and an antiseptic mouthwash and gargle is of great value, especially when tonsils and throat congestion tend to aggravate the symptoms. Elimination of the bowels can be regulated with mild laxatives. A soft diet including broths, gruel, soft-boiled eggs, and custards, but especially liquid foods, is given while the temperature is about normal. Hot compresses, more soothing than cold, applied locally will make the patient more comfortable, as will sponging with hot water and keeping the face warm and protected from chills.

Isolation of all mumps patients is now recommended. Those persons who nurse them should keep away from their faces, since most infections come from the nose and mouth, and it is also advisable to wear a mask in the sickroom.

Fortunately, few persons die of mumps. The rare but dreaded complications usually develop as the swollen glands in the face subside. Pain and swelling may evolve in the testes of the male and, on rare occasions, in the ovaries and breasts of the female. A form of meningitis may result and middle-ear congestion may lead to deafness. Other exceptional complications which may occur in both sexes are pancreatitis, optic neuritis, facial paralysis, and permanent enlargement and dysfunction of the parotid gland.

In 1945, researchers, adapting the mumps virus to eggs, developed a mumps vaccine. It is not particularly significant for children who have not reached puberty, since mumps in children is usually mild, and therefore routine immunization is not recommended.

muscle cramps. *See* CRAMPS.

myasthenia gravis. A chronic disease of the nervous system, affecting the voluntary muscles and rendering them exceedingly weak and exhausted when they are used. The muscles of the eyes, face, neck, throat, tongue, and lips are especially involved, but others, like arm and leg muscles, may be affected later. In many cases, the person with myasthenia is so fatigued that she cannot hold anything in her hands, keep her eyes open, or even feed herself.

The development of the disease is gradual, but its onset may also be sudden. Early symptoms are general debility, weakness of one or the other voluntary muscles, double vision, difficulty in swallowing and chewing and talking.

Remission of the disease may occur for longer or shorter periods—as, for example, during pregnancy. In some cases, however, myasthenia gravis may prove rapidly fatal, and before the new treatments were developed was almost always fatal.

Myasthenia gravis usually begins in adulthood, but cases of affected babies have been known. Women are generally attacked in the early thirties and before the age of forty, much more often than men, whereas the incidence is higher in men in the later periods of life.

Medical science is still not certain of the cause of myasthenia. It may be stimulated by a deficiency in the transmissive connection between nerves and muscles. Enlarged thymus glands have been found in some sufferers and thus the disease has been associated with overactivity of the lymphatic tissues of the thymus gland. In young patients removal of the thymus gland has brought encouraging results. Some physicians have used X-ray treatment for the thymus gland, with some success. Most cases of myasthenia are helped by a drug, Neostigmine, which is administered first intravenously and later by mouth. In most cases this drug acts rapidly. Special exercises are used to strengthen the muscles of a patient. Sometimes Neostigmine is combined with potassium choloride, ephedrine sulfate, and other drugs.

myocardial infarction. *See* CORONARY THROMBOSIS.

myomectomy. Surgery which removes uterine fibroids but preserves the uterus.

myopia. Nearsightedness, an optical defect.

myxedema. A constitutional disorder, usually due to degeneration or absence of the thyroid gland, because of disease or surgical removal. The incidence of myxedema is much higher among adults between thirty-five and forty-five, principally women, than other age groups. The condition, therefore, has been called "acquired cretinism." Cretinism is a condition due to thyroid deficiency which is characterized by stunting of physical and mental development of children.

Juvenile myxedema, which usually afflicts children around puberty, is treated as a form of cretinism. Generally it is not as serious in its mental and physical consequences if treatment is instituted early enough.

Symptoms of myxedema develop slowly and many months may pass before they are distinct enough to be easily diagnosed. Some of the more significant symptoms are absence of perspiration, loss of hair, decay of teeth, general weakness, thickening of the skin of the nose and its mucous membranes, swelling of the lips, abnormal sensitivity to cold, a stiff walk, pronounced hoarseness, and often mental abnormalities.

Before treatment with thyroid was introduced, the chance of survival was usually low. The milder form of the disease can now be cured by administration of sufficient and graduated doses of thyroid gland extract.

Strict surveillance and hospitalization may be essential in the early period of treatment because of possible pronounced changes in the general condition of the patient during prolonged treatment with thyroid. Symptoms may disappear, one after another, after a short time, and the physical change in the patient's appearance will be remarkable. Continued administration of small doses of thyroid gland during the lifetime of the patient has been found essential to sustain the im-

provement. *See also* CRETINISM; THYROID GLAND.

nail biting. A behavior problem common among children and not unusual among adults. Children often put their fingers in their mouths unconsciously—for example, while reading a book or watching a motion picture when they are apparently calm. High-strung children will usually succumb to biting their nails more easily than calm ones. The reasons for a person to bite her nails are varied, including tenseness, lack of manual activity, or emotional disturbance. Scolding, nagging, threatening, shaming, or applying bad-tasting ointment or mechanical restraints to the fingers will aggravate rather than help overcome nail biting. More successful is an appeal to the pride or vanity or maturity of the girl. Sometimes a change in the parents' general attitude toward the child will make her feel more secure and subsequently stop biting her nails.

nails. The nails, located at the end of the fingers and toes, are elastic horny plates, composed of cells with abundant quantities of keratin, the basis of all horny tissue. They are thin, flattened, and slightly rounded at the edge. Concealed in the skin are the roots of the nails and the producer of the nails, the matrix. The thin and therefore white "half-moon" or lunula extends into the visible part or body of the nail. Average healthy fingernails grow about 1/30th of an inch a week and toenails about a fourth this speed. A healthy nail is pinkish, smooth, and naturally shiny. Temporary ridges or spots may be evident even in healthy persons.

Abnormal conditions in the strength, texture, color, brittleness, and growth of nails are indicative of the state of health of the body. Dark brown or blue spots may result from some undesirable condition, possibly an infection or inorganic poisoning. Pale and soft nails may occur from a deficiency of calcium, and nails with a bluish tinge sometimes indicate poor circulation. White spots are usually due to minor injuries or pressure, and repair, as in most nail conditions, is rapid if the matrix is not destroyed.

narcolepsy. Recurring sudden attacks of irresistible sleep. In some cases it may be accompanied by a cataplexy, or tonelessness of the muscles. Here the person has spells of muscular weakness, often following anger, laughter, fright, or a startling noise. The knees may give way and the person fall to the ground, but without loss of consciousness.

Narcolepsy occurs in persons suffering from certain brain diseases, and has also been known to develop after serious injury to the head. Some cases have been associated with tumors involving certain portions of the brain. In other instances, excessive sleepiness or ease of falling asleep has been part of a mental condition.

Narcolepsy usually occurs in people who are rather undynamic and lethargic. The person with narcolepsy generally manages to stay awake while working at something that interests her, but when left alone or when lying down she quickly falls asleep. Persons with narcolepsy have even been known to sleep while standing in a bus. Narcolepsy is sometimes also associated with a condition of hunger called bulimia. Few people die of narcolepsy, unless as a result of an accident.

In treatment of narcolepsy, amphetamine, or Benzedrine, has been found useful in preventing the attack of sleep. People who are subject to certain forms of heart symptoms, such as palpitations, tremulousness, and internal tension, as a result of taking Benzedrine may take Dexedrine. In especially severe cases of cataplexy, potassium chloride is given. These drugs are powerful and should never be used unless prescribed by a doctor.

nearsightedness. *See* EYE; MYOPIA.

neoplasm. An abnormal growth of body tissue. It may be benign or malignant.

nephritis. Inflammation of the kidneys. Like Bright's disease, with which it is often considered synonymous, this term actually covers not one but a group of disorders with similar symptoms. Albumin is almost always present in the urine. Dropsy is another condition in which a breakdown in the excretory system of the kidneys causes the retention of liquid and swelling in various parts of the body.

Several different kidney disturbances are distinguished, each with a special technical name, a few of which are acute and chronic glomerulonephritis, chronic pyelonephritis, and arteriolar nephrosclerosis.

Nephritis is a condition made more

severe by pregnancy. Spontaneous abortion is common. The treatment is bed rest in a hospital with careful observation.

Nephritis is a major health problem. More than 100,000 people annually die of nephritis in the United States. This is 7 per cent of all deaths, making it the fourth greatest cause of death.

The discovery of albuminuria, or albumin in the urine, is a symptom which must not be regarded lightly, because nephritis is detected most easily and quickly by the discovery of albumin in the urine, which may have grave consequences. Albuminuria, which may be found during a general medical examination, must always be followed immediately by further study. Albuminuria by itself does not necessarily or inevitably point to nephritis. It may be found in persons who do not have other symptoms and in many whose kidneys are affected but not sufficiently to justify a diagnosis of nephritis.

The first symptom of nephritis may be detection of albumin in the urine or a vague feeling of illness or minor disturbances of other functions, such as a slight elevation in blood pressure. Unusual fatigue and listlessness, diminished appetite and headaches may be manifest. As the disorder progresses, a typical train of events usually ensues. The sight is slightly disturbed. The need to urinate at night may interrupt sleep. Weight may be either lost or, with waterlogging of tissues, gained. Gradually more serious symptoms appear, including nausea, sometimes diarrhea, vomiting, and enlarge-

ment of the abdomen due to fluid associated with lung and liver congestion. As the condition becomes more severe, unconsciousness and convulsions may supervene.

Acute nephritis or glomerulonephritis ordinarily has a rapid course, but if treatment is sufficiently early and adequate, fatality is rare. Typically a disease of young adults and of children, this is the form of kidney disorder most frequently called Bright's disease; the exact cause is unknown. Secondary effects of infection elsewhere in the body caused particularly by streptococci are frequently suspected to be the primary source. The kidneys themselves, however, are not infected nor can the specific organisms be found in them. Toxic substances such as certain metals can incite acute nephritis.

When kidney inflammation is suspected, the urine should be examined without delay. If albumin is present it will collect and coagulate when tested with heat or strong acid. In nephritis, examination of the urine will also show red blood cells and tiny molds of the minute tubes in the kidneys, which may be composed of any of numerous substances; these are called hyaline, granular or blood casts, or some other name. Urine tests are essential not only as an initial diagnostic aid but also to trace the progress of the disease. Acute nephritis may persist for a few weeks or some months, but usually terminates in eight to ten weeks.

Acute nephritis was formerly considered a fatal disease. Actually, however, about 90 per cent of those who have nephritic symptoms get well, with prompt diagnosis and adequate treatment. The other 10 per cent tend to become eventually chronically nephritic.

Rather than a specific remedy, treatment of nephritis demands adherence to certain basic procedures which assist the body to overcome the disease. The primary objective is elimination of the condition before it becomes chronic. Usually the acute disease is amenable to treatment, whereas a full return to normal from the chronic type is infrequent.

When acute nephritis eventually becomes chronic, a transitional stage, called nephrosis, may intervene. The manifestations include reduced amount of urine, high urine albumin, general edema, and fluid in the abdominal and chest cavities. This may persist for weeks or years, and is best treated in a hospital where the complicated tests of internal conditions on which prescription of treatment depends can be made most easily and satisfactorily.

Any person whose urine has revealed albumin should have a general medical checkup at least once a year. The kidneys possess great reserve power. Even when substantial parts of them no longer function the remaining healthy portions maintain a necessary minimum activity. *See also* KIDNEYS.

nephrosis. Any degeneration of the kidney without signs of inflammation, one of the commonest chronic diseases of children and one of the least understood. It produces serious disturbances of other bodily functions as well as that of the kidney. The fluid that should be passed on through the kidneys to the bladder for disposal is instead distributed throughout the body, causing swellings called edema. The face is so badly swollen that the eyes are almost closed. The stomach may be distended to about twice its normal size and the swelling extend down to the feet.

Frequently a few days or weeks or months after the illness is first observed, the child will pass a large quantity of urine and her swelling will disappear within a few days. This is known as diuresis and it may occur spontaneously and frequently throughout the course of the disease, although there is no consistent pattern. The edema-free period following diuresis may last only a few days, several weeks, or even months, or it may be permanent. Complete recovery rarely occurs in less than two years after the onset of the disease and sometimes much longer. Why nephrosis disappears has not yet been explained. A low-salt diet and ACTH or cortisone seem to have been the prime factors in helping some patients. Formerly approximately 50 per cent of all nephrotic children died. New methods of treatment have reduced this rate to some degree. Many of the deaths have not occurred as a direct result of the disease, but from peritonitis or other infections to which these children are highly susceptible. Today these infections are usually controlled by antibiotics.

After the child has returned from the hospital, every possible precaution should continue to be taken against infections, since even tonsillitis may lead to fatal complications. The psychological well-being of the patient is also significant, and her life should be as normal as possible. *See also* KIDNEYS.

nervous breakdown. A popular, inexact term which covers a wide variety of mental disorders. Any form of mental or emotional difficulty, from the mildest anxiety state to the most severe form of insanity, can be called "nervous breakdown" by the layman. Since the term is so broad as to elude definition, it is never really applicable to any condition.

nervous system. The entire nervous apparatus of the body. It controls all muscular movements, both voluntary and involuntary; is responsible for thought processes; regulates such body functions as circulation, respiration, digestion, and elimination; and conducts pain and other sensations to the brain.

Certain drugs, like bromides and the new tranquilizers, may diminish the activity of the nerve cells. Other drugs can increase activity. Similar effects are produced by the toxins of various disease germs. In some cases nerve cells may be killed. Physical injury can also damage nerve tissue.

Nerve cells weakened by inflammation may recover if the damaging cause is removed, but nerve cells that are destroyed, as in poliomyelitis, cannot be replaced.

Sclerosis is the name given to a fibrous change of the supporting tissue in the brain or spinal cord. Nervous tissue may be converted into a fibrous mass, and may also be damaged by pressure from tumors from within or from tumors or other swellings in adjoining tissue.

Poor nutrition may weaken nerve tissue. Degenerative softening of nervous tissue is caused by deprivation of the blood supply. Disorders of the endocrine glands may also upset nerve cell metabolism. If a nerve is blocked, loss of sensation and paralysis and wasting of muscles ensues. Diseases affecting the brain are dangerous to the nerve centers. These include centers for the heart, respiration, blood pressure, and others. *See also* ATAXIA; BRAIN; MULTIPLE SCLEROSIS; NEURALGIA; NEURITIS; PARALYSIS; POLIOMYELITIS; SCIATIC NEURITIS; SPINAL CORD; SYMPATHETIC NERVOUS SYSTEM.

neuralgia. Means pain in a nerve, and the term implies that the pain is felt along the nerve or the part of the body supplied by it without any corresponding physical changes.

There are many different types of neuralgia, depending on the nerve involved. Nerves especially apt to become irritable and produce severe pain are the brachial nerve in the arm, the intercostal nerves running between the ribs, the nerves of the scalp, and the sciatic nerve. The fifth cranial nerve, also known as the trigeminal nerve, which supplies the forehead, face, and jaw, is most often affected with neuralgia. The nerve may be so sensitive that even a cold current blowing on the face or a light touch of a finger to the face causes stabbing pain.

In severe cases of neuralgia, or when medical treatment fails, a surgical operation which destroys the nerve roots usually gives permanent relief and involves little risk, even for elderly persons. In neuralgia affecting any nerve, the doctor first determines the nerve area involved and then takes steps to prevent the sensation of pain from traveling along that nerve. To do this, he may use sedative drugs, inject local anesthetics or alcohol, or treat the nerves with X-rays. Diagnosis is more difficult in those cases in which the sensations of pain are mental rather than physical in origin. *See also* TIC DOULOUREUX.

neuritis. Inflammation of a nerve or of a nerve sheath. In neuritis, pain and tenderness are felt over an area supplied by the particular nerve affected. It may be limited to one nerve or affect several, as in multiple neuritis or polyneuritis. Neuritis of the optic nerve can cause temporary or even permanent blindness.

Other symptoms of neuritis include loss of feeling or disturbance of sensation and sometimes paralysis, so that it is impossible to move the affected area. Many different causes of neuritis are recognized. Some types result from frostbite, dislocation, poor posture in sleep, drugs or injections, cold or radiation treatment. Neuritis occurs in cases of chronic alcoholism, arsenic or lead poisoning, with or following diabetes, in infectious diseases like diphtheria or malaria, in rheumatism and occasionally in influenza. It can also be present in cases of nutritional deficiencies, especially when vitamin B is deficient, as in beriberi.

Treatment of neuritis depends on the doctor's diagnosis of the underlying cause, and the treatment is directed toward removing that cause. For relief of pain, analgesic drugs and barbiturate sedatives are given. Limiting movement of limbs and providing rest, followed by moderate movement, is helpful. During the acute phase, heat also helps to alleviate pain. Other specific measures, such as diet adjustment, which may include vitamin B supplements, may be prescribed by the doctor as the individual case demands. *See also* SCIATIC NEURITIS.

neurosis. An emotional disorder, but without a severe accompanying personality change. It refers to the type of adjustment a person has made to situations which she unconsciously feels may cause her anxiety. The type of adjustment constitutes the nature of the neurosis. The cause is usually attributed to the existence within the person of an emotional conflict, contradictory desires, usually of a highly complex nature.

Several types of neurotic reaction can be identified, all of which are an attempt by the person to shield herself from her inner conflict. In the depressive reaction, the person experiences a general sense of physical and mental inertia, marked by an attitude of general pessimism, self-deprecation, and self-absorption. The neurotic depression is provoked by seemingly nothing, or if it is a response to a particular event—for example, the death of a friend—it becomes exaggerated and lengthy and eventually seems to exist for itself.

Amnesia is an extreme type of dissociative reaction. Here the person loses awareness of who she is for a time, in order to protect herself from some unpleasant situation. She literally refuses to be herself. Unlike delirium states, a person who has suffered from amnesia can recall under hypnosis events which occurred during the time, although consciously she cannot.

In conversion reaction, the person, rather than face a painful situation, imagines that she has some physical disorder, such as blindness or inability to move one arm. Since she usually has no knowledge of body function, the symptoms she describes are often inaccurate. This used to be called hysteria.

In phobic reaction, the person develops an intense fear of some particular thing, such as water or cats. This object becomes a substitute or symbol for her inner anxiety and since she can usually avoid the object, she can thus avoid her anxiety.

These and other neurotic reactions constitute an elaborate defense which the person sets up to protect herself from acknowledging some inner emotional trouble. They operate as safety mechanisms which allow the person to cope with and adjust to her environment. Thus she stays in contact with reality, as opposed to a psychotic person, who undergoes severe personality disorder and loss of contact with reality. *See also* AMNESIA; INVOLUTIONAL MELANCHOLIA; MANIC-DEPRESSIVE PSYCHOSIS; PARANOIA; PSYCHOANALYSIS; SCHIZOPHRENIA.

nevus. A congenital discoloration, a birthmark.

night terrors. Children sometimes experience nightmares which are intensely disturbing to them. Physical factors, such as indigestion, intestinal worms, adenoids, or febrile disorders, may be the cause; but more often night terrors occur in emotionally disturbed children, and if they recur, the child should probably receive psychiatric help.

nipple. The small protuberance on the breast from which, in females, the milk glands discharge. It contains erectile tissue and is surrounded by a brownish or pink area called the areola.

During pregnancy, nipples should be washed well with soap and water. If excessively dry, they may be massaged with cold cream or lanolin. During nursing, they may become sore and cracked due to the infant's chewing.

node. A protuberance or swelling, a knot or knob.

noma. A very serious form of gangrene of the vulva or the cheek. It requires immediate attention.

nosebleed. *See* EPISTAXIS.

nursing. Care of the sick, wounded, or infirm. Good nursing in sickness can hasten recovery, prevent complications, and perhaps even save a life. Often just keeping the patient as comfortable as possible and in good spirits is of great significance.

The nurse may help select and prepare the room where the patient will be, seeing that it is clean and properly ventilated, with all excess furniture and decorations removed. She will make the bed each day, and in between keep it smooth and tidy. In most cases she will wash the patient once a day with warm water and soap, washing and drying only one part of the body at a time, with the rest covered. If the patient cannot be completely washed each day, his face and arms should be kept clean. The teeth and mouth should be cleansed several times a day. As in a hospital, the usual time for full toilet is in the morning, about an hour before breakfast.

The temperature of the sickroom should be moderate, and kept as even as possible. Good ventilation is essential; if windows are opened, a screen should be used to prevent air from blowing directly on the patient. *See also* BED SORES; CONVALESCENCE.

nymphomania. The excessive desire of a woman for sexual gratification. This manifests itself in an insatiate urge for sexual intercourse. Since the causes of the condition are emotional, psychotherapy is necessary.

obesity. A condition in which excessive fat is stored in the body, due to a positive energy balance. Usually obesity comes from overeating. Far less common is obesity resulting from an organic disease or deficiency which occurs because of disturbance of the pituitary or thyroid glands. Obesity also results from changes in the secretions of the sex organs, as occurs in pregnancy and in menopause.

A tendency to obesity seems inherent in certain races and in families, but for the most part it is individual and directly related to the rate of intake of food and the use of that food to supply energy to the body. The unused food is stored as fat and deposited in parts of the body which usually are first to show excessive fatness, such as hips, stomach, breasts, and buttocks. Fat may also be stored around important internal organs—for example, the heart and liver—and interfere with the proper functioning of the organs.

As well as being unattractive and uncomfortable, obesity is dangerous to health, especially in middle age and thereafter, when it is increasingly difficult to correct. An obese person tends to fatigue and shortness of breath; there is a strain on the joints of the feet and legs, with a consequent predisposition to flat feet and to osteoarthritis of the knees and lower back. Heart disturbances, diseases of the pancreas and kidneys, gall bladder and certain cancers are more common in the fat person, as well as diabetes, which presents special problems among obese persons. The mortality rate in surgery is higher and the general life span is shorter.

In the great number of cases, the body weight can be reduced by modification of the diet. Foods containing starches and sugar are limited and fats virtually eliminated. Emphasis is placed on fruits and vegetables, which may be eaten in large quantities to give a feeling of satiety and supply vital mineral salts and vitamins without adding large numbers of calories. Drastic reducing diets, or "fad" reducing diets are seldom satisfactory for any length of time and a diet which can be sustained over a long period should be selected. Gradual reduction of weight is better than rapid reduction and usually not more than two pounds a week should be lost.

A reducing program that includes drugs or reducing salts should never be undertaken without the advice of a doctor, since drugs, such as amphetamine, which discourage appetite have a stimulating effect which may cause insomnia, and thyroid extract, unless obesity is directly related to thyroid deficiency, may produce serious effects on the heart and nervous system.

The biggest problem in weight reduction is sustaining the weight loss. In many cases the person gradually gains back the pounds lost. To be able to maintain the correct weight often requires a whole new attitude toward food, a re-education of taste. The emotional factors relating to obesity have received special study and it has been discovered that many fat people eat as a compensation for some dissatisfaction in their lives.

olfactory sense. The sense of smell, which depends on the system of nerves and specialized tissue known as the olfactory nervous system.

oligospermia. A cause of infertility in men, usually the result of their occupation. Jobs which expose men to strong chemicals or X-rays may cause defective sperm.

omentum. A large membrane covering the lower part of the stomach and hanging down in apron fashion over the coils of the intestine. It is part of the peritoneum, the membrane lining the interior of the abdominal cavity and surrounding the contained soft organs, and is a storage place for fat. The omentum

may be involved in hernia and require surgery. *See also* PERITONITIS.

onychia. Inflammation of the matrix of the nail, resulting in the loss of the nail. *See also* NAILS.

oophorectomy. Surgical removal of the ovary because of inflammation or for similar conditions.

ophthalmia. Severe inflammation of the eye, especially the conjunctiva, the mucous membrane covering the anterior part of the globe of the eye. *See also* CONJUNCTIVITIS; EYE; PINKEYE.

optic nerve. The second cranial nerve connecting the retina of the eye with the brain. It conducts the sensory impulses of sight. *See also* EYE.

orchitis. Inflammation of the testicles, the sex glands of the male (the prefix "orchi-" refers to the testicle). The condition is characterized by swelling, pain, and a sensation of heaviness in these organs. Various infectious organisms, including those of gonorrhea, syphilis, or tuberculosis, may cause orchitis. In many cases of mumps, in young men from fifteen to twenty-five years of age, the infection spreads to the testicles.

orgasm. The climax of sexual excitement, during which the sense of pleasure is at its height. It is followed by a period of relaxation and a feeling of fulfillment. In the female, ejaculation of fluid may or may not take place. However, the inability to come to climax may be overcome, being largely due, in many cases, to mental causes rather than physical. In the normal male, ejaculation of semen accompanies an orgasm. *See also* IMPOTENCE.

orthodontia. The branch of dentistry

concerned with malocclusion, or deviation from normal alignment of the teeth.

Orthonovim. Brand name for one of the oral contraceptives.

osteitis. Or ostitis, inflammation of the bone. In common practice, osteitis refers to inflammation of the dense shafts of long bones, the spongy portion of the ends of the long bones, or the tissue of the short or flat bones.

Tuberculosis is a common cause of osteitis, but it may also be produced by various organisms, such as the staphylococci. Some degree of osteitis will also be found in such bone disorders as osteomyelitis.

Paget's disease, also known as osteitis deformans, begins in the bone marrow, spreads to other portions of the long bones, and also affects the skull. The sacrum, pelvis, and lower extremities are also involved. The long bones lengthen and thicken, often becoming twice their normal size. At the same time, they soften and become bowed where weight is placed on them. The skull grows progressively larger.

Outside of neuralgic pains and headache, the health of the person is unaffected. The disease generally occurs between the ages of forty and sixty, and is rarely fatal. However, other complications such as spontaneous fracture, secondary anemia, and bone sarcoma may cause death. Paget's disease is of unknown origin, and no positive treatment for it has as yet been found.

osteomyelitis. Certain pus-forming germs, and sometimes those of tuberculosis, pneumonia, or typhoid fever, produce infection in the bones which is known as osteomyelitis. Though the germs may enter from infected tissues close to the bone, usually they are carried by the bloodstream.

Osteomyelitis may appear in any bone of the body, but is more common in the leg and arm bones. The greatest danger arises when this infection attacks the jawbone.

Osteomyelitis in its early stages often gives an inflamed and swollen appearance at the point of infection, and a blood test will reveal an increase in the number of white blood cells. Fever and rapid pulse are also present, pain is felt in the bone, and sensitivity in the diseased area is likely to be great.

osteopathy. A system of treatment of disease by manipulation of bones, joints, and other body tissues. It is based on the theory that the body is a mechanical organism whose structures and functions are co-ordinate and interdependent and that a disturbance of either constitutes disease. The theory also holds that when the structure of the body mechanism is normal, environmental conditions favorable, and nutrition adequate, the body is capable of making its own remedies against disease and other toxic states.

otitis. Inflammation of the ear which can involve the outer ear, the passage to the drum and the outer surface of the eardrum itself, and the middle ear. Rarely is the innermost ear affected in this type of inflammation. Otitis can be acute or chronic. *See also* DEAFNESS; EAR; MASTOID.

otosclerosis. A chronic disorder of

the ear in which spongy bone forms in the capsule of the labyrinth of the ear and the small bones lose their power to conduct sound. The exact cause of otosclerosis is unknown. Tests have been made to determine whether or not it is hereditary, due to vitamin deficiency or to failure of glandular function, but none of these has been conclusive enough to establish the underlying cause.

Otosclerosis affects women more often than men. Frequently the first sign is an annoying ringing in the ears, and a gradual and progressive loss of hearing. It may affect only one ear at first, but eventually both ears become involved. Sometimes enough hearing is retained for the person to follow ordinary conversation, but in other cases it is necessary for her to use a hearing aid or learn to lip read.

Various types of treatments are used in otosclerosis, including careful control of diet, vitamin supplements, drugs to allay the ringing sensation, glandular extracts to correct glandular failure, and surgical procedures. One positive treatment is the Lempert operation in which a window is drilled from the outer healthy bony structure into the inner ear. Fenestration, as this method of surgery is called, has been successful in a great number of cases, but is usually only possible when the nerves are unimpaired. Another operation, sometimes called the Rosen operation, restores movement to the stapes, one of the three small bones which make contact with the eardrum. *See also* DEAFNESS; EAR.

ovarian pain. Ovarian pain is actually uterine pain that is referred. It sometimes follows childbirth or abortion and may reflect a disorder in the ovary.

ovaries. The two sex glands of women. They lie in the lower part of the abdomen and perform two essential functions: they germinate the female reproductive or egg cells, one of which passes through the Fallopian tube to the uterus every month; and they provide internal secretions or hormones which influence most feminine physical characteristics and which are related to the reproductive process.

The hormone estrogen determines the familiar feminine attributes; it causes both external and internal sex organs to grow to adult size and the development of the typical figure with lines softened by a layer of fat under the skin.

The other hormone secreted by the ovaries, progesterone, causes changes in the uterus and prepares it to receive the fertilized egg cell. Progesterone is secreted approximately for only a week, or a little more, each month after the egg cell has been released by the ovary.

The female phenomenon, menopause or change of life, is bound intimately with the discontinuance of these hormones. When ova are no longer released each month progesterone is no longer developed. Gradually the estradiol diminishes and finally ceases. Estrogen normally is produced from the second until approximately the fifth decade. Endocrine disorders can cause changes in younger women similar to those of menopause.

Removal of the ovaries because of infection or for some other reason results in the termination of the hormones and causes definite bodily changes regardless of age. One of the great advances in medicine has been the discovery of the exact chemical character of the hormones and the method of extracting them from natural substances or of manufacturing them artificially. Now these are substituted for those hormones lost. The removal of one, or part of one, ovary has no such effects.

One of the principal disorders of the ovary is the formation of cysts, sacs which contain liquid material of glandular origin of various kinds which may grow to considerable size. If the cyst remains small, difficulty may not ensue, but if it enlarges it must be removed surgically.

The ovaries may be affected by growth other than cysts, such as tumors and cancers. Since the physician cannot ascertain the exact nature of such a growth by external examination, an operation is usually necessary in order to determine the type of growth involved and the proper course to be pursued.

Infection may reach the ovaries through the Fallopian tubes, the passages which each month ordinarily carry the egg cell into the uterus. Gonorrhea, streptococcal and tuberculous infections are common. Fever and pain as well as swelling may be relieved quickly by application of heat or cold, with a hot-water bottle, heating pad, or ice pack. Sulfa and antibiotic drugs used under the doctor's direction usually are effective. However, the infection may not respond to treatment and the removal of the ovary or the Fallopian tube by surgery may be necessary.

Another ovarian disorder is caused by strain, stretching, and twisting of the tissues which fasten the ovary to the abdominal wall. The affected ovary may stop functioning temporarily and as a result its blood supply may be interrupted or the ovarian ligaments themselves, as they are called, may be involved. Surgery is sometimes required to correct this condition.

ovulation. The process in which the egg or ovum is released from the Graafian follicle of the ovary. In the sexually mature female, ovulation occurs every twenty-eight days. This cycle ordinarily produces only one egg at a time; infrequently it produces two or more eggs which can result in multiple birth. Following ovulation the egg enters the Fallopian tube where fertilization by the male sperm takes place following intercourse. If fertilization does not occur, the egg undergoes degeneration and a new cycle begins. Failure to ovulate results in sterility. *See also* CONTRACEPTION; MENSTRUATION; OVARIES; STERILITY.

ovum. The egg cell which, when fertilized, is capable of developing into an organism similar to its parents. Maturity is simultaneous with ovulation and occurs approximately two weeks before the next menstrual cycle.

oxygen. A colorless, odorless, gaseous element which constitutes about one-fifth of the volume of the atmosphere. Formerly used by physicians only in life-and-death emergencies, today oxygen is used frequently in the treatment of many diseases.

Among modern mechanisms employed are the incubators for premature infants as well as oxygen rooms and oxygen tents. Many of these devices involve the danger of fire and explosions unless they are supervised by experts.

Generally speaking, oxygen is prescribed for all patients who either cannot breathe easily, or who, for some reason, are suffering from a limited supply of air. Such a need arises, for example, in pneumonia or carbon monoxide poisoning.

ozena. Or atrophic rhinitis, a disease affecting the mucous membrane of the nose and characterized by an extremely offensive odor. A gradual degeneration of the nasal membrane is followed by discharge of matter and formation of large foul-smelling crusts. The sense of smell is affected so that the person himself is unaware of the odor coming from the nose. The interior of the nose is dry and the internal structure so affected as to make the airway through the nose unusually wide. Continuous coughing and hacking to clear the passages of the crusts which get into the throat also occur.

Ozena, which was once quite common, especially among young girls, has largely disappeared. However, ozena may affect children in whom an early nasal infection has gone untreated and atrophy of the nasal membrane followed by symptoms of ozena may result from negligence.

Paget's disease. Two separate and distinct disorders are named Paget's disease. One of the disorders is osteitis deformans, a disease of the bones, which is discussed under osteitis, and the other is Paget's disease of the nipple.

Paget's disease of the nipple is a cancer of the breast. It generally affects only one breast and is manifested by redness and dryness of the nipple, cracks and ulceration. The nipple is usually tender and frequently there is an abnormal discharge. Cancer of the breast is ordinarily detected a year or two after the nipple is affected, which in most cases is considered an early warning sign. *See also* BREAST; CANCER; OSTEITIS.

pain. A disturbed sensation, causing suffering or distress. Pain is produced by irritation of the trunk, root, or terminal of a sensory nerve. Nerve endings in the skin are also sensitive to touch, heat, and cold as well as pain. Pain may be considered a protective mechanism in that it directs attention to some disturbance in the body.

Pain varies with the cause and among different people, some persons being more sensitive to it than others. Pain may be described as boring, gnawing, cutting, burning, throbbing, and in other ways. The description of the type of pain often helps to determine its cause—for example, a throbbing pain is associated with suppuration. The situation or point of origin is an even better indication of its cause. However, the area of the pain may be misleading, as in the case of a referred pain in the temple resulting from a bad tooth, or a pain in the back of the shoulder caused by irritation of the liver. The system whereby pain originates in the nerve endings and is channeled into the spinal cord and up into the brain may also cause pain to be felt in tissue that has been removed—as, for example, a pain in a leg which has been amputated.

Pain which is entirely mental in origin is called psychogenic pain. Frequently it is vague and irregular and the person often exaggerates in describing it. The pain usually disappears when the mental cause has been erased. *See also* ACUTE ILLNESS, ACUTE PAIN.

palate. The roof of the mouth. It is composed of the hard palate and a soft palate. *See also* CLEFT PALATE.

pallor. When the physician notices extreme paleness in a patient, his examination will be for anemia.

palsy. *See* PARALYSIS AGITANS.

pancreas. One of the vital organs of the body, ranking in importance with the liver. It is situated in the abdominal region, behind the stomach, close to the liver and gall bladder with which it shares a common duct leading into the duodenum, the first part of the small intestine. The pancreas is about six inches long, yellowish in color, soft, with a head, body, and tail.

The pancreas performs two distinct functions. The first is to secrete the pancreatic juice into the intestinal tract. This fluid is one of the chief chemical aids in digestion, containing certain enzymes essential in the digestion of starch, proteins, and fats. The pancreas also acts as an endocrine gland, secreting insulin directly into the bloodstream. Insulin is valuable in the regulation of blood sugar levels and in the conversion of sugar into heat and energy.

Insulin is produced by the part of the pancreas known as the Islets of Langerhans, groups of specialized cells found scattered throughout the organ. A disorder of the pancreas which cuts down the production of insulin results in the disease known as diabetes mellitus. Tumors may also develop in the Islets of Langerhans and cause an overproduction of insulin. This combined with an insufficiency of blood sugar gives the symptoms of an overdose of insulin and may include coma, convulsions, or periodic attacks of fatigue and shortness of breath. Surgery to remove these tumors is the most effective method of controlling the condition.

The pancreas may be affected by infection of the gall bladder, the bile duct, or stomach, and jaundice may result from such inflammation. If cancer is involved, it may also produce jaundice.

Acute damage of the pancreas may occur from direct invasion of the organ by bacteria, or by blockage of the pancreatic duct resulting in the retention of powerful digestive ferments. Violent symptoms may develop suddenly in the abdomen, including severe pain, vomiting, hemorrhage, paleness, and shock.

While surgery was once the first step in treating acute pancreatic infection, current management resembles that practiced in other hemorrhagic acute gastrointestinal disorders. The patient is put to bed and blood transfusions are given. Intravenous feeding is begun and continued until the acute stage is passed. Surgery is avoided in this stage, and pancreatic secretions are inhibited by nasal suction from the stomach. Drugs to relieve pain are given, and in some cases blockage of the nerves is effected. When the condition warrants, the patient is placed on a bland diet, as in cases of duodenal ulcer. *See also* DIABETES; INSULIN; JAUNDICE.

papilloma. Growths like small tumors. Ovarian papillomas sometimes reach large size and must be removed surgically.

paralysis. Temporary or permanent loss of muscle function, sensation, or voluntary motion, usually caused by injury to nerves or destruction of nerve cells which control the function of the affected muscles or muscle tissue. An example of paralysis is the cutting of a motor nerve, as may happen in injury to the wrist or forearm. The muscles supplied by the nerve cease to function and begin to degenerate. Unless the cut ends are successfully joined together by surgery and unless nerve fibers grow into the old nerve trunk, these muscles will be permanently inactive.

Damage to nerve cells or fibers may be caused by disease, pressure, or destructive injury to the brain or spinal cord, any of which may produce partial or total paralysis of several muscles. Paralysis due to brain damage is most likely to be a stiff or spastic type, and paralysis due to damage to the cells in the spinal cord is generally a limp flaccid kind.

Specific terms are used to describe various types of paralysis. Paralysis of both arms and both legs is called quadriplegia. Paralysis of one side of the body is hemiplegia. Diplegia is paralysis of similar parts on each side of the body. Monoplegia is paralysis of a single arm or leg or a single muscle or group of muscles, such as those on one side of the face. Paralysis of both legs is paraplegia.

As well as being caused by injury to the brain, spinal cord, or nerves, paralysis can be brought about by embolism, thrombosis, or brain hemorrhage, known as apoplexy or stroke. Tumors and various progressive diseases and degenerations can affect the spinal cord and produce various types of "creeping paralysis." Various forms of neuritis affect the muscle through the nerves and cause a temporary paralysis. Paralysis which is mental in origin occasionally occurs, as in hysteria. *See also* APOPLEXY; CEREBRAL PALSY; PARAPLEGIA; POLIOMYELITIS; STROKE.

paralysis agitans. A disease distinguished by muscular weakness and trembling of parts of the body at rest. Scientifically the condition is known as paralysis agitans, and it is also called Parkinson's disease or shaking palsy. The disorder is typically one of elderly people, striking mostly persons in their sixties and seventies. On rare occasions brain inflammation, such as encephalitis, may cause a similar disturbance.

Paralysis agitans ordinarily affects first a single arm or leg, then the second limb on the same side, and finally those on the other side. Often an arm first betrays symptoms by losing the typical swing that accompanies walking, and the face begins to lack its customary expressiveness and changes slowly or not at all with passing moods. Involvement of the limbs is followed by that of the trunk muscles, which gives the body a stooping posture. Steps become shorter and more rapid and develop into a combination of a shuffle and run. The rate at which the disease advances varies in different persons. Often it progresses slowly, leaving the health good in other respects. Intervals as long as a year may occur between the phases of development from one limb to another.

Changes in the brain, in other nerve tissue, and in blood vessels of the brain have been observed in association with paralysis agitans.

Treatment of paralysis agitans is usually limited to relief of symptoms, to efforts to keep the patient comfortable, to maintaining his general health and thus to endeavoring to retard the progress of the disease.

Drugs of the belladonna type reduce rigidity; they may be administered in various ways to give relief. Baths and massage relieve the tensions in the muscles and are soothing to the skin.

Operative procedures have been developed which diminish the circulation of blood to the areas in the brain concerned with the tremors. Success has been reported in many cases of paralysis agitans.

paranoia. A rare psychosis characterized by delusions of persecution and often hallucinations, usually of an auditory type. Contact with reality is still maintained, but it is distorted. The paranoid person feels that a person or group is persecuting her, perhaps trying to kill her. Often this intense fear and suspicion is combined with excessive but unrealized ambitions and delusions of grandeur. The paranoid person blames the "persecutor" for her failure. In the true type of paranoia, one thing becomes the "persecutor," rather than the person being suspicious of everything, and this thing dominates the person's life.

paraplegia. Paralysis of the lower limbs, due to severe injury to the spine or spinal cord. It may result from a severe blow to the spinal cord, fracture or dislocation of the spinal column, or from bullet or knife wounds.

parathyroid glands. The four small glandular bodies attached to the back of the thyroid gland in the neck, two lying on each side. Together they are about the size of a small bean and are the smallest glands of internal secretion.

The function of their secretion or hormone is to regulate the use of calcium and phosphorus in the body. When the glands are underactive and the quantity of the secretion deficient, the amount of calcium in the blood drops and the amount of phosphorus increases, eventually producing tetany, a spontaneous muscle spasm. Overactivity of the glands results in withdrawal of too much calcium and phosphorus from the bones, rendering them soft and fragile.

When tetany occurs as a result of underaction of the parathyroids, the muscles have a tendency to go into painful prolonged spasms; tingling, numbness, and sometimes twitching may accompany the spasm. The forearms and hands are most often affected; the throat is the most troublesome part. The muscles eventually become abnormally sensitive to stimuli. People with tetany frequently are subject to nervousness and emotional depression. Tetany often results from inadvertent removal of the parathyroid glands, which are so small that they can be unknowingly removed or destroyed during a surgical operation on the thyroid gland.

paresis. Persons who have had syphilis over a period of time sometimes develop in later years a condition known as paresis. It is also called general paralysis, general paresis, general paralysis of the insane or dementia paralytica, or paretic neurosyphilis. The syphilis has infected the brain and coverings of the brain, resulting in a tissue damage sufficient to cause paralysis and mental disturbance. Paresis is three to five times more frequent in men than women. *See also* SYPHILIS.

Parkinson's disease. *See* PARALYSIS AGITANS.

Parry's disease. A name given to toxic goiter. It is also called Graves' disease and Basedow's disease. *See also* GOITER.

parturition. The act of giving birth to a child. *See also* PREGNANCY AND PRENATAL CARE.

patch test. An allergy test in which a small patch of adhesive containing a substance to which a person may be sensitive is applied to the skin. The appearance of redness and inflammation is considered to be positive proof of such sensitivity. *See also* ALLERGY.

pediatrician. A specialist in children's diseases. His special field is called pediatrics.

pediculosis. *See* BODY LICE.

pellagra. A dietary deficiency disease, once prevalent in the United States, especially in the South. It is due to malnutrition and is caused by a diet deficient in, among other essential vitamins and minerals, nicotinic acid or niacin, which is absolutely vital for growth and health of the human body. Symptoms of pellagra are chiefly inflammation of the mouth, redness and soreness of the tongue, secondary cracking of the skin and ulceration around the mouth. The skin of the back of the hands and the forearms may become red and thickened, and the neck and chest are sometimes similarly involved. The alimentary tract is affected and diarrhea, vomiting, and loss of appetite appear. Other symptoms may be headache, irritability, anxiety, muscular weakness, and—in extreme cases—melancholia and dementia.

pelvis. A basin-shaped ring of bones at the base of the trunk, joining the spine and the legs. The gaps in the skeletal structure are filled with muscles and membranes, actually forming a closed basin.

The female pelvis may be deformed from birth or as a result of disease, presenting special problems in childbirth. The obstetrician measures the dimensions and capacity of the pelvis of a pregnant woman to determine whether or not difficulties will be encountered in parturition, the act of giving birth. This is known as pelvimetry, or measurement of the pelvis.

The pelvis is the most variable part of the human skeleton but it is almost always larger in diameter in the woman than in the man.

pemphigus. An acute or chronic disease of the skin, characterized by the appearance of large blisters which develop in crops or in continuous succession.

The chronic form of pemphigus, pemphigus vulgaris, was formerly fatal in a large number of cases, but is now successfully treated with ACTH and cortisone, and fatality almost never occurs. The disfiguring and annoying skin lesions which the disease produces are now also successfully treated.

penicillin. An antibacterial drug.

Penicillin is used against germs which cause pneumonia, meningitis, gonorrhea, boils, common throat infection, and various staphylococcal diseases. It is also extremely effective in treatment of syphilis, replacing most of the earlier remedies. Subacute bacterial endocarditis, formerly fatal in a great number of cases, has been found to be controllable by penicillin. Penicillin is also used for trench mouth, rat-bite fever, and other infectious diseases.

The discovery of penicillin led to the development of streptomycin, Aureomycin, and many other antibiotics which have helped enormously to combat a great number of infectious diseases. *See also* ANTIBIOTICS.

penis. The male organ of copulation, which also contains the urethra which carries urine from the bladder to the outside of the body. *See also* CIRCUMCISION; TESTICLES.

peptic ulcer. An ulcer is any sore or break in the surface usually of the skin or mucous membrane, resulting from destruction of the underlying tissues or from loss of the covering layer of tissue. Peptic ulcer, commonly known as "ulcers," is a chronic condition in which the lining of the stomach or duodenum, the first part of the small intestine, is inflamed as a result of the action of digestive juices on the mucous membrane.

Peptic ulcers are found four times as often in men as in women, and ten to twelve times as often in the duodenum as in the stomach. They usually occur in definite locations which are bathed freely or regularly in gastric juices. Thus the upper part of the duodenum, which receives partially digested food along with a certain amount of gastric juice as it is sent to the intestines, is a place where peptic ulcers are particularly apt to develop.

Pain, the outstanding symptom of peptic ulcer, usually occurs at certain regular times and is relieved by eating. Constipation is another common symptom. Nausea, vomiting, loss of appetite, and even anemia may occasionally be symptoms. Unfortunately most persons suffer symptoms over a period of five to eight years before seeking medical advice.

pericarditis. An acute or chronic inflammation of the pericardium which covers and encloses the heart; it is caused by infection in the heart, or from infections in other parts of the body, from rheumatism, or wounds or tumors in the heart.

perineum. The part of the female body between the external genitals and the anus. In childbirth, these tissues are subject to great pressure and often tear and must be sewn up by the obstetrician. To prevent tearing during delivery, the doctor often makes an incision of the appropriate length in the perineum, which is later sewn and permitted to heal. After the delivery, the application of analgesic ointments and other preparations, as well as sitz baths, are helpful measures in healing the torn or incised perineum.

peritonitis. Inflammation of the peritoneum, the membrane which lines the abdominal cavity. The peritoneum can be affected by many disturbances and inflammation is the most serious. Occasionally peritonitis is the result of direct injury to the abdomen, but usually it is a byproduct of infection of one of the organs lying within the peritoneum, or of infection of the blood.

Acute peritonitis develops rapidly and a physician should be consulted as soon as possible. Death can result within a few hours or days following the onset of peritonitis.

Peritonitis is the most serious complication of appendicitis and may also follow the rupture of an ulcer of the stomach or intestine. Infection and pain begin almost simultaneously, the pain being most intense at the point of infection. A generalized feeling of acute illness follows as the body absorbs the poisons from the infection. The temperature rises, the abdomen is sensitive to touch, the abdominal wall is rigid, and vomiting begins. *See also* APPENDICITIS.

pernicious anemia. *See* ANEMIA.

perspiration. Or sweat, the fluid, largely water, excreted by the sweat or sudoriferous glands, situated beneath the outer surface of the skin with ducts opening into them. The chief function of sweating is to regulate body temperature. As moisture evaporates, heat energy is absorbed and in the process the surface on which evaporation takes place is cooled. Sweating is one of the main methods by which the body maintains the constant temperature vital to health and life.

pertussis. *See* WHOOPING COUGH.

perversion. Maladjustment of the sexual life in which satisfaction is sought in ways deviating from the accepted norms.

pessary. A ring of plastic usually tried to help hold in place a prolapsed or displaced uterus. They are most frequently used for elderly patients who are not good surgical risks.

pharyngitis. *See* PHARYNX.

pharynx. The area in the throat between the mouth and the opening of the esophagus or gullet. It functions as a resonating organ in speech. A group of semicircular muscles in the pharynx also help in the swallowing of food. The pharynx is generally divided into the nasal pharynx, extending to the nose, and the laryngeal pharynx, leading to the larynx and trachea.

The mucous lining of the pharynx may be affected by acute or chronic inflammation as the secondary effect of a severe cold, sore throat, or acute tonsillitis. It may also be infected by streptococci, as in septic sore throat. In most forms of acute pharyngitis the infection attacks suddenly, and the mucous lining becomes swollen, purple, and glazed, and covered by thick mucus. The uvula may swell and the tonsils also be seriously affected. Sometimes the swelling is severe enough to interfere with breathing; and fever, coughing, and a feeling of fatigue may develop.

phenolphthalein. A drug used as a laxative in constipation.

phenylketonuria.—PKU. An inborn error of metabolism which damages infants so that they become mentally retarded. This can be detected by a urine test. The feeding of the missing substance can correct the condition.

phlegmasia. Also known as white leg or milk leg. A swelling, usually of the lower limbs, usually during the lying-in period. The treatment is to elevate the limbs, to eat an extremely simple diet, and have complete bed rest.

phlebitis. Inflammation of a vein, accompanied by swelling and pain. When infection and clotting occur, the condition is thrombophlebitis. Blood vessels that are swollen and knotted are often described as varicose.

Any illness which slows the blood circulation and which entails a long period of lying down may induce formation of clots in the blood vessels of the legs. After such an illness, when the person walks, clots may form, the legs swell and become blue, and even lameness result. To relieve this type of phlebitis, the foot of the bed is elevated and the legs kept free of pressure with a bed cradle. The legs may also be wrapped in soft cotton and placed on a pillow when the patient is sleeping, or a semielastic bandage worn. Moderate exercise is sometimes helpful. Recovery usually occurs in about ten days.

phthisis. An old term used for tuberculosis or any disease characterized by emaciation and loss of strength, especially diseases of the lungs. *See also* TUBERCULOSIS.

pigmentation. Coloration of the skin; it is determined not only by the amount and nature of the pigment in the epidermis, but also by the color of the blood and the size of the blood vessels, especially those which are close to the surface.

The skin of a light-haired person contains little pigmentation, so that the blood shows through rather clearly. In a brunette, the pigmentation is heavier and the blood less visible. When the skin is almost black, the blood underneath is virtually invisible.

Flushing of the skin, a special aspect of skin pigmentation, is due to a temporary enlarging of the blood vessels close to the surface of the body, set off by certain nerves, and is provoked physiologically—by direct exposure to the sun, for example—or psychologically by emotional experiences such as embarrassment or confusion. *See also* FRECKLES; LIVER SPOTS; MELANOSIS.

piles. *See* HEMORRHOIDS.

pilonidal cyst. A pilonidal cyst develops from an improperly formed glandular organ, found under the skin at the end of the spine, which contains hair follicles and which secretes sebaceous and other fluids that have no outlet. This causes formation of a cyst, which may become infected and cause pain. The cysts seem to occur most frequently in men between the ages of twenty and forty-five.

pineal gland. An organ, about the size of a pea, located in the head near the lower part of the brain. Its function, although considered vital in the human system, is not clearly understood. Researchers have discovered a hormone which is secreted from the pineal gland, but thus far its function is not completely known. One hormone is melanotonin, concerned with pigmentation.

Enlargement of the pineal gland may crowd the passage through which the cerebrospinal fluid flows out of the brain into the spinal cord. When the canal is closed entirely, the brain fluid, seeking escape, creates such pressure that death may result.

Tumors of the pineal gland are rare, and in young boys cause development of sexual organs to adult size and function. They do not have the same effect on young girls. A pineal tumor in an adult woman may cause menstruation to cease, and in an adult man may provoke the sex glands and testes to degenerate.

Although surgical removal of the pineal gland is not often advisable, because of the high mortality rate, in some cases permanent cure has been achieved by this means. Radiation therapy may bring a temporary cure.

pinkeye. An inflammation of the conjunctiva, the tissue which covers the inner surface of the eyelid. It may be caused by a germ often carried on towels or on soiled hands. The eyes become red and the eyelids swollen and puffy. Often the eyelids are stuck together with pus when the person awakens from sleep. Medical treatment varies, depending on the type of germ involved. A similar appearance, called vernal conjunctivitis, may develop as the result of allergy. *See also* CONJUNCTIVITIS.

pinworm. *See* WORMS.

pituitary. The most important gland of the endocrine system, or glands of internal secretion. This gland secretes substances into the blood which are carried to organs in other parts of the body where they exert significant effects. Thus, the endocrine system regulates many of the most important of the bodily functions. These include growth, sexual development, defenses against emergencies and disease, and many metabolic processes. The pituitary performs an unusual number of these and, in addition, controls other endocrine glands. Endocrine secretions are called hormones.

The pituitary is divided into two distinct portions: the anterior and the posterior. The anterior is much more important, having a profound role in bodily growth, the development and activity of the adrenal cortex, the sex glands, the thyroid, and the pancreas. The posterior is related especially to water retention by the kidneys.

The mechanisms involved in control of growth are not fully understood, but the significance of the pituitary in the process is well established. The growth hormone, if excessive during childhood and adolescence, will produce giants, and if insufficient, dwarfs. If pituitary overactivity occurs later in life when the principal bones have lost capacity to grow further, those of the extremities—the head, hands, and feet—may enlarge, resulting in a condition called acromegaly. The face may assume a coarse look and the tongue grow. Usually due to a pituitary tumor, acromegaly can be treated by surgery or X-ray.

When the pituitary is removed from an immature animal, its long bones soon cease to expand and its total size and weight remain smaller than normal.

Another function of the pituitary is the stimulation of the sex glands to maturity. This occurs at puberty, until which time the pituitary growth hormone controls growth. When the sex glands, under the pituitary stimulus, develop to a point of secreting the full amount of their own hormones, the growth hormone ceases to affect increase in height. The pituitary continues throughout life, however, to secrete growth substance, but its function after the attainment of physical maturity is not yet fully understood.

When pregnancy occurs, a hormone related to the female periodic cycle becomes superfluous for the time being and is excreted in the urine. The Aschheim-Zondek test for pregnancy is based on this fact. In this test, immature rabbits or mice are injected with urine from the patient. If the hormone is being excreted and is present in the urine, the animals mature in a few days which signifies that the person is pregnant. This test achieves 98 to 99 per cent accuracy.

Slow sexual development in young people and reduction of fertility because of underactive testes or ovaries in adults can be treated by extracts of pituitary gland containing the sex-stimulating pituitary hormones.

One of the most significant pituitary secretions is ACTH, the initials of the term adrenocorticotrophic hormone, which means that the substance has a special affinity for the cortex or outer part of the adrenal gland. Since the adrenal cortex is greatly involved with meeting stresses of practically all kinds which the body bears, the function of the pituitary substance which stimulates it is particularly significant. ACTH is now used, with much the same effect as cortisone, an adrenal-cortical hormone, to relieve several diseases, including arthritis, asthma, hives, and exceptionally high fever.

When the pituitary is removed, the adrenal glands degenerate. Degeneration of the adrenals also causes Addison's disease, which was formerly fatal. Now the lives of patients with such disorders may be extended by use of hormones derived from the adrenal cortex.

Other pituitary substances are associated with the secretion of milk and the activity of the thyroid gland.

The posterior pituitary is connected with retention of water by the kidneys. Many nerve fibers connect it to the section of the brain involved in regulating weight, sleep, muscular coordination, and emotional activity. It affects the system of involuntary muscles when these are inactive and so is sometimes used in aiding childbirth and stimulating the bowels. The posterior pituitary also is involved in controlling blood sugar.

General pituitary inactivity renders a person dull and slow, in mind as well as body. Sleep occurs easily and fat accumulates. In young children this inactivity retards both mental and sexual development. Overactivity of the pituitary induces a variety of symptoms.

Other pituitary functions include a relationship with the parts of the pancreas producing insulin, which regulates body utilization of sugar, and another relationship with the thyroid gland. When the pancreas is removed from an animal, sugar appears in its blood and urine, since sugar cannot be used properly without insulin. If the pituitary is also removed, these symptoms are relieved. Removal of the pituitary with the pancreas left intact causes a diminution of sugar.

A pituitary secretion partially controls the thyroid, and deficient thyroid activity leads to pituitary enlargement. The thyroid is enlarged, in turn, by administration of the pituitary hormone related to it. Pituitary deficiency tends to lower the basal metabolism which functions closely with the thyroid. The pituitary also influences the parathyroid glands which are involved with the body's use of calcium.

A possible relationship between the pituitary and growth, and the processes which lead to cancer is being investigated. Cases have been recorded in which a cancer of the prostate gland and of the breast have been controlled by removal of the pituitary.

Among the most serious disorders which involve the pituitary is Cushing's disease, in which a tumor in the anterior lobe causes, among other symptoms, obesity of the abdomen, face, and buttocks. Atrophy, or degeneration, of the anterior lobe in adults results in Simmond's disease, characterized by extreme emaciation. In rare cases of Froehlich's syndrome, the anterior lobe is so affected as to produce extreme obesity and infantile sexual organs. *See also* CUSHING'S SYNDROME.

placenta. The organ in the uterus through which the fetus is fed, and which acts as its lung and kidney. It also protects the fetus from infection and secretes several birth hormones. At birth it is about one-sixth of the baby's weight.

placenta previa. A placenta that is situated mostly or partially in the lower uterine cavity. It may cause a sudden painless loss of blood after the twenty-eighth week of pregnancy. The main danger of this is prematurity. The treatment is to conserve the blood supply and prevent anemia.

platelets. Also called thrombocytes. *See* BLOOD.

pleurisy. A group of symptoms produced by inflammation or infection of the pleura, the lining of the chest cavity covering the inside of the chest wall, the top of the diaphragm, and the outer side of the lungs.

The most common sources of pleurisy are pneumonia, tuberculosis, and influenza. The first signs are usually pain, which may become severe on taking a deep breath, a cough, fever, and rapid shallow breathing. In some cases, a quantity of fluid is effused. This accumulation is known as pleurisy with effusion or "wet" pleurisy. Sometimes a large amount of pus is formed by secondary infection, producing a condition known as empyema which is extremely serious and requires immediate care.

In the form called "dry" pleurisy, which almost always follows an acute case of pneumonia, pain appears over the site of the infection and with a stethoscope the doctor can hear a sound of rubbing inside the chest cavity. When the underlying infection is cured, the pleurisy disappears.

pneumonia. An inflammation of one or both lungs. Many types of pneumonia have been distinguished, but usually when the word pneumonia is used without qualification, lobar pneumonia, in which one or more entire lobes are infected, is implied, and the causative organism is the pneumococcus. Other organisms may also produce pneumonia, such as the streptococcus and staphylococcus, which may cause bronchopneumonia.

The symptoms of a typical case of pneumonia may follow a slight cold or infectious disease or may appear suddenly without warning. A shaking chill may be followed by a sharp stabbing pain on the side of or in the chest, with coughing and expectoration of brown or bloody sputum. The pulse is rapid, the cheeks flushed, temperature rises sharply, and weakness and even prostration, headache, nausea, vomiting, and diarrhea sometimes ensue.

poisoning. Any substance which is capable of producing a harmful or deadly effect can be considered a poison. For most such substances there is both a safe dose and a poisonous dose, the severity of the effect depending on the amount taken and on the age and physical condition of the person involved.

poliomyelitis. An inflammation of the anterior horn cells in the gray matter of the spinal cord. It is caused by a virus, the smallest living material. Viruses differ from bacteria mainly in that they cannot move by themselves and cannot live outside a living body. The virus of infantile paralysis, or poliomyelitis, as it is more properly called, is one of the smallest known. Man is affected almost exclusively, although monkeys may be infected.

Poliomyelitis can exist in one of three forms. Many people have had poliomyelitis without realizing it, having contracted a mild case which rendered them immune to further attacks. Poliomyelitis may cause only a little diarrhea, stomach upset, cold, or muscle aches, which last for a few days. This is known as abortive poliomyelitis. If temporary paralysis of arms or legs occurs, the condition is known as nonparalytic poliomyelitis. The third type, paralytic poliomyelitis, may cause lasting damage or death if respiratory muscles are involved.

Epidemics of poliomyelitis usually occur during the warm months, July to October in the United States, and February through April in Australia. The virus is present in the nasopharynx and bowel movements and may be spread by sneezing, coughing, or by contamination of water or food with sewage. The poliomyelitis virus affects the cells of the spinal cord, brain, and other nervous tissue, leading to the familiar paralyses. Adults as well as children may be affected. Symptoms may be vague at first and include fever, headache, spasms of the arms, neck, thighs, and weakness. Treatment, which is not yet wholly satisfactory, consists of exercising the affected muscle groups to prevent withering and shrinking from lack of use; employment of the iron lung to carry on respiration when the respiratory or breathing muscles are damaged, and other such supportive measures.

Countless numbers of children have become permanent cripples as a result of polio, and many adults and children have died from it.

The development of the Salk and Sabin poliomyelitis vaccines have been a particular blessing to all parents and children. The vaccines can produce immunity to the poliomyelitis virus, and this may last for many years. The Salk vaccine is produced by growing virus on the tissue of the kidneys of monkeys. The virus is then denatured, or killed, making it safe for injection into human beings. Even though denatured, the vaccine can cause the human body to produce resistant substances, or antibodies, to poliomyelitis. The Sabin vaccine is taken orally and contains living attenuated virus. All human beings should be vaccinated.

polycythemia. A disease of unknown origin in which the production of red blood cells in the bone marrow is greatly increased. The average number of red blood cells is about five to six million per cubic millimeter of blood. In polycythemia, the number may reach as many as fifteen million red blood cells per cubic millimeter of blood. Usually white blood cells and platelets increase also, adding to the viscosity of the blood and affecting its flow to the brain and other parts of the body.

The symptoms in polycythemia may include dizziness, severe headache, and a feeling of fullness in the head. In some cases, fainting occurs and numbness and tingling in the hands and feet. The person may feel irritable and sluggish and have occasional spells of amnesia. Sometimes the vision is disturbed and there is a constant ringing in the ears. The spleen becomes greatly enlarged in order to act as a storage reservoir for the increased production of blood cells. The person's skin often has a bluish cast because of the prominence of small veins.

polyhydramnios. An excess of amniotic fluid during pregnancy.

polyp. A non-malignant tumor which

hangs by a pedicle or stalk from the surface of a body cavity. Polyps vary widely in structure and nature, depending on their location. In the ear, a polyp consists of granular tissue caused by chronic irritation. A nasal polyp contains a soft overgrowth of mucous membrane and generally indicates disease of the underlying bone tissue. A rectal polyp is usually a glandular tumor. Polyps are frequently found inside the sinuses as inflammatory growth on mucous lining. A gastric polyp is a non-malignant tumor in the stomach.

Surgery is generally employed to remove polyps. In the nose, the base must also be excised after the polyp has been removed. Sometimes polyps occur in groups in the large intestine and must be removed and the entire area excised because of the danger that one may have become malignant. Electric current is often used to remove polyps in the urethra. Polyps on the walls of the uterus may not require treatment unless they endanger health. Rectal and gastric polyps also may become malignant and should therefore be removed.

postpartum hemorrhage. A hemorrhage which occurs after childbirth. A serious condition and one in which the physician employs emergency measures.

pre-eclampsia. An abnormal condition of pregnancy with symptoms of raised blood pressure, headaches, abnormal weight gain, and swelling. In the early stages the patient has a vague lassitude and a feeling of malaise, with mild headache, slight nausea, and spots in front of the eyes. Later symptoms are dizziness, throbbing headache, stomach pain, and blurring of vision.

pregnancy and prenatal care. Pregnancy is the state of a woman from conception to childbirth, usually 280 days. During this time, many changes take place in the body of the prospective mother. While the greatest changes take place in the organs immediately concerned with childbirth, every organ is influenced by pregnancy. When pregnancy occurs, the uterus becomes thickened and enlarges with the growth of the prospective child. The breasts begin to develop as early as the second month and in young women who are having their first baby as early as the second or third week. A greater tenderness and fullness of the breasts and a darkening and enlarging of the nipples is apparent. Various glands of the body are affected by pregnancy and produce greater amounts of secretion. The whole rate of chemical changes, measured by basal metabolism, is also likely to be increased.

Certain definite signs indicate to the doctor that a woman is pregnant. In the majority of cases, the regular menstruation disappears after the woman has conceived, and will not recur again during pregnancy. Disappearance of menstruation in a woman whose menstrual periods have always been regular usually indicates that she is pregnant. There are cases, however, in which a woman has had one or even two discharges of blood from the uterus after conception, but the quantity and duration are usually much less than normal. More frequent urination is often a sign of pregnancy. Some women will experience a feeling of sickness, nausea, and vomiting, especially in the morning. These symptoms usually develop during the second month and rarely last past the end of the fourth month, and many variations occur in their appearance, intensity, and duration. Some women are troubled several times a day, and in rare instances the sickness takes place only at night when the woman goes to bed.

Many women become increasingly emotional during pregnancy, with feelings of peevishness, fretfulness, irritability, unreasonableness, and depression. Other women, on the contrary, feel unusually cheerful. The craving for unusual foods is a manifestation of the emotional changes that may occur, as is a change in daily habits. A woman who has been exceedingly clean and meticulous may suddenly become careless and slovenly.

When the expectant mother is twelve to fourteen weeks pregnant, her abdomen will begin to enlarge. At the end of sixteen weeks the enlargement of the abdomen will seem pronounced to her, although other people probably will not notice it for another month. The womb continues to enlarge in order to give room to the growing fetus. Between the sixteenth and eighteenth weeks she is likely to feel a faint fluttering, which is called "quickening." This symptom is not a certain one, because things can occur inside the abdomen that resemble the movement of the fetus

but actually stem from other causes. Women who are excessively worried about being pregnant frequently imagine that they feel movements.

Some signs of pregnancy are so positive that they leave no doubt. One is an X-ray picture which shows the presence of the prospective child. Another is its heartbeat, which is audible between the eighteenth and twentieth weeks and occasionally earlier. Laboratory tests are almost infallible. The Aschheim-Zondek tests ("rabbit tests") are highly reliable in diagnosing pregnancy. They are, however, expensive and only required in unusual cases.

Once the condition of pregnancy has been established the expectant mother should talk to the doctor about prenatal care, for her health must be the best possible during pregnancy. Any disease or ailment she has must be known to the doctor to avoid further possible complications for mother and child. Prenatal care is especially significant if she is diabetic or has heart disease.

Fees should be decided in advance in a frank discussion with the doctor or obstetrician. If the child is to be born in a hospital, arrangements for reserving a bed for confinement should be made well in advance. Some families find that hospitalization and sickness insurance cover most of the expenses. However, financial limitations need not and must not limit or prevent prenatal care. Most hospitals offer classes which instruct expectant mothers, and fathers, in the care of the baby. The prospective mother should also discuss with her doctor whether or not her new baby is to be breast fed or formula fed. If breast feeding is recommended, the doctor will advise her in the care of her breasts.

The expectant mother will see her doctor usually once a month, unless unusual symptoms arise, and more often during the later days of pregnancy. During these visits, he will make a complete physical examination, which includes blood pressure and urine, to determine whether inflammations or diabetes are present. He makes accurate measurements of the organs concerned in childbirth and thus is able to anticipate difficulties which might arise. He examines her blood, one of the blood tests establishing whether or not the blood contains the rhesus factor. Blood containing the rhesus factor is Rh positive, blood which does not is Rh negative. If the baby's blood is Rh positive and the mother's is Rh negative, the baby may be born with anemia and require a blood transfusion at birth.

At each visit, the doctor will ask the pregnant woman about symptoms, since certain symptoms may indicate complications. He should always be informed of persistent headaches, bleeding from the vagina, undue swelling of the hands and feet, leakage of water from the vagina, blurred vision, abdominal pains, serious vomiting, fainting spells, scanty urine, and excessive gain in weight. If necessary, he will then determine the cause and significance of these symptoms in or-der to anticipate and, in most cases, prevent serious complications.

The best way to help prevent complications in labor or delivery is to maintain good health and stamina throughout the period of pregnancy by proper diet and strict attention to the rules and advice of the doctor. The food supply for the baby reaches it through the blood vessels which connect with the mother. If her diet is deficient, food cannot be extracted from her tissues and organs for its growth. Her food intake should be regulated with the needs of the growing child. A good general rule for her is to eat the foods she usually eats, provided she has had a proper diet, but to make certain that she receives sufficient milk, and more fruits and vegetables than she ordinarily would. She should particularly watch her supply of vitamins and such mineral salts as calcium, phosphorus, iron, and iodine. Milk and milk products provide most of the essential calcium, but the doctor may recommend additional calcium in the diet.

Iron is absolutely vital for the building of red blood cells. That many babies are born slightly anemic indicates that the diet of many pregnant women is deficient in iron. They should be sure to eat plenty of iron-containing foods and, if necessary, take extra iron prescribed by the doctor.

Of the mineral salts, iodine is of great significance. A lack of sufficient iodine in the diet may influence not only the mother's thyroid gland but that of the prospective child.

She also requires more protein. Meat is one of the best sources of not only protein but also the B vitamins, such as thiamine, riboflavin, and niacin. Fish, poultry, and eggs also supply protein.

Fats, particularly butter, cream, and cheese, provide vitamin A and should be included in the diet. Sugars and starches, including whole-grain cereals, bread, and potatoes, are needed to provide materials for energy. But since fats, sugars, and starches also supply a substantial amount of calories, they should not be eaten in large quantities. Fried or greasy foods, heavy sauces and dressings, and rich pastries and pies should be avoided.

The pregnant woman should get regular moderate amounts of sunshine, if possible. If not, additional vitamins, A and D, may be prescribed in the form of cod liver oil. Fresh fruits and vegetables, particularly citrus fruits and tomatoes, supply vitamins A, B, and C.

The nausea and vomiting that occur during the early months of pregnancy are sometimes helped by eating small amounts of food every two and a half hours rather than three daily meals. Various new remedies, such as Bonamine, compazine, Dramamine, and Marezine, are available to relieve continuous vomiting.

During the months before the child is born, the pregnant woman should wear comfortable clothing, and be careful not to wear elastic garters that constrict blood vessels and aid development of varicose veins.

Although the pregnant woman's mental condition cannot affect her child's physical condition, she should nonetheless avoid nervous irritation, undue fatigue, and excess emotional reactions, not only for her own benefit but also for the sake of those about her.

Medical care and advice are particularly desirable during the last four or five weeks of pregnancy. Her condition for the confinement will be rechecked. Meanwhile the baby has grown to such a size that it cannot twist and turn in the womb any longer. It has settled into the position of delivery, normally with its head downward. If the doctor finds that these developments are slower than desired, he may attempt to correct the position by manipulation. He will also establish whether or not the space for passage of the baby is satisfactory. He will decide when a Cesarean section is necessary.

A rigid or special program of self-care is seldom necessary for the pregnant woman, but there are some hygiene rules she would do well to follow. She should, of course, keep herself well groomed. Social activities can and should be continued on a moderate scale. Pregnancy is no reason for becoming dull and unattractive. As a rule, shoes with one- or 1½-inch heels are better than higher-heeled shoes which make it more difficult to stand or walk comfortably and thus give an awkward appearance. The doctor may prescribe a maternity corset to relieve stress and strain on the abdominal muscles. It should be well fitted and preferably made of a non-elastic material. Brassieres which lift the breasts upward and inward and do not flatten them are recommended.

The pregnant woman always needs ample sleep and rest, in a well-ventilated room, and especially during the last few weeks. An afternoon nap is desirable. If she cannot sleep, just lying down is beneficial. If she has difficulty resting, the doctor may give her some medication to promote relaxation.

During pregnancy, small amounts of a liquid called colostrum, which later is followed by real milk, may exude and form on the nipples. It must be removed by soap and warm water to avoid irritation.

The pregnant woman should visit her dentist early in pregnancy and follow his instructions for care of her teeth.

She can continue to bathe during pregnancy, although many doctors prefer showers or sponge baths to tub bathing during the last month or two. The best temperature for the water is between 85° and 90° F., even for those who are accustomed to cold or lukewarm baths. Unusual types of baths, like Turkish and Russian sweat baths, ocean baths, or cold showers, should never be taken except on the advice of the doctor.

The amount and kind of exercise that the pregnant woman takes depends primarily on her previous habits, but she should never exercise to the point of fatigue. As soon as she begins to feel tired it is a good time to stop. Walking is the best exercise, except in bad weather. It stimulates deep breathing, brings more oxygen into the lungs and blood, and assists in proper elimination. She should always walk slowly and avoid crowds. Two miles daily is an average amount of walking. Although sun is beneficial, she should avoid too much exposure.

Strenuous activities which require lifting, excessive stretching or reaching are to be eliminated. Particularly undesirable are running, tennis, swimming, skating, skiing, and horseback riding. During the early months of pregnancy, dancing may be enjoyed, but the pregnant woman should avoid crowded dance floors where she can be bumped and pushed.

If she likes to drive, short drives can be continued, avoiding rough roads and bouncing. During the last few months, traveling should not be undertaken if possible.

As the birth of the child approaches, all arrangements for its coming can be checked, such as accommodations, clothing, bassinet or bed, diapers or a diaper service. If there are other children in the family, arrangements for their care should be made.

If this is the woman's first baby, it is essential to be able to recognize the beginning of labor. Slightly painful contractions of the womb will be the first sign. They begin in the lower part of the abdomen and soon spread to the front of both sides. After some time these contractions become more frequent and pronounced. A few drops of blood mixed with mucus may appear or, in some cases, water may flow at the onset of labor.

At the first sign of labor, the

woman should notify her doctor, since the time for confinement may have come. A woman bearing her first child, a primipara, usually has a more lengthy labor. When the contractions start to come every few minutes, the birth is approaching. After the first baby, labor, in most cases, will be shorter so that particular care of the time element must be taken. There is no cause for concern if labor does not begin according to expectations. A few days', even ten days', difference in calculation is not unusual since not all pregnancies take the same course.

premenstrual tension. Before the beginning of the menstrual period, a woman may become restless, irritable, highly emotional, and unable to concentrate. It has been suggested that this is caused by estrogen retention. There are now specific drugs on the market to relieve the symptoms of premenstrual tension.

presbyopia. A form of farsightedness in which objects close to the eye may be seen only with difficulty. Farsightedness is a change which normally comes with advancing years. First showing itself when the person is, perhaps, in her forties, presbyopia becomes progressively more acute until approximately the age of seventy-seven.

prickly heat. Medically called miliaria, an acute inflammatory skin rash, characterized by acute itching, which occurs when the skin fails to adapt itself to an increase in temperature and humidity. Heat rash, as it is also called, affects children more frequently than adults.

Newcomers in a tropical locality will often cease to suffer from prickly heat as soon as their bodies have become adjusted to the new environment.

primigravida. A woman who is pregnant for the first time.

primipara. A woman who has delivered one child.

progesterone. A female hormone produced after ovulation. It is involved in the maintenance of normal pregnancy. It also relaxes the muscles of the stomach, the intestinal tract, leg veins, kidney, pelvis, ureters, and rectum. These effects may be the cause of such disturbances of pregnancy as morning sickness, heartburn, constipation, varicose veins, and hemorrhoids. It is used to prevent abortion when there has been a history of miscarriages.

Enovid, and other formulas of synthetic progesterone, and estrogens are widely used to prevent conception.

prolapse. The dropping of an internal body organ from its normal position, or the protrusion of the lining of a body cavity through a natural opening, or of an organ through a wound.

At childbirth, the stretching of the supportive tissues of the uterus may produce prolapse of the uterus, in which the womb falls from the normal position and the cervix is pushed far into the vagina. Symptoms are a bearing down sensation and, in the bladder, stress incontinence—a condition when the patient loses control whenever she laughs, sneezes, or coughs. Severe prolapse can cause the womb to push the cervix through the vagina. This may provoke complications which require surgery. To correct prolapse by other than surgical means, various types of pessaries may be used, depending on the nature of the prolapse.

Prolapse through wounds occurs in the case of the bowels or the lung, when the abdominal or chest wall is penetrated. Another example of prolapse may be associated with a perforated corneal ulcer, where there is danger of prolapse of the iris.

prostate. An organ in the human male located at the neck of the urinary bladder, surrounding the first part of the urethra, the passage through which urine is excreted from the bladder.

The prostate is partly glandular and partly of muscular tissue. It produces a substance called prostatic fluid which is an important part of the semen, the material that transports the male sperm cells into the female during intercourse. Prostatic fluid is produced constantly and escapes through the urine. During sexual excitement it increases in volume and is discharged into the urethra and thus into the semen at the time of ejaculation. The exact function of the prostatic fluid is not known, but it is believed to be related to the survival of the sperm in the female vagina.

The most frequent disorder of the prostate is its gradual enlargement in men over fifty. Sometimes this is first noticed in increasing difficulty of urination; in other cases the first sign may be desire, even during sleep, to urinate more often.

As the condition develops, a residue of urine tends to remain in the bladder. Eventually this will begin to decompose and irritate the whole bladder, leading to inflammation. One recourse now widely employed is the use of a catheter to assure complete evacuation, another is surgical removal of part or all of the prostate, and a third means is the use of glandular substances which restrain its overgrowth.

protein. One of a group of complex nitrogenous substances of high molecular weight which are found in various forms in animals and plants and are characteristic of living matter. In the chemical makeup of the body, proteins occupy a significant place, being essential in the maintenance of tissue and also a valuable source of energy. In the process of digestion, the complex proteins, which are largely giant molecules, split into simpler forms and finally into amino acids. *See also* EDEMA; VITAMINS.

Provera. A synthetic female hormone used to prevent spontaneous abortion.

Provest. A female oral contraceptive.

pruritis. *See* ITCHING.

pseudocyesis. False pregnancy. In certain cases a woman's abdomen may enlarge and menstruation may stop and she may think she is pregnant when she is not. The condition has occurred in women extremely anxious to have children. It is sometimes due to an abnormal mental state in which the woman imagines she has had sexual intercourse with a man she would like to have as husband or lover. Men have been accused of being father of an unborn child or guilty of fornication or adultery because of this.

When treated by anesthesia the enlargement of the abdomen disappears.

psittacosis. Commonly called "parrot fever," a disease not only of parrots, parakeets, lovebirds, canaries, pigeons, ducks, and other birds, but one also readily transmitted to human beings. Occasionally the infection is spread from one infected person to another.

psoriasis. A chronic inflammatory skin disease, and one of the ten most frequent skin ailments. It affects both men and women, and usually appears after the age of fifteen. It is non-infectious, but some families seem to have a tendency to it.

The cause of psoriasis is unknown. Numerous theories have been advanced, but as yet no cause has been definitely established. Some doctors believe it is of nervous origin, others think it may be related to difficulty in digesting fat, or to certain germs and viruses.

The first sign of psoriasis is generally an eruption of pinhead-size, bright red spots which group to form larger ones, finally becoming great patches of reddened skin. The healing begins from the center and leaves a red or reddish brown stain. Also characteristic of psoriasis are thick, silver-white scales. When they are removed, small bleeding spots remain. There is seldom any itching nor is general health affected.

Eruption is usually on the elbows, knees, and backs of the arms and legs; occasionally the chest and abdomen are involved. Sometimes the lesions become infected and form pus. Fingernails and toenails and the palms of the hands and soles of the feet may be affected also.

psychiatry. The branch of medicine that treats mental and emotional disorders.

psychoanalysis. The method developed by Sigmund Freud to determine the patterns and motivations of human personality in order to treat various emotional disorders. Many persons, among them Jung and Adler, have worked in this field, modifying and changing the Freudian psychoanalytic method, so that many types of psychoanalysis are now practiced. The technique is used in the study and treatment of a wide variety of emotional problems, particularly the neuroses.

Typically the patient in psychoanalysis meets with her analyst a minimum of two one-hour periods a week, and talks as freely and fully as possible about anything she chooses. The patient comes to realize more and more what in her past and present life is relevant and significant and to discuss that. Gradually the psychoanalyst and patient come to recognize the roots and patterns of the patient's attitudes and actions. The goal is to create within the patient both an intellectual and emotional awareness of why she thinks and acts as she does. Often an intellectual grasp of the problems precedes an emotional grasp—i.e., she may *know* that she drinks to excess when she is worried, but still not have reached the point where this knowledge will serve to help her. Since neuroses have origins which reach far back into the patient's life, the patient often devotes a large part of her attention to early childhood and adolescence.

Psychoanalysis can take from months to years, the patient deciding when she no longer needs the services of her psychoanalyst.

psychoneurosis. An emotional disorder caused by an individual's desires that conflict with her own or society's idea of what is "right." Most psychoneuroses do not show outward abnormal behavior but appear as emotional reactions in the form of physical disease. They are characterized by conditions known as neurasthenia, hypochondria, hysteria, or compulsive states in which the patient repeats certain words or acts completely against her will.

psychosis. A severe mental disorder, which manifests itself in abnormal behavior, reactions, and ideas. The person is no longer able to cope with the demands of her environment. A psychotic person differs from a neurotic person in that the neurotic person has succeeded in making an adjustment to her environment, the nature of the adjustment usually constituting the neurosis. *See also* MANIC-DEPRESSIVE PSYCHOSIS; NEUROSIS; PARANOIA; SCHIZOPHRENIA.

psychosomatic disorders. Illnesses which result from the interaction of mind and body. The emotional factor in sickness has been recognized since ancient times. However, our understanding of the role of emotional factors and their interrelationship with organic diseases

has only recently advanced to the point that psychosomatic medicine is now a recognized and widely used term as well as a definite branch of medical science.

Psychosomatic disorders may result from multiple causes where the emotional stimulus is combined with other factors, such as a physical predisposition. In ailments like asthma or colitis, for example, the site of the difficulty may be physically predisposed, while the immediate source is emotional in origin.

Psychosomatic disturbances may take place in any of the involuntary organs of the body, including the digestive tract, the respiratory region, the heart and circulatory systems, the genitourinary system, the endocrine glands, and the skin.

Certain forms of allergy are also greatly influenced by emotional factors. In some instances chronic cases of asthma have been helped by psychotherapy. *See also* NEUROSIS; PEPTIC ULCER.

ptomaine poisoning. *See* FOOD POISONING.

puberty. The period of life when a person becomes functionally capable of reproduction. In temperate climates it usually occurs between the age of twelve to fifteen in girls and from thirteen to sixteen in boys.

In girls, menstruation begins, the breasts enlarge, and hair occurs in the pubic and axillary regions.

In boys, hair appears on the face and chest, under the axilla, and in the pubic region. There is a change of voice, an enlargement of the penis, and the appearance of erection and erotic dreams with ejaculation. In addition to the physical changes, profound psychological alterations and adjustments occur in both sexes.

puerperal. Relating to childbirth. It may be used to describe any time between the last stage of labor and the period approximately six weeks later when the pelvic bones have returned to their normal position.

puerperal sepsis. Childbed fever. An acute infection of the genital tract following childbirth. Long labor and manipulation predispose to infection. Before treatment with sulfonamides and penicillin the mortality in puerperal fever was very high, the disease being the major cause of maternal deaths.

pulse. The intermittent change in the shape of an artery due to an increase in the tension of its walls following the contraction of the heart. The impulses which the beating of the heart sends through the arteries can be felt at various places on the surface of the body. The artery usually selected for examination of the pulse is the radial artery lying over the radius bone at the wrist. A finger is placed on this artery and the number of beats per minute recorded. A machine which measures pulse rate has also been developed.

In adults, the number of pulsations per minute varies from 67 to 72. In infants, the rate is 120 to 140 in the first few weeks of life, slowing gradually to 100 to 120.

Excessive rapidity of pulse rate is called tachycardia, and excessive slowness is called brachycardia. In fever, the pulse rate increases from 8 to 10 beats per minute for each degree of temperature rise above normal. After exertion the rate increases but usually returns to normal within a few minutes.

Normal pulse is regular, the beats occurring in the same intervals. In auricular fibrillation, the pulse is extremely irregular. The force of the pulse may also vary in disorders associated with a depressed physical state and with certain ailments of the blood vessels. *See also* ARTERIOSCLEROSIS; BLOOD PRESSURE; HEART.

purgative. *See* CATHARTICS.

purpura hemorrhagica. A condition caused by a decrease to below normal in the number of blood platelets, which are factors in coagulation. When a shortage of blood platelets occurs, bleeding will begin almost spontaneously, particularly from the mucous membranes in the nose and mouth. Bleeding underneath the skin is frequent, giving the appearance of bruises.

In many women, a lessening of the platelets occurs at menstruation.

Purpura hemorrhagica is seen most frequently in persons between the ages of twelve and twenty-five, although it may occur at any age. The condition may develop gradually so that the onset cannot be determined accurately. Some acute cases are so severe that there is danger of bleeding to death within a few days or weeks. In others, the condition may be chronic, varying in severity throughout the person's life.

pus. The thick, creamy, yellowish product of inflammation, found in abscesses. It consists chiefly of serum and white blood cells. The color varies with the causative micro-organism. A discharge containing or forming pus is called purulent.

pyelitis. An inflammation of the pelvis or lower part of the kidney. In pregnancy, chills, fever, and pain between the hips and ribs may be indicative of pyelitis. *See also* KIDNEYS; NEPHRITIS.

pyelonephritis. The most common type of kidney infection, involving both the pelvis of the kidney and the kidney itself. *See also* KIDNEYS; NEPHRITIS.

pyemia. An infection due to the presence of pus-producing germs in the bloodstream and the formation of abscesses where these organisms lodge. *See also* BACTEREMIA.

pylorus. The valve which releases food from the stomach into the duodenum and into the small intestines. Ulcers may form in the pylorus with subsequent scarring and constriction. Babies are sometimes born with an enlargement of the muscles which form the pyloric valve. This causes obstruction of the passage of food and spasms which result in vomiting. The child will lose weight rapidly since she cannot retain food. The usual treatment for a congenital malformed pyloric valve is a surgical division of the muscle.

pyorrhea. Usually refers to an inflammation of the gums and outer covering of the roots of the teeth when it reaches the purulent stage. It is easier to prevent than cure and rarely occurs when good general care is taken of the teeth and gums. Beginning with tender, bleeding gums the inflammation advances until the teeth become loosened from the supporting gum. The dentist follows a regular course of treatment. If started early enough, treatment is effective, but when there is extensive bone loss and shifting of teeth in their sockets little can be done, and removal of the teeth affected is advised in order to save the rest. *See also* GINGIVITIS; TEETH.

Q fever. Often called nine-mile fever, an infection which resembles influenza or virus pneumonia. It is caused by a rickettsial organism, a micro-organism smaller than bacteria but larger than a filtrable virus, and is transmitted to man by ticks that live on infected animals.

Q fever begins with fever, headache, chills, malaise, and weakness. Mild cases last a few days, but more severe attacks may persist for two to three weeks; the condition usually ends in complete recovery. Treatment ordinarily consists of good nursing care and use of appropriate drugs early in the course of the illness.

Q fever can be acquired by contact with infected milk or dairy products, and proper pasteurization of milk is a significant factor in preventing the spread of Q fever.

quarantine. The limitation of freedom of movement of persons or animals who have been exposed to a communicable disease, for a period of time usually equal to the longest incubation period of the disease to which they have been exposed. The word quarantine comes from the Italian word for forty. During the Middle Ages, ships were detained for forty days before entering port in an attempt to avoid spread of the plague.

quickening. The first feeling of fetal movements by a pregnant woman. These first noticeable movements of the unborn child usually appear during the sixteenth to eighteenth week of pregnancy.

quinsy. A sore throat caused by an abscess in the tissues around the tonsils. Pain is generally localized on one side. The person has great difficulty in swallowing and talking, the breath becomes unpleasant, the tongue thickly coated, and the sense of taste and smell may be affected and almost lost.

Rest in bed is imperative and the physician will prescribe antibiotic drugs at once to relieve pain and control infection. Sometimes he will incise the abscess to release the accumulation of pus. *See also* TONSILLITIS.

rabbit fever. *See* TULAREMIA.

rabies. Or hydrophobia, an acute infectious disease of animals, caused by a filtrable virus, and transmitted to other animals and human beings by the bite of an infected animal. It occurs in dogs, cattle, horses, wolves, cats, bats, and other animals. The dog is most often attacked by rabies, as well as being the most frequent transmitter of the disease to human beings.

The first signs of rabies in a dog are irritability and restlessness, followed by difficulty in swallowing and paralysis, which makes the mouth hang open and causes drooling of saliva. In the final stages of rabies, an infected dog will howl, snap, run about, and bite. Eventu-

ally it becomes paralyzed, has convulsions, and dies. The disease rarely reaches the last stages, since the animal is usually spotted before and disposed of.

radiation. The therapeutic use of roentgen rays or radium. The term is also used to denote divergence from a common center of sensations and stimuli.

radium. The rays which radium gives off have an effect on the growth of human tissue, and radium has been effectively used in treatment of skin diseases of various types, including cancer, tumors, growths on the skin, and in hemorrhage and infections.

rale. A French word meaning rattle and referring to the various sounds that are heard in the lungs when the doctor examines them with a stethoscope. Many adjectives have been employed by doctors to describe these sounds, such as coarse, medium, fine, moist, and dry.

rectocele. Protrusion of the rectum into the vagina associated with prolapse of the uterus.

rectum. The lowest segment of the digestive tract, about six to eight inches long, terminating in the anus or lower opening through which solid waste matter is evacuated from the body. The large intestine, immediately above the rectum, first acts on the indigestible residue which remains when food has been digested and passes it on into the rectum. When this occurs, the body, by a specific mechanism, indicates to the brain that expulsion of the waste through the anus is ready. This is the urge for movement of the bowels. *See also* DIGESTIVE SYSTEM.

red blood cells. *See* BLOOD.

reflex. An involuntary movement or reaction to a stimulus, removed from the point of action. Many reflex actions take place in the body as part of its ordinary functioning or in connection with disease. The knee jerk, an example of a reflex action, is absent in many diseases of the brain and spinal cord. The oculo-cardiac reflex is a slowing of the heartbeat that follows compression of the eyeball. A slowing of five to thirteen beats per minute is the normal decrease. When a substance is put on the back of the tongue, the swallowing reflex takes place. Laughter is a reflex to tickling, and when an infant starts on hearing a loud noise, a startle reflex is provoked.

relapsing fever. One of a group of specific infectious diseases caused by spirochetes; it is characterized by recurring attacks of high fever. The disease is transmitted by the bite of ticks, lice, and sometimes bedbugs.

Usually relapsing fever begins with sudden chills followed by a fever which may go as high as 105° and remain at a high level for several days, and headache and weakness may occur. At the crisis there is often danger of collapse. After a few days the patient suddenly recovers, but in a week or so will again be ill.

reproduction system. The human reproduction system consists of the generative apparatus.

Anatomy. In the male the scrotum, or bag, contains the two testicles. These produce not only the sperm cells, which fertilize the female egg, but the cells which give a man his secondary sex characteristics, the deep voice, beard, heavier bones, narrow pelvis, rough skin, and flat breasts.

Each testicle has a long tube which leads to a separate semen reservoir. The sperm cells pass through these tubes to the semen reservoirs, in which there is a sticky white fluid provided by the neighboring prostate gland. This combination is known as semen.

In sexual intercourse, the external organ, the penis, becomes rigid and is inserted by the male into the female's vagina. At the climax of this relationship, the semen is shot through the penis into the vagina, close to the opening into the womb.

The ovaries of the female resemble the testicles of the male. The female egg cells originate in the ovaries and pass into the Fallopian tubes, which resemble the semen reservoirs in the male. The eggs remain in these tubes a few days and then, unless fertilized, go down into the womb, or uterus. The uterus is a small empty organ which can be greatly expanded. From there the cells leave the body by way of the vagina during the female menstrual period.

The entrance to the vagina resembles a small pair of vertical lips. Outside these is a larger pair of lips which encloses not only the entrance to the vagina but also the mouth of the urethra, through which urine is expelled, and, in front of that, the clitoris. The clitoris is a small fleshy projection which, in sexual excitement, may become erect, like a tiny penis. The external female sex organs are known as the vulva.

Conception. In intercourse, the sperm cells are deposited near the mouth of the womb. These sperm cells may travel further, enter a Fallopian tube, where one of them may meet with and fertilize one of the female egg cells. At once, by process of self-division, the egg cell will begin to grow.

Leaving the Fallopian tube, this fertilized egg cell fastens itself to the inner wall of the womb. Soon, between the wall and the cell, the placenta develops. This is the channel of communication between mother and child, but the blood of the two never intermingles. Each, in the placenta, will have its own separate blood vessels. Other materials, however, such as fluids and gases, are passed from mother to child through the walls of these blood vessels, a process known as osmosis, which permits the mother to supply the child with such essentials as food, water, and oxygen. The child may also use this channel to rid itself of waste.

The placenta, together with membranes developed during pregnancy, is eliminated after the birth of the child, in the "afterbirth."

The new human being may be said to exist as soon as the sperm cell has fertilized the egg cell, at which time the sex is determined. Every cell in the body of a female contains two chromosomes, or sex determiners, whereas each cell in the body of the male has only one. However, when the female pro-

duces egg cells, only one determiner will be found in each. When the male develops sperm cells, half of them contain one determiner each, while the rest do not contain any. If the sperm cell which fertilizes the egg cell happens to contain a determiner, the result will be a fertilized egg cell with two determiners and the child will be female. However, if the fertilizing sperm cell does not contain any determiner, the child, possessing only the one determiner, will be male.

As yet, there is not a scientific means of determining, before birth, whether or not the child is male or female. *See also* CERVIX; CONTRACEPTION; OVARIES; PREGNANCY AND PRENATAL CARE; TESTICLES; UTERUS.

reserpine. A new alkaloid drug which has proved useful against high blood pressure and in relieving the symptoms of acute mental disorders. The substance is derived from rauwolfia serpentina, a root from which extracts have been used in India for many centuries for a variety of medical purposes. Reserpine is a specific substance isolated from the root and believed to be the active principle to which the therapeutic effects are due. *See also* BARBITURATES.

respiratory diseases. Those disorders which affect the act of breathing with the lungs or the apparatus, the organs, tissues, and membranes, involved. The respiratory system in the human being is chiefly composed of two lungs and the air passages which lead to them. *See also* COMMON COLD; LUNGS; PNEUMONIA; TUBERCULOSIS.

retina. The light-receptive layer and terminal expansion of the optic nerve, the eye. Vision is accomplished through the passing of light rays through the human eye to the nervous tissue at the back of the eye, called the retina. A serious disorder of the retina is detachment of the retina, a condition in which small areas of the retina separate from the underlying coats, usually as the result of injury, infection, or tumor and, sometimes, as a result of a disease, such as tuberculosis. An operative procedure has been developed in retinal detachment.

Inflammation of the retina is called retinitis, which may be due to infection, hemorrhage, or other types of injury. Sometimes it is associated with inflammation of the kidneys or hardening of the blood vessels.

Retinoblastoma is a malignant tumor of the retina, occurring in infancy or early childhood. In some instances tumor of the retina is present at birth. This disorder rarely occurs in persons more than ten years old. *See also* EYE.

retrodisplacement. A term used to describe shifting of the uterus backward in the abdomen.

retrolental fibroplasia. A form of blindness that occurred only among premature babies. Medical detective work finally showed that keeping the babies under oxygen twenty-four hours a day was the cause. Babies are now under oxygen only a few hours at a time and the condition has been eliminated.

rheumatic fever. A febrile disease characterized by painful migratory arthritis and a predilection to heart damage leading to chronic valvular disease. It most frequently attacks young people between the ages of six and nineteen and, although no longer the leading cause of death in this age group, is among the foremost health problems. In at least one-fifth of all cases of rheumatic fever the most serious associated condition is the attack on the heart. Rheumatic fever usually appears following infections of the nose and throat, but it may also be associated with ear infection, scarlet fever, St. Vitus' dance and other similar ailments related to streptococcal infection.

Pain and the other symptoms can usually be controlled by a doctor. The detection of the first signs of the heart disease associated with rheumatic fever is difficult. The obvious signs of heart damage, such as irregularity, rapidity, pain, changes in size, and accumulations of fluid in the heart sac, appear later. When the heart enlarges and its action is impaired, the sounds of the heart change and the pulse generally reflects the condition of the heart. Also typical of rheumatic condition are nodes which appear under the skin and an outbreak of rash.

The valves of the heart may be affected. Small nodules form on the valves and interfere with normal function. The nodules eventually disappear, leaving scars and causing the valve to develop unusually large numbers of blood vessels. If attacks of rheumatic fever recur, the patient may develop hardening of one of the valves. The blood is also affected. The white cells increase with the infection and the sedimentation rate of the red blood cells mounts, receding as the patient improves. Sometimes infection of the kidneys and the intestinal tract or severe pain similar to that of an attack of appendicitis accompany rheumatic fever.

Drugs of the salicylate group are especially useful in controlling such symptoms as fever, pain, and swelling in the joints. However, although these drugs do relieve the painful symptoms, they do not cure the disease itself. ACTH and cortisone have been lifesaving in controlling inflammation.

When the heart is especially involved, extra care must be taken to avoid every possible strain. Continuous bed rest, for weeks or even months, for the duration of the active stage is absolutely imperative.

Unfortunately rheumatic fever has a tendency to recur after it has apparently gone. The doctor must determine, after the active stage has passed, whether or not the heart has been permanently damaged, and the person must continue to be reexamined at regular intervals to make certain that new activity has not begun and that he is in good health. For example, every sore throat should be treated immediately with antibiotics and sulfonamides.

Since complete bed rest, preferably outdoors in an open pavilion or on a protected porch, is so vital, children with rheumatic fever are best cared for in special sanatoriums where they may remain as long as necessary under the best possible conditions of ventilation, rest, sunshine, and nutrition.

The vast majority of children with rheumatic heart disease can and should attend regular schools and engage in a normally active life. In many large cities special schools are maintained for children with handicaps of the heart.

rheumatism. An overall term used to indicate diseases of muscle, tendon, joint, bone, or nerve resulting in discomfort and disability. About 7,500,000 people in the United States are affected by it, which makes it the most widespread chronic disease and ten times more frequent than tuberculosis, diabetes, or cancer. Of those affected, 400,-000 are completely helpless; 800,-000, despite treatment, are partly crippled; and the rest have chronic pain and discomfort. Rheumatism has been called one of the principal health problems in the United States.

The most common form of rheumatism is rheumatoid arthritis. Other forms are degenerative joint disease, spondylitis, bursitis, fibrositis, myositis, neuritis, lumbago, sciatica, and gout. These are all primarily afflictions that affect persons after the age of forty. Rheumatic fever, which often involves the heart, is essentially a disease of childhood, attacking children between the ages of five and fifteen. *See also* names of specific diseases mentioned above.

Rh factor. *See* BLOOD TYPES.

rhinitis. Any inflammation of the nasal mucous membrane. One of the chief forms is the common cold. Rhinitis is largely the result of infection, but may be due to sensitivity to various substances. *See* *also* COMMON COLD; HAY FEVER; OZENA.

rhinophyma. A form of acne, involving the blood vessels and sebaceous glands in the nose, which results in swelling and formation of great nodules. Rhinophyma is a disfiguring condition, sometimes called "toper's nose" or "whiskey nose." Little can be done to alleviate it, except by plastic surgery.

rhinoplasty. A plastic operation on the nose.

rhythm method. A means of preventing pregnancy by avoiding intercourse during those days of the month when the female is ovulating. Ovulation ordinarily takes place between 12 and 16 days after the beginning of the previous menstruation. Since there are numerous variations of this cycle, the method has been refined in a manner by which the woman takes her temperature when she suspects ovulation has begun. Temperature increases slightly during ovulation.

riboflavin. The scientific term for the vitamin commonly called vitamin B_2. A deficiency of riboflavin may produce general body weakness and various skin disorders. The tip and margin of the tongue become sore and inflamed, painful cracks and fissures occur at the corners of the lips, and the face becomes greasy and scaly. The eyes are particularly sensitive to riboflavin deficiency and the cornea becomes cloudy and ulcerated, the mucous membranes inflamed, and the vision may be permanently impaired.

rickets. A deficiency disease that affects infants and children and is characterized by a failure of cal-

cium salts to be deposited in sufficient quantity in growing cartilage and newly formed bone in the body. Deformities and other symptoms result from the failure of the bones to develop properly; they include growth of nodules on the ribs, development of potbelly, and bending bones. The child with rickets often sits with his thighs slightly spread apart, with one leg crossed over the other. The hands are placed on the floor or on the thighs, to assist the backbone in holding the body erect. The pull on the tissues by the muscles and the ligaments plus the softness of the bones cause bending, so that bowlegs and knock-knees are characteristic. Rickets also leads to delayed eruption of temporary teeth, and to deformities of the unerupted permanent teeth.

Since rickets is caused by insufficient amounts of vitamin D, calcium, and phosphorus during the age when growth is rapid, and since the failure to receive sufficient amounts of one vitamin is likely to be associated with the failure to receive sufficient amounts of other vitamins and minerals, treatment involves a proper diet which includes them.

rickettsial diseases. Illnesses caused by one of the rickettsial organisms. Rickettsiae are a family of microorganisms which have characteristics in common with both the filtrable viruses and true bacteria. Under the microscope they have many shapes, but most of them resemble tiny rods.

The rickettsiae are transmitted from man to man by an intermediate host, usually blood-sucking ticks, lice, or fleas. They generally pass into the bloodstream of man through the bite of the insect, but infection may also be caused by excrement of the insect deposited on the skin.

The organism is responsible for at least four groups of diseases in human beings: typhus fever, the Rocky Mountain spotted fever group, scrub typhus, and Q fever. A person who has had a disease in a particular rickettsial disease group will have complete immunity to other diseases of the same group but will not be immune to those of the other groups.

roundworm. *See* WORMS.

rubella. Another name for German measles. *See* GERMAN MEASLES.

Rubin's test. By injection of gas or air into the Fallopian tubes, the doctor can find out if they are open and can permit passing of an ovum. Closure of tubes may be a cause of sterility.

rupture. *See* HERNIA.

sacroiliac. The joint at the base of the spine, between the sacrum and the ilium. There is no movement normally in this joint but in pregnant women it becomes movable, allowing the pelvis to tip slightly during labor.

sacrum. A triangular-shaped bone formed by the five sacral vertebrae fused together at the lower end of the spine. Inflammation of the joint between the sacrum at the back and the pelvis at the front produces pain which is sometimes mistaken for sciatica.

sadism. A sexual perversion in which

a person derives pleasure from inflicting cruelty or pain on others. The word sadism is derived from the Marquis de Sade, a Frenchman who lived about 1800 and wrote several books about sexual cruelty.

St. Vitus' dance. *See* CHOREA.

saliva. The opalescent, tasteless, weak alkaline fluid secreted chiefly by the salivary glands which open in the mouth, under the jaw, in front of the ear, and under the tongue. The lining of the mouth also secretes saliva.

Salk vaccine. *See* POLIOMYELITIS.

salpingitis. Inflammation of the uterine or Fallopian tubes, due to infection. *See also* FALLOPIAN TUBES.

sarcoma. Malignant tumor, most frequently involving non-epithelial tissue, which includes fibrous and connective tissue, cartilage and bone. Cancer in the skin, arising from the layers below the epidermis, occurs only in children. Sarcoma of the nerve cells is known as fibroneurosarcoma. It is also found in lymphoid and fatty tissue. Sarcoma may be detected and diagnosed by microscopic examination of a piece of the tumor, a procedure called a biopsy. *See also* CANCER.

scabies. Popularly known as "the itch," or "seven-year itch," follows invasion of the skin by the microscopic itch mite, which is no more than a fiftieth of an inch long, and whose scientific name is *Acarus scabiei.*

Several areas of the body seem to be favored by the mites. Most often they burrow on the inside of the fingers, near the webs. Other locations are the insides of the toes, the ankles and knee joints, the front of the armpit, the breasts of girls and women, and the outer sex organs of boys and men. The face never seems to be attacked.

The body becomes sensitized to the insects and intense itching results. Numerous blisters may form, and scratching may result in infection.

To rid the body of the itch mites, the most effective treatment includes bathing in hot water every day, followed by the use of sulfur ointment. For patients sensitive to sulfur, ointments containing other drugs, including benzene hexachloride which is less irritating than sulfur, may be prescribed.

Underclothing and bedding must be changed daily until all danger of further hatching of the eggs is removed. Extreme care must be taken that the infested person not infect other persons with whom she comes in contact.

scarlet fever. An acute infectious disease characterized by a scarlet skin eruption. It occurs most frequently in fall or winter, and in children between the ages of five and twelve. Children less than one year old seldom contract it, probably because they have received antisubstances in their blood from the mother which afford protection.

The period of incubation is approximately three days following contact with an infected person. The symptoms are a painful sore throat, chill, nausea, and vomiting. The pulse rate increases, the temperature may rise as high as 104°, and the child may suffer a severe headache.

The rash first appears in pinpoint spots of bright red, usually on the chest and neck, and then gradually over the rest of the body. Although this rash attacks the body more often than the face, the face often shows red spots, if only because of the high fever. Although the rash may continue only two or three days, it will take a week or more before the skin regains its normal color. Ten days to two weeks after the onset of scarlet fever, peeling of the skin begins. Large pieces of skin may come away from the feet and hands or drop off in scales, and other parts of the body can be affected, such as the teeth, fingernails, and sometimes the hair. The tongue develops a pitted scarlet appearance which gives it the name strawberry tongue.

Although scarlet fever often proves to be a relatively mild infection, it may have serious complications. The kidneys are frequently involved, or the ears, glands, and joints, so that this disease can do serious damage.

Treatment demands that particular attention be given that as little effort as possible be placed on the kidneys and heart, since they are already receiving from the toxin itself an attack almost greater than they can endure. Ordinarily the patient is required to remain in bed at least three weeks and must be protected from chill and cold. Sponge baths of tepid water may be given. A mild gargle may relieve sore throat, and one of the newer antibiotics will be even more effective. Reactions of the heart and kidneys and ears must be carefully watched. Occasionally when the ear is infected the ear drum is punctured so that the pus can be drained before the internal ear is involved.

Since the advent of sulfa drugs and penicillin, serious complications from scarlet fever have become rare.

schizophrenia. A severe mental disorder, a major psychosis, which involves a loss of contact with reality and a temporary or permanent disorganization or disintegration of personality. "Schizo" means splitting, "phrenia" means mind, and the term refers to a splitting away of the mind from reality. Schizophrenia is the most common form of mental illness and one-fourth of all hospitalized mental patients fall into this category.

The schizophrenic person rejects the outside world and turns to her own self-created world. Her actions are made in accordance with this imagined world and so are difficult to interpret. Her speech may be garbled and unintelligible and her actions completely inappropriate to her external situation, since they are motivated by her fantasy world and her inability to perceive reality in the normal way.

Schizophrenia is not one disease but rather a set of complex symptoms which encompass many forms of mental disorder. The causes are extremely difficult to treat. Factors which would appear pertinent in some cases do not apply to others. The schizophrenic is a person who has apparently been unable to find a way of adjusting to some painful situation and so has rejected the outside world in favor of her own inner version. Organic factors are also believed to be related to schizophrenia.

In the past few decades, understanding and treatment of schizophrenia has greatly improved and the rate of partial or complete recovery is higher. Expert psychiatric care is essential, preferably as soon as possible.

sciatica. *See* SCIATIC NERVE; SCIATIC NEURITIS.

sciatic nerve. The large long nerve which supplies the muscles of the thigh, leg, and foot and the skin of the leg. It runs the entire length of the leg with many branches and subdivisions. The nerve can be irritated or compressed at any point. *See also* SCIATIC NEURITIS.

sciatic neuritis. Also frequently called sciatica, inflammation of the sciatic nerve, the longest nerve in the body, which passes from the lower part of the spinal column downward to the leg along the rear of the thigh. True sciatica is sciatic neuritis, and pain is felt in the thigh and other areas associated with the sciatic nerve. The part of the spinal cord where the nerve originates may be disturbed, for example, by a slipped or ruptured disc, or by an inflammation in the vertebral bones. An abnormal condition in a nearby blood vessel may cause it to press on the nerve. Acute and prolonged constipation is sometimes responsible because the accumulation in the bowel exerts pressure on the nerve or because the body absorbs unexcreted toxic substances to which the nerve reacts. External conditions or occurrences may precipitate a sciatic disturbance, such as a bad fall or severe contortion of the body, or prolonged exposure to cold and dampness.

Diagnosis of the specific cause of a particular case of sciatic neuritis demands the attention of a skilled physician. The pain is only a symptom and the source of it must be determined before proper treatment can begin.

scleroderma. A disease in which all the layers of the skin become hard and rigid. A serious affliction, scleroderma attacks women more often than men, usually between the ages of twenty and forty. Localized scleroderma often appears and disappears spontaneously in children.

Before the disease becomes apparent, the victim may for some time have complained about alterations in the circulation of her blood. Soon the hands and feet take on a bluish tinge, which changes later to white or yellow. At the same time the tissue itself becomes increasingly hard and rigid. Eventually both arms and legs—and even the entire body—may become hard as stone.

Almost nothing is known about the cause of scleroderma. Obviously serious damage is done to the tissues, as well as to the superficial blood vessels.

sclerosis. A hardening of part of the body due to overgrowth of fibrous tissue. The term is applied particularly to hardening of the nervous tissue from atrophy or degeneration of the nerve elements, and to thickening of the arteries caused by growth of fibrous tissue and deposits of fatty substances and cal-

cium salts. *See also* ARTERIOSCLEROSIS.

scoliosis. *See* SPINAL CURVATURE.

scurvy. A nutritional disorder caused by a lack of vitamin C. It is characterized by extreme weakness, spongy gums, and a tendency to develop bleeding under the skin and from the mucous membranes and bone coverings. *See also* VITAMINS.

seasickness. *See* MOTION SICKNESS.

sebaceous cyst. *See* WEN.

seborrhea. A functional disease caused by excessive secretion of the sebaceous or oil-producing glands in the skin. The condition may vary widely, from nothing more than dandruff, the commonest form, to seborrheic dermatitis, in which the whole scalp and sometimes the face and other parts of the body develop a greasy kind of crusting and scaling, accompanied by red irritated areas.

In some cases, dandruff begins in childhood as a simple scaling of small white bits of skin from the scalp and then continues as a mild annoyance for many years. Often, however, the process gradually becomes more and more involved with greasy discharges from the scalp and skin of the face, and "oily" seborrhea may develop, sometimes with so much discharge that drops of oil actually collect on the skin.

Treatment of troublesome dandruff should be under a doctor's direction, but the person who has seborrhea will find that more than the usual participation by the patient is required. Success depends largely on her willingness to take frequent shampoos, massage the scalp with prescribed lotions and ointments, and brush the hair daily.

The doctor has other measures which he uses to shorten the treatment time. A new preparation, derived from selenium, has proved effective against many of the annoying symptoms.

semen. The male fertilizing fluid.

senescence. The process of aging. As people grow older, their bodies undergo changes. The cells of the body begin to lose their power of repair, and the glands tend to function less efficiently. Digestion becomes disturbed, and the senses of taste, smell, sight, and hearing often weaken or begin to fail. In the aging process of the human body, the condition of the blood vessels is the most significant single factor. Hardening of the arteries, the wearing out of the muscular tissues of the blood vessels, and heart failure are the result of degenerative changes in the tissues. As the consequence of these changes, the body may either lose bulk or become corpulent. The bones are harder and more brittle, the hair grays and often falls out, the capacity for muscular and mental effort decreases, and diseases affecting the circulatory system, heart, kidneys, lungs, and other organs begin to manifest themselves.

Within the limits imposed by aging, medical science can do much for these disorders, and older persons should be examined by a doctor at frequent intervals.

Many of the changes in the vision of older persons are due to changes in circulation, including hardening of the arteries. The pupil of the eye becomes smaller and less movable, and the color of the eyes becomes lighter. The lens of the eye grows and increases in weight throughout life, and a reduction in elasticity promotes the condition known as presbyopia, which is due to a loss of accommodation in the lens. Sometimes a cataract, typical of old age, forms. The exact cause is not known, and the decision whether or not to remove a cataract depends on many factors related to the person's mental and physical condition, as well as the actual condition of the eye.

The eyelids of an older person develop wrinkles, and she seems to cry more easily, sometimes suffering from an excess of tears. This is often due to relaxation of the tissues of the eye, which do not hold the material as well as do the tissues of younger persons. With surgical advances, techniques have been developed for maintaining the normal relationship between the tissues and overcoming the excess of tears.

Like the rest of the body, the teeth and jaws are subject to change in old age. The jaws change shape and the teeth tend either to fall out or require extraction. Artificial dentures often replace the loss of teeth.

The functioning of the digestive system becomes less efficient as a person grows older, and frequently a simpler, more easily digested diet is preferred. Three meals a day should still be eaten, but they can be smaller. The diet, of course, should continue to be balanced, and vitamin or mineral supplements taken if necessary. Less protein is required for tissue repair, although foods which supply energy are still essential in sizable amounts.

During late maturity, a thorough physical checkup is a wise precaution against disease in old age. Many maladies to which older persons are subject result from chronic diseases which occurred years before. The diseases that take the greatest toll of life among the aged are heart diseases, cancer, and cerebral hemorrhage. Other afflictions are arthritis, rheumatism, diabetes, prostatic enlargement, kidney diseases, hardening of the arteries, high blood pressure, and nervous and mental conditions. *See also* GERIATRICS; SENILITY.

senility. The extreme stage of cerebral arteriosclerosis, which produces in the aged symptoms approaching dementia. The mind of the senile person becomes feeble and she may be so confused that she requires constant care and attention, and cannot be left alone. This condition is also marked by extreme forgetfulness. In such moments, she may begin to do something in one part of the house and and then suddenly go off to another room, forgetting what she had started out to do. In other instances, the senile person may wander away from her home and walk confusedly about, not even having presence of mind to ask directions.

Often the rest cycle is reversed, and the senile person sleeps during the day instead of at night. She will be active all night, moving about from room to room while the rest of the household sleeps. At daybreak, drowsiness sets in and she may sleep and doze the rest of the day.

In the most advanced stages of senility, all touch with reality may be lost and symptoms of dementia manifested. Coherent communication with others becomes impossible and helplessness, incontinence, and loss of brain function are noted. At this stage, hospitalization is often the best solution, and a large percentage of beds in mental institutions are devoted to senile persons.

In treating senility, the doctor will check and prescribe accordingly for high blood pressure, overweight, and diabetes. Any correctable illness or condition will also be treated, including diet deficiencies and anemia, both fairly common among senile persons. In most cases, the teeth and digestion of the aged will be in such poor condition that a bland diet of chopped meats and strained and puréed vegetables will be advised. An effort should be made to cater to the special tastes and preferences of the individual, who may be "cranky" about her food. In treating the reversed sleep cycle, a combination of a mild stimulant in the morning and a moderate sedative at night is effected in most cases, although the situation may be fairly difficult to control. Tranquilizing drugs, among other measures, have been found effective in treatment of the extremely confused. Much remains to be learned and done in the care and treatment of senility. *See also* GERIATRICS; SENESCENCE.

septicemia. Another word for bacteremia or blood poisoning. In obstetrical cases infection of retained placenta or blood clots may take place within the uterus and lead to septicemia. *See* BACTEREMIA.

septic sore throat. An acute infection of the throat caused by an organism, streptoccocus hemolyticus. It is the most severe of all sore throats, and serious complications may ensue if treatment is not prompt.

sex. Whether male or female, is determined by the chromosomes, the glands, the structure of the body, and psychologically by the manner of rearing. Some people incline toward both sexes even in structure.

shingles. *See* HERPES ZOSTER.

shock. The condition caused by acute failure of the peripheral circulation, the circulation of the blood in the veins and in the capillaries farthest from the heart. The essential functions of the body are diminished. Shock may occur during times of great emotional stress, injury, pain, sudden illness and accident, such as burns, and has been one of the most difficult emergencies to confront physicians.

sinuses. Cavities or channels within bones. Those in the head which connect with the inside of the nose by narrow passageways sometimes cause trouble. The sinus in the cheekbone is called the antrum, the one above the eyes is the frontal sinus, and deeper behind the nose is the ethmoid sinus, which is actually a series of small sinuses, varying from three to more than fifteen in some cases.

The membranes of the sinuses are susceptible to infection. If the opening of the sinus into the nose becomes blocked, the infectious matter will cause symptoms of sinusitis, which include headache, pain, and, when the infection is absorbed into the body, high fever. An ordinary cold may end in a few days, but if the sinuses become infected the symptoms may last for many weeks. Eventually the sinus disorder may become chronic, with an increase in the intensity of the original infection.

sleeping sickness. *See* ENCEPHALITIS.

sleeplessness. *See* INSOMNIA.

slipped disc. The backbone as an integrated system is so designed and put together that it breaks only under the most extraordinary and violent shocks. It can support a weight far larger than that of the body of which it is a part, and can move this body in practically any direction. In addition, the backbone is capable of a range of movements extending from a stevedore's lift to an acrobat's contortions and a ballet dancer's delicacy and discipline.

The intervertebral disc, a little cushion of cartilage that lies between every second vertebra of the spinal column, makes all this possible. The center of each disc is composed of a special material called nucleus pulposus, which tends to move about slightly in correspondence to movements of the body. These discs cushion the body and especially the head against direct impact of the shock of walking which a solid bone would transmit. They also permit an ease and degree of rotation of the vertebrae which would otherwise be impossible.

Occasionally a disc is displaced during common experiences of everyday life. An automobile accident may throw a sudden and excessive shock on the spine and cause an injury at first not apparent. A bumpy airplane landing may have the same effect. Many forms of athletic exercise involve some risk of injuring a disc. Activities such as gymnastic work which subject the spine to frequent sharp heavy shocks while the back is in an unusual position tend to do this most frequently.

The detection of a dislocated disc is not a simple matter and may require prolonged study. The injury is not apparent through simple exploration with the fingers. X-ray and careful review of the symptoms will help the doctor make a diagnosis.

Rest, wearing braces, and surgery are all alternative remedies for the condition. The doctor's judgment alone can determine the best treatment.

smallpox. Or variola, a contagious infectious disease, often fatal, with fever followed by a papular eruption which produces pitted scars. The introduction of vaccination, developed by the English physician Edward Jenner in 1796, and the more recently improved techniques for quarantine and isolation have brought smallpox almost completely under control and it is now comparatively rare.

The incubation period is generally eight to twelve days. Smallpox begins with violent headache, chill, pain in the back and limbs and a high fever, and, in children, convulsions and vomiting. Within three or four days small reddened pimples appear over the face and wrists and spread rapidly to the arms and chest. These form blisters in a day or two and in about eight or nine days begin to dry, leaving a blackish crust. The face swells and feels irritated and the rash, particularly on the face, can be agonizing. The eyelids may be swollen shut. After three or four weeks the crusts fall off and the characteristic pitting scars or pockmarks of smallpox remain.

Complications caused by bacterial infection result in bronchopneumonia, conjunctivitis, or more serious damage to the eyes or middle ear.

The immunity gained by vaccination is temporary and vaccinations must therefore be repeated at five-to seven-year intervals. The first vaccination is generally given between the ages of three months and one year and is repeated between the ages of seven and eleven years, especially if an epidemic is present or if travel is planned to areas where the disease is more common than in the United States. *See also* IMMUNITY; IMMUNIZATION; INFECTIONS; VACCINATION.

smegma. A glandular, ill-smelling secretion found under the labia minora in the female and under the prepuce of the male penis. Since the prepuce is removed during male circumcision, circumcised males secrete little or no smegma. In those groups which regularly practice male circumcision, there is little if any cancer of the female cervix.

sneezing. A natural reflex action involving a deep intake of breath followed by closure of the glottis; the mechanism is similar to that of a cough. A violent expiration effort ensues, the glottis opens, a blast of air is sent out through the nose, taking with it mucus and other material. Frequently the eyes water immediately following a sneeze.

snoring. The rough, audible sound made by breathing through the nose in such a way as to cause a vibration of the soft palate. The noise made by snoring is due to the intermittent passage of air at places in the mouth where there may be partial obstruction. Adenoids sometimes cause snoring, especially in children.

somnambulism. A sleep or sleeplike state during which walking or other activities are performed. It is fairly common in children. In adults it is rarer and of more serious significance. Usually sleepwalking stems from some conflict in the mind which is unresolved and continues to stimulate the person even during the period of sleep. Usually when the person's doubt or fear is removed—which, in serious cases, may require psychiatric help—the sleepwalking ceases. A person awakened during sleepwalking is usually perplexed and distressed. He should not be criticized or scolded, but consoled and returned to bed.

sore throat. Inflammation of the pharynx, called pharyngitis, or of the tonsils, called tonsillitis. In a common cold, the soreness is usually in the back wall of the upper throat and affects the nasopharynx and the palate. *See also* COMMON COLD; LARYNGITIS; PHARYNX; QUINSY; SEPTIC SORE THROAT.

Spanish fly. *See* CANTHARIDES.

spasm. An involuntary sudden contraction of a muscle. The usual cause is irritation of the nerve cells or nerves which supply the muscle. A sustained contraction is called tonic. Contraction and relaxation rapidly alternating produce clonic spasm. A general spasm over the body is a convulsion or fit. Massive spasms are characterized by sudden movements which involve most of the body musculature and last from a fraction of a second to several seconds. They may affect infants and young children. The commonest form of spasm is one in which the limbs and trunk are suddenly flexed, followed by relaxation. Similar attacks may occur in series.

Almost anyone can at some time have a muscle spasm. Sudden chilling of the body during swimming may cause a muscle spasm, or whenever the circulation of the blood in any part of the body is greatly diminished sudden involuntary contractions may occur. Disorders in the nervous system—for example, the death of a nerve cell in the interior portion of the spinal cord—may result in paralysis of the muscles with spasm of the opposing muscles.

Sometimes children develop habit spasms—not to be confused with chorea or St. Vitus' dance. The movements of habit spasm are quicker and always repeated in the same way, whereas the movements of chorea are irregular and variable. Spasms in children may sometimes occur as a result of distress, such as fear of punishment.

Whenever a spasm of the muscle

occurs, examination by a doctor is necessary to determine the source. If it is a condition affecting the nerves, medical or surgical management may be required. In some instances, injection of one of various substances around the nerves of the area involved is the only treatment to stop a spasm. *See also* CHOREA; CONVULSION; TIC DOULOUREUX.

sperm. The male germ cell.

spina bifida. An essential step in the development of the human embryo before birth is the growing together of two sides of the original channel in the back, thus forming the space where the spinal cord will lie. Failure of these to grow together results in a structural condition known as spina bifida, meaning literally a split spine.

This condition occurs in approximately one in every 1000 births, but the specific form of the defect always varies. Ordinarily spina bifida will be only a gap in the coverings which should enclose the spinal cord. In other instances, however, one or more vertebrae may be absent. This deformity may be accompanied by a bulge in the sheathing of the spinal cord projecting to the exterior, as in a hernia. This creates in the back a bulbous body filled with liquid.

Some cases of spina bifida are accompanied by what is called hydrocephaly, derived from words meaning water and head. In this condition the fluid which is normally required within the membrane containing the brain increases inordinately in quantity because of interference with circulation and drainage, and the skull bones expand to compensate. The size of the head becomes grossly disproportionate to that of the body.

Immediate medical attention should be given to every such case. Exposure of any part of the nervous system, as occurs in spina bifida, is extremely serious. Surgical repair will benefit at least half the children affected by the condition but must be undertaken as early as possible to obtain the greatest benefit. The elimination of the bulge in the back often will accomplish much for the patient.

If the condition is left unattended, the distortion of the spinal nerves and the strain to which they are subjected will disturb their function. When the abnormality occurs in the lower spine, the defect may cause paralysis of the legs and loss of normal control over bladder and bowel action. If the nerve supply of the skin is inadequate, ulcers may develop.

spinal cord. The relatively large branch of nervous tissue that extends from the brain down through the vertebrae. The brain and the spinal cord together constitute the central nervous system.

spinal curvature. The spine is one of the most fundamental structural elements of the body and forms a basis around which other essential parts are arranged. Seen from the side, the spine has a modified S shape, giving it a springiness and elasticity that protect the delicate organs in the head and elsewhere from constant bumps and shocks. Seen from the front, it is a straight line. When this line loses its straightness and becomes a looplike curve, either to the right or to the left, the resulting condition is scoliosis, or curvature of the spine.

spleen. A large, ductless, glandlike organ which lies in the upper left part of the abdomen, just below the diaphragm and toward the rear of the body.

The functions of the spleen have significant relationships to the character and circulation of the blood and to resistance against disease.

At times the spleen contracts, discharging a quantity of blood into the general circulation. Therefore, when an animal or human being exercises intensively, the spleen is believed to maintain the proper volume of blood circulating in the blood vessels.

Enlargement of the spleen is a disorder of variable sources. Sometimes enlargement is due to splenic destructive activity against worn-out blood cells and disease-creating organisms which are retained within the spleen. Sometimes a fatty material enlarges the spleen. Enlargement of the spleen appears in several major infectious diseases, among them malaria.

An enlarged spleen is not always explicable, and if an adequate cause is not ascertained the organ must be removed. In such cases a lymphoma or tumor of lymphoid tissue may be responsible. In certain specific diseases, such as purpura hemorrhagica or thrombocytopenia, a clotting disorder of the blood, removal of the spleen is considered beneficial. In the case of Banti's disease, splenectomy is not generally recommended. The spleen is not essential to life—as is, for example, the liver—and its removal rarely produces adverse effects.

sprains. Injuries in the area of a joint, in which a sudden movement or a fall will stretch or overstrain connective tissue fibers belonging to the ligaments, muscles, or tendons so that they are torn or ruptured. Fluid or blood then gets into the joint. Sometimes a sprain is so severe that a bone is broken. For this reason every severe sprain should be X-rayed. The opening of the football season and the onset of winter produce a sudden increase in the number of sprains, particularly of the ankle.

sprue. A feverless chronic disease. Sprue comes from the Dutch word that describes an inflammation of the mouth. The disease, known for more than two thousand years, is generally considered to be a tropical ailment, although it will occur in persons who do not live in the tropics. Both tropical and nontropical sprue are probably nutritional deficiency disorders of the small intestine, marked by impaired absorption of food elements, particularly fats. However, the exact cause is unknown.

Symptoms of sprue are diarrhea, cramps, and distended stomach due to gas.

squint. Or strabismus, failure to focus both eyes on the same point. In the most common form, one eye looks toward the object while the other is turned from it.

There are many kinds of squints, caused by a large number of disorders and diseases in the eye, the muscles that move it, the nerves supplying them, and the brain which controls and co-ordinates the nerve impulses.

Treatment is generally effective, but requires the co-operation of the patient. When a child has a squint, sympathetic attitudes on the part of his family and persons around him can be of great help.

stammering. *See* STUTTERING AND STAMMERING.

Stanford-Binet test. The Stanford-Binet "I.Q." or Intelligence Quotient test is a revision of the Binet-Simon tests which were originally conducted in France by two French psychologists, Binet and Simon.

No test has yet been developed which can conclusively measure someone's intelligence, but many different methods have been tried, with varying degrees of success. The Stanford revision of the Binet-Simon test is one of the most widely used at present.

sterility. The incapacity to produce children, is a complex phenomenon involving a variety of factors. Chief responsibility may be borne by the woman, the man, or both. Even when one or the other is specifically accountable, sterility may apply only to a given set of circumstances; in another situation the same person might not be sterile. Because of its variability, sterility may properly be regarded as characteristic of a particular union of two persons, rather than of either the man or the woman separately. Scientists have determined that circumstances pertaining to the marriage relationship may cause sterility.

Medical statistics indicate that men are responsible for 30 to 40 per cent of all instances of childlessness. Diagnosis of the condition and endeavors to correct it demand first an examination of the husband. If the results indicate that he is responsible, the general physical condition of the wife is determined. A frequent cause of sterility in men is some disorder associated with the male germ cell, the sperm, one of which must fertilize an ovum, or female egg cell, before conception occurs. These male cells are produced in the testes, the two male sex glands, and stored in the seminal vesicles, higher in the body.

Such disorders may involve various organs or tissues. The glands may not produce sperm cells even though otherwise the man appears to be sexually normal. The sperm cells produced may be weak or malformed, so that they cannot function properly and carry the fertilization process to the final stage. Furthermore, there may be insufficient numbers of them; although only one sperm can fertilize a given egg cell, a normal male provides three to four million of them on each ejaculation. Any of these conditions may be responsible for the woman's failure to conceive, and the doctor has means for testing to find out whether or not such a condition is present.

Conditions in the woman which prevent conception are even more varied than in the man. Among the simplest are infection, inflammation, or injury of the parts of the body involved. Sometimes the cause is blockage of a passage through which the sperm cells should travel. Occasionally congenital deformities of the sexual organs may cause such occlusion or otherwise render conception impossible. In a few instances the uterus may be undeveloped or missing entirely.

A frequent cause of sterility in women is some irregularity in the system of glands of internal secretion, the endocrine glands, or of their products, the hormones. The sex glands are a significant part of the whole glandular network, and a mishap in the latter can affect the female sexual cycle at one of several points, making conception difficult or impossible.

Other conditions which can induce sterility include faulty diet, a subject not yet thoroughly understood, and emotional or mental disturbances which can react upon physical factors.

That a woman has not attempted to prevent conception and still has not conceived does not necessarily mean that pregnancy is impossible for her. The condition may continue for years and then terminate in a normal pregnancy and delivery.

Complete physical examination of both husband and wife by a doctor is essential for the couple who seem sterile and wish to correct it. Such an examination will include studies of sperm cells of the husband and examination of the wife's sexual organs to determine their condition and whether or not the necessary tubes are open and functioning properly. A complete record of the sex experiences of both husband and wife is also imperative. The cause or causes that the physician finds operative will determine the recommendations. Often a previously sterile couple can achieve conception by careful use of knowledge of the alternating periods of fertility and infertility in the female, regulated by the menstrual cycle. When a disease has closed one or both of the Fallopian tubes within the woman, attempts to free them by surgery or forcing a passage of air through them are only rarely successful.

steroids. Most hormones are chemically steroids. This includes ovarian, testicular, and adrenal hormones such as estrogen, follicle stimulating hormones, progesterone, gonadotropin, and androgens.

stomach. The portion of the alimentary tract, the digestive tube, which extends from the lower end of the esophagus or gullet, the canal extending from the pharynx to the stomach, to the beginning of the duodenum or first part of the small intestine. The normal stomach is J-shaped with a bulge above and to the left of the junction with the esophagus. The shape varies according to its fullness or emptiness and the position of the person.

Various congenital deformities may affect the stomach, such as enlargement of the muscle of the pyloric valve. Gastroptosis or dropped stomach may occur later in life. Surgery is generally successful in correcting congenital abnormalities when they are known.

Inflammation of the lining of the stomach is a common disorder, occurring in various forms and at any time throughout life. Peptic ulcers are another common stomach disorder, resulting from action of the gastric juices on the stomach wall.

An increase in the amount or concentration of gastric juice causes acidity.

Cancer of the stomach is responsible for a great number of deaths each year in the United States. It usually occurs in late middle age and more often in men than women, men past forty-five being the most frequent victims. Cancer of the stomach is of several types, including ulcerating cancer, tumor growing in the stomach cavity, and a diffuse thickening of the stomach wall. Loss of weight, appetite, and general normal health are symptoms of stomach cancer, but unfortunately the cancer is often too far advanced before it is detected to be effectively treated and may have spread to regional lymph nodes and other organs. Because of the danger of stomach cancer, any form of stomach "upset" after middle age should receive immediate medical attention. If the cancer is discovered soon enough, an operation to remove the cancer with a portion or even all of the stomach can be successful in curing the condition, and so it is imperative that it be diagnosed at the earliest possible time. Cancer of the stomach is too often a hopelessly fatal disease because of a late diagnosis. See also DIGESTION; FISTULA; FOOD POISONING; GASTRITIS; INDIGESTION; PEPTIC ULCER.

stomach ache. See ABDOMINAL PAIN.
stomach ulcer. See PEPTIC ULCER.
streptococcus. A genus of bacteria which grows in chains, resembling tiny strings of beads when viewed under the microscope. Streptococcus germs are present in infections such as erysipelas, scarlet fever, subacute bacterial endocarditis, puerperal fever, subacute sore throat, streptococcus throat, and certain forms of enteritis and rheumatic fever.

streptomycin. An antibiotic drug. It is similar to penicillin in its antibacterial action and method of manufacture, and has been found particularly effective against many disease-producing germs that penicillin also attacks. In addition it is a powerful agent against some diseases that are not affected by penicillin, such as tularemia, a severe infectious disease acquired in handling infected rabbits.

Streptomycin is also effective in treating certain types of blood and urinary infections which are not helped by other drugs. Reports indicate that it may cure tuberculous meningitis, and it has been successfully used in diseases produced by the common colon bacillus. Pneumonia, streptococcus infections, staphylococcal penumonia, and staphylococcal meningitis are among the many diseases in which streptomycin has been effectively used.

Streptomycin is taken orally or injected directly into the bloodstream, as the condition dictates. In cases of meningitis, it is injected into the spinal fluid. See also ANTIBIOTICS.

stress incontinence. A condition in which a woman cannot hold her urine while on her feet or when she coughs, sneezes, or takes any exercise.

striae. Atrophica or gravidarum. Narrow scars on the abdomen caused by stretching during pregnancy or obesity. They are red immediately after childbirth but gradually change to silver in color.

stroke. A sudden and severe seizure or fit of disease. The term is generally used for apoplexy, and in connection with sunstroke and heatstroke. *See also* APOPLEXY.

stuttering and stammering. Spasmodic speech defects, resulting in a sudden check in the flow of words, or a rapid repetition of a consonant or consonants with which the person has difficulty. Usually the difficulty is with the sounds *p, b, m,* and *w,* which are sounds made by the lips. The stutterer or stammerer does not, however, always have difficulty with the same sounds. Her emotional state at the time of speaking may be a factor in how she speaks.

Stuttering or stammering are almost never due to any organic weakness, either in the organs used in speaking or in the nerves and nerve centers which control them. Physical factors may, however, sometimes aggravate it. The doctor will first make sure that inflammation of adenoids, abnormal length of uvula, abnormal size of the tongue, and improper development of the mouth are not involved.

Often children who stutter develop behavior changes; a fear of appearing ridiculous produces a subsequent lack of confidence. Persons naturally left-handed but trained to use their right hand stammer more frequently than others, and males more often than females. Anyone acutely embarrassed or terrified is likely to stammer, until her emotion is under control. Stammering is usually an expression of self-consciousness, shyness, or fear. In an eager youngster, however, it may be nothing more than failure to keep up with her rapid flow of thought; words and thoughts are conceived faster than they can be expressed. Stammerers almost always can sing and talk to themselves quite fluently.

Because stuttering and stammering are primarily conditions which have emotional causes, treatment is directed toward the person's mental conflicts. When the conflict is resolved, the person will probably regain self-confidence and the speech defect disappears. The person with a speech defect may benefit from special speech correction classes. A class is often preferable to personal instruction since the person will be encouraged by the progress of others and the realization that she is not alone in her problem. Her family and friends must be patient, tolerant, and confident; anger and impatience will only aggravate the situation.

sty. *See* EYE.

suffocation. *See* ASPHYXIA.

sulfonamide drugs. "Sulfa" drugs, are derived from or are compounds of sulfonamide, and their introduction into medicine marked a turning point in the treatment of disease. Among the sulfonamide drugs are sulfadiazine, sulfapyridine, Gantrisin, Kynex, and others. These drugs act effectively on diseases caused by staphylococcus, meningococcus, streptococcus, and organisms of the dysentery group.

Before sulfa drugs, treatment of such diseases as lobar pneumonia and spinal meningitis depended on serums, which were only moderately successful. Management of infections of the middle ear was so ineffective that loss of hearing and mastoiditis often followed. Treatment of gonorrhea depended on repeated and frequently unsuccessful urethral injections. The use of sulfa drugs virtually revolutionized treatment of these and other conditions.

suppuration. Refers to the formation of pus.

sweat. *See* PERSPIRATION.

sympathetic nervous system. Autonomic nervous system, supplies and exerts a regulatory activity to most of the involuntary organs of the body—glands, heart, blood vessels, for example—and involuntary muscles in the internal organs.

The blood supply to any part of the body can be increased by interruption of the sympathetic nerves that pass to that part. In hypertension, sympathectomy—cutting off the sympathetic nerves by surgery —is sometimes employed to increase the flow of blood into the abdominal area and lower limbs and thus decrease the blood pressure. Currently drugs are preferred to surgery to block the sympathetic nerves. Interruption or treatment of the sympathetic nervous system has occasionally been used in heart conditions such as angina pectoris, in cases of severe pain involving the urinary tract, to control serious disorders of the sweat glands, and to aid movement of the bowels.

The sympathetic nervous system is responsible for the physical sensations that accompany emotion. For example, suppressed resentment may cause overactivity of the muscles and glands of the stomach, and actual pain can result. In some psychotic or neurotic conditions, the system is involved and changes can occur in affected organs.

syncope. A brief unconsciousness during which the person falls to the ground. Young women, especially, are said to faint from excitement, exhaustion, or inadequate ventilation.

syndrome. A set of specific symptoms which occur regularly in the same combination and constitute a specific disease. Dozens of disorders are known as syndromes, a large number of them bearing the name of the first doctor to note the syndrome, connect it with the underlying disease condition, and call attention to it. Well-known syndromes are Cushing's syndrome, indicating tumor in certain parts of the brain; Korsakoff's syndrome or psychosis, associated with chronic alcoholism; and Addisonian syndrome, a condition caused by insufficiency of the adrenal glands.

synovitis. Inflammation of the synovial membranes, those membranes which line the joints. The chief manifestation is an outpouring of fluid into the joint cavity. It may occur as a reaction to injury or as a result of infection somewhere else in the body.

"Water on the knee" is a typical instance of synovitis. A combination of rest and gentle pressure from bandaging will help to induce absorption of the fluid. *See also* JOINTS AND JOINT DISORDERS.

syphilis. A contagious venereal disease which can infect any of the body tissues. It is characterized by a variety of lesions, of which the chancre (primary lesion), the mucous patch, and the gumma are the most distinctive.

The vast majority of adult cases of syphilis are acquired through sexual contact. Treatment usually seems to render the infected person incapable of transmitting the disease, but there is some evidence that persons presumably cured can still infect others.

A few hours after exposure, the syphilis spirochete penetrates the skin or mucous membrane and enters the bloodstream and tissues. The "hard chancre," the primary stage of the disease, does not appear until ten to ninety days later, three weeks being the average time. Usually the chancre is found on the genitals or in the mouth, but it may appear elsewhere and occasionally not at all. The fluid from the chancre is highly infectious.

Even without treatment, chancres generally disappear in ten to forty days, and the secondary stage, small raised red areas on the skin or small mucous patches in the mouth or on the reproductive organs, begins two to six months later. Generally lymph nodes throughout the body become enlarged. These lesions of secondary syphilis heal by themselves in three to twelve weeks, but may recur later.

The third stage of syphilis develops almost immediately after the secondary symptoms have disappeared, or, in some cases, may be delayed for years. Ulcerlike draining lesions appear on the skin; hard nodules or gumma occur in the internal organs or tissue under the skin. The blood vessels and heart are often damaged and the lungs may be affected during this stage.

Syphilis is the only venereal disease that may be acquired congenitally by the passing of the spirochete from the mother to the unborn child. Syphilitic infection may cause abortion or stillbirth. Infants who are born with syphilis may soon die; or, if they survive, may later develop blindness, deafness, paralysis, deformities, or even mental disturbances. Because of these terrible consequences, every prospective mother should be examined for syphilis so that, if she does have it, treatment can begin immediately. Even if treatment is delayed until the fourth or fifth month of pregnancy, the child may still be born healthy. If, however, treatment has been inadequate or absent, the newborn child should immediately be given penicillin. The amount given to children depends on the age the treatment begins; children over two years receive the same dose as adults.

Usually the first symptom of syphilis is a sore at the point where the germ has entered the body. The doctor makes his diagnosis by studying the material from the sore under a microscope.

When the syphilis germ enters the body, it multiplies quickly and gradually invades every organ and tissue, certain germs being limited to certain parts of the body, and syphilis can therefore imitate a wide variety of diseases.

Current treatment of syphilis with penicillin and other antibiotics has largely replaced former methods of treatment. These drugs can halt the spread of the disease within a few days. Penicillin is used not only for early syphilis but to alleviate the symptoms of neurosyphilis and in congenital syphilis.

It cannot be too strongly urged that anyone who suspects that she has syphilis see a doctor immediately. Some people through false shame or modesty permit the disease to spread to a critical point before seeking medical aid. The fact that a person has once had syphilis should always be mentioned when she later sees a doctor or dentist for other reasons, since it may furnish a clue to treatment. *See also* CHANCRE; PARESIS.

syringe. An instrument used to inject fluid beneath the skin or into a cavity. It consists of a nozzle, barrel, and plunger or rubber bulb. There are various special types of syringe, the rectal syringe, and the urethral syringe.

tabes. A wasting or degeneration. Although there are many types of tabes, the word usually designates tabes dorsalis, also known as locomotor ataxia, a disorder of the nervous system resulting from syphilis.

talipes. Any one of a variety of deformities of the human foot, especially those of congenital origin, such as clubfoot. *See also* CLUBFOOT.

tampon. A plug, usually of lint or cotton, to absorb secretions or arrest hemorrhage in a body cavity.

A trademarked product called Tampax is much used in menstruation.

tapeworm. *See* WORMS.

tear glands. The little indentation at the inner end of the eye is known as the tear gland and serves as a kind of reservoir for tears. From this reservoir several small tubes, called tear ducts, carry the tears to the eyes.

Another tube, the nasal duct, carries a similar fluid to the nose. For this reason, whenever a person sheds tears, she will also find it necessary to blow her nose.

teat. The nipple of the mammary gland.

teeth. The calcified organs supported by sockets and gums of both jaws. Their chief function is to grind food into small enough pieces to be easily swallowed and digested. The teeth help to form words and also give expression. Their loss is usually associated with old age, and loss of teeth in a young person may require a major emotional adjustment. Sound teeth contribute to health, while decayed teeth and diseased gums permit germs to enter the body. Thus the teeth may become focal points of infection and lead to other disorders.

The process of cutting teeth is ordinarily called teething or dentition. There are two dentitions; the first produces the primary teeth, also known as the deciduous, temporary, or milk teeth, and the second produces the permanent teeth. There are twenty primary teeth: four incisors, two canines, and four molars in each jaw. The incisors are the front cutting teeth; the two in the middle are called central incisors, and those on either side are called lateral incisors. Outside these are the canine teeth which are sharp, pointed, and able to tear food. Beyond the canines are the molars or grinding teeth. The arrangement of teeth is the same in the upper and lower jaws and on the right and left sides.

The second, permanent set of teeth contains thirty-two teeth. Twenty of these gradually replace the primary dentition, which starts at about six or seven years of age and finishes at about twelve years or older. This dentition begins with the appearance of the first permanent molars, and afterward other permanent teeth are cut, including the central and lateral incisors, the first and second premolar, the canines, and the second molar. The premolars which replace milk molars have two cusps on the crown and are also known as the bicuspids. The third molar teeth, the wisdom teeth, may appear between the ages of seventeen and twenty-five or later, or not at all.

The first teething is sometimes painful and the gums swollen, hot, and tender. The child may be generally upset, and colds, earache, and fever are not uncommon during this period. The second dentition rarely causes any trouble, with the exception of aching which may accompany eruption of the wisdom teeth.

Sometimes malocclusion, or irregularity in placement of teeth, may be found in the deciduous and the permanent dentitions. A special branch of dentistry, orthodontia, has been developed to correct malocclusion, and the earlier the condition reaches the attention of the specialist the quicker and more effective the treatment will be.

Total or partial anodontia, or lack of teeth, is rare. Rickets may be the cause of delayed dentition or malformation of teeth. Premature eruption of teeth has little significance, except that it may cause discomfort to a mother who is still nursing.

Mottling and discoloration may occur during formation of teeth, and is caused by excess fluorine in the drinking water or the food. Occasionally the child's teeth are malformed or incompletely calcified. These conditions should be treated by a dentist.

A small amount of fluorine in drinking water, about one part per million, has been found to help protect teeth against decay. Fluoridation of water has been tried successfully in many communities and is approved by all leading scientific organizations in medicine and dentistry.

Unless teeth are adequately cleansed, tartar may form about the neck of the tooth and lead to infection of the gums, to pyorrhea and other disorders, and to diseases of the mouth. Food may adhere in spaces between the teeth and ferment, and acid substances attack the enamel and cause dental caries or tooth decay. *See also* DENTAL CARIES; FLUORIDATION; ORTHODONTIA; PYORRHEA; VINCENT'S ANGINA.

temperature. The degree of intensity of heat of a body, especially as measured by the scale of a ther-

mometer. The normal temperature
of the human body is 98.6° F., with
occasional variations during the
day, amounting to no more than
one degree. The temperature is generally slightly higher toward evening, when it may be 99.1°, and in
early morning it may fall to about
97.3°.

An early morning temperature in
women of 98.8° or 99° occurs in
relation to ovulation. In this way
the rhythm method shows periods
of fertility and infertility.

tendon. Or sinew, a fibrous band of
connective tissue which unites a
muscle with another part of the
body, and transmits the force exerted by the muscle. *See also* BUR-
SITIS.

teratoma. A tumor composed of fetal material or other abnormal tissue.

testicles. Or testes, the two male sex
glands which hang outside the body
in a small sac of skin called the
scrotum. They perform two significant functions: they produce both
the male reproductive cells, the
sperm, and the male sex hormone,
the internal secretion which causes
the body to assume the attributes
of masculinity.

Both sperm and so-called interstitial cells originate within the testes,
the tubular structures known as
seminiferous tubules. When the
sperm cells mature, they migrate
to one of the two seminal vesicles
located near the urinary bladder,
where they remain until used. The
interstitial cells remain in the testes,
occupying the spaces between the
tubules, and produce male sex hormones.

The hormone known medically as
testosterone has been extensively
studied and found to have many
effects in the body. Appearing in
quantity only as puberty approaches, it evokes growth of the
sex organs to their adult size.
Stronger and heavier male bones
and muscles are dependent on the
testosterone, which also causes the
vocal cords in the larynx to enlarge, resulting in the characteristic
low pitch of the male voice, and
prompts the growth of body hair.

Testosterone has a definite effect
on emotional and mental development, influencing adult interest in
sex, and ideas and attitudes usually
identified as adult and masculine.

The body may contain at least one
other male sex hormone, if not
more, but this has not as yet been
scientifically established.

The term eunuch signifies a male
deprived of the testicles or of the
external male genitals. Such men
tend to lose many or most typically
male characteristics.

The testicles normally descend
from within the body to the scrotum by the time of birth. However,
this does not always occur. Since
the internal temperature of the
body is too high to permit the organs to produce sperm cells, the
glands cannot develop and function
properly. Therefore, when the
testes do not descend, some of the
male characteristics may be latent.
Treatment by hormones alone may
be sufficient, but often surgery is
indicated to correct this condition,
called cryptorchism. *See also* OR-
CHITIS; REPRODUCTION SYSTEM; UN-
DESCENDED TESTES.

tetanus. Or lockjaw, an infectious disease, often fatal, which especially attacks the muscles of the neck and lower jaw. This disease is caused by the tetanus bacillus, a germ which ordinarily infests the intestines of cattle, horses, or men, and which is also found in the earth. The germ invades human beings primarily through wounds. Since it thrives best without oxygen, it is found most abundantly in deeper wounds, especially those which contain soil or foreign refuse.

About seven days after the invasion of the germ, the person infected is likely to feel a kind of pulling pain in the wound. This is accompanied by a spasm of the muscles. She may develop chills and fever, a painful headache, and probably a general feeling of irritability. Stiffness is first evident in the muscles of the jaw and neck, and a series of violent convulsions and spasm may soon follow. Sometimes occurring as frequently as every minute, these spasms may be so extensive that every muscle in the body is involved.

The tetanus bacillus engenders an exceedingly strong poison which may be fatal. Prevention of the disease consists of injecting an antitoxin under the skin as soon as a wound has been inflicted. The wound is then opened wide, thoroughly cleaned of foreign matter, and cleansed with antiseptic. *See also* IMMUNIZATION.

tetany. *See* PARATHYROID GLANDS.

thermometer. In medicine, the instrument used to take the temperature of the body. In the United States, the Fahrenheit scale is most frequently used, usually graduated between 94° and 110°. The normal body temperature, 98.6°, is generally indicated by an arrow. The centigrade thermometer is used in Europe.

throat. The inside of the throat includes the larynx, or voice box, the pharynx, the upper part or fauces, which is the space surrounded by the soft palate, a group of muscles used in swallowing, the palatine arches and the base of the tongue. On the outside, the front part of the neck is also described as the throat.

A sore throat is an inflammation of part of the throat. Inflammations are manifested by redness, swelling, and excessive discharges of mucus due to many different sources. Most common is exposure to cold, an extension of inflammation from the tonsils, adenoids, or the nose.

One form of sore throat, pharyngitis, may be an entirely separate disease or the symptom of another ailment, such as scarlet fever, influenza, measles, or smallpox.

Excessive use of tobacco, exposure to large amounts of dust, smoke, irritating fumes, and sudden changes in temperature or excessive dryness and similar atmospheric conditions may cause irritation of the throat. Persons who are sensitive to certain food substances frequently react with blisters on the tissues of the throat, which become infected and produce irritations and inflammation. Swelling and inflammation of the throat may produce pain in the ears, because of blocking of the tubes which pass from the nose to the ear. A sense of fullness or obstruction, with much spitting and hawking, can also develop.

In "strep" throat, which is septic sore throat caused by the streptococcus germ, a membrane, a thin layer of tissue, sometimes appears in the throat, the glands may swell, and the temperature may rise as high as 105° F. Penicillin generally cures this condition. *See also* LARYNGITIS; QUINSY; SEPTIC SORE THROAT; SORE THROAT.

thrombosis. A clot formation inside a blood vessel; the clot is called a thrombus. Thrombosis is caused by failure of the mechanism in the blood which keeps it fluid. Such a disorder usually occurs in veins in which the flow of blood is slowed, as in a varicose vein of the leg, or in a leg vein of a person who must lie in bed for a long time. In some cases, thrombosis is associated with bacterial infection in the area affected, or in an actual inflammation of the vein, as in thrombophlebitis. Thrombosis may also occur in narrow arteries through which the blood passes with difficulty, but arterial thrombosis is much rarer than venous thrombosis.

Thrombosis does harm by obstructing the flow of blood to and from the part supplied by the vessel and as a source of traveling fragments of clots, or emboli. An embolus is especially dangerous when it affects the lung, and there is always danger of sudden death.

Thrombosis is often the source of stroke, although a stroke caused by thrombosis is less dramatic and severe than one from an embolism or with hemorrhage. Strokes from thrombosis have a better chance for recovery, but some permanent disability usually persists.

A clot in the main vein of a limb produces swelling. For example, a clot in a main vein of the leg, deep in the upper calf, will cause a swelling of the foot and ankle and probably most of the leg below the obstruction. The amount of harm done depends on what area the artery supplies and whether or not there are alternative routes for the blood. If there is no alternative route, all the living cells which compose the part supplied will die. The effect is exactly the same as that of an embolism or of complete blocking and obliteration of the artery by progressive hardening and narrowing.

Thrombosis is treated by certain anticoagulants, including heparin, dicumarol, and others, and in some cases surgery is employed to remove clots and help restore the flow of blood to the affected parts. Anticoagulants together with proper massage and exercise have been particularly effective for patients with swollen legs due to thrombophlebitis when infection is not a complicating factor. In some cases of varicose veins, a thrombus may change into fibrous or scarlike tissue and the inside of the tube is obliterated. In this way a natural cure is sometimes effected. *See also* APOPLEXY; COAGULATION; CORONARY THROMBOSIS; EMBOLISM.

thrush. A fungus infection of the mouth in infants and occasionally older persons. White spots form, then become shallow ulcers. Frequently fever and gastrointestinal disturbance are present. It is most frequent among bottle-fed babies. The fungus may spread to the buttocks, groin, and other areas of the body.

thumb sucking. In a healthy, happy baby, thumb sucking, if practiced in moderation, is normal and may be ignored. The child will discover new amusement with the passage of time. Persistent thumb sucking, authorities claim, may lead to malocclusion of the teeth. If the child ceases sucking his thumb before the age of five, however, this malocclusion has a tendency to cure itself.

To cure a persistent thumb sucker is not easy. Painting the thumb with a bad-tasting medicine or forcing the child to wear a mitten have not been successful methods and are not recommended. The source of the habit lies in some kind of emotional disturbance or sense of insecurity. To cure thumb sucking, therefore, the source of the habit should be found. *See also* CHILD CARE.

thymus gland. A gland located in the chest near the heart. This gland has an unusual part in the development of the body. Instead of growing like the rest of the physical structure, the thymus is largest during the first eight or nine months of life and after the second year normally shrinks almost to the point of disappearance and is replaced by other types of tissue.

If the gland does not shrink and its size and activity continue, the results can be serious. Occasionally, especially in infants, the gland enlarges so much that it interferes with circulation and breathing, because of its proximity to the heart and windpipe. X-ray treatment is often beneficial to reduce such an enlargement. Persons may develop thymic enlargement so suddenly, apparently in response to some stress or shock, that death results. This type of growth occurs in the condition called status lymphaticus, which is rare.

The person whose thymus gland has failed to shrink has a "peaches and cream" complexion and, if male, will probably not have to shave, or infrequently. Such persons seem younger than their actual age. They lack body hair and may be subject to low blood pressure and fatigue.

In premature cessation of functioning of the thymus, aging seems to occur before the usual time, and blood pressure is apt to be high and body hair excessive.

The thymus is apparently implicated with development of the skeleton, the sex glands, and with metabolism of calcium, and also concerned in formation of resistance to disease and sensitization.

thyroid gland. One of the most significant of the endocrine glands, which produce secretions that regulate many basic processes of the body, the thyroid gland lies in the front part of the throat along the windpipe.

The thyroid secretion, thyroxin, is involved in the process of oxidation which occurs within the cells and by which the tissues generate the energy they require. Its importance is indicated by the serious consequences of excessive or deficient amounts of it in the body. A child born with insufficient thyroid activity becomes a cretin, physically undergrown and mentally an idiot. Thyroid deficiency in later life causes physical and mental coarsening and dulling. Excessive thyroid produces general restlessness, speeds up the heart, and may have other untoward effects. Both hyperthyroidism, too much thyroid, and hypothyroidism, too little, can be successfully treated.

The thyroid is susceptible to a variety of diseases, the most common being simple goiter, usually due to a lack of iodine. In Graves' disease, or exophthalmic goiter, overactivity of the thyroid causes a popeyed appearance and other serious symptoms. Tumors too, of lesser or greater malignancy, may affect the thyroid. Surgical removal is indicated for most types of thyroid cancer. X-ray and radium treatment and radioactive iodine have also been beneficial in certain cases. A number of infectious and non-infectious diseases of the thyroid also respond well to treatment. *See also* BASAL METABOLISM; CRETINISM; GLANDS; GOITER; HYPOTHYROIDISM.

tic douloureux. Or trigeminal neuralgia, one of the more common neuralgias or paroxysmal pains, usually beginning in the middle life and occurring more frequently in women.

The attacks occur without warning, in violent, knifelike darts of pain. The face is twisted in spasms and there is a free flow of tears and saliva. The seizure lasts only a few seconds and may clear up spontaneously, with varying periods of relief. The pain may involve the first or ophthalmic division which includes the forehead and eye, the second division around the nose, or the third or side of the mouth. The second and third branches seem to be more frequently affected. The pain does not spread to the back of the head or across to the other side of the face. The attacks tend to increase in acuteness and extent and as the condition becomes worse the periods of freedom from pain become shorter. The seizures often are influenced by seasonal changes and occur more frequently during spring and fall. Pain may be prompted by touching the affected side of the face, by exposure to cold, washing, eating, drinking, or talking, and emotional tension or fatigue intensify the attack.

Treatment consists largely of measures to relieve individual attacks. Nicotinic acid and trichlorethylene inhalations give temporary relief. A drug called Tegretal has been helpful.

The operation consists in cutting the branch or branches of the trigeminal nerve which carry the pain to the affected area of the face. In those cases in which the eye is involved and the first branch is cut, the patient is given special instruction in care of the eye, since sensation in this area is affected when the nerve is cut and the patient is unable to detect the presence of foreign bodies in the eye.

tongue. The movable muscular organ attached to the floor of the back of the mouth. Its chief functions are to help with chewing and swallowing food, with taste, and to form sounds in speech.

Normally the tongue is pinkish

white in color, moist and clean; a tongue that is dry, dark, and furry indicates disease. Among the most common of peculiar sensations that disturb persons is a burning painful tongue.

When no apparent physical cause exists, purely mental reasons are thought to be responsible—for example, a woman in menopause who is worried about developing cancer might experience a burning tongue.

Sometimes the tongue is inflamed through contact with edges of rough teeth, or ill-fitting false teeth. Frequently burning tongue is associated with difficulties of the digestive system. In such cases, the doctor will want to make a complete examination, which includes blood tests as well as checking the digestive system.

In a few instances, burning, and even ulcers, of the tongue have been found to be caused by the fact that different electric potentials have been used to fill teeth on opposite sides of the mouth. In a condition called glossitis, the tongue itself is infected and may have superficial or deep abscesses. The tongue may be subject to cancer or other specific diseases.

tonsillectomy. *See* TONSILS.

tonsils. Masses of spongy lymphoid tissue located at the sides of the throat in the entrance to the digestive and respiratory tracts. They frequently become infected, with such symptoms as swelling, inflammation, pain, soreness, difficulty in swallowing, enlargement of the glands of the throat, fever, a rapid pulse, and general illness.

The person affected with tonsillitis should be put to bed and the doctor called. Ice packs or hot compresses may be applied about the throat and neck to relieve pain. The doctor will take steps to combat fever. Early administration of drugs, particularly antibiotics, greatly reduces the possibility of serious complications or aftereffects, which can include deafness, kidney disease, rheumatic fever and other heart ailments.

Extraction of diseased and enlarged tonsils and adenoids, which interfere with breathing, is usually beneficial not only in removing a source of infection but also in improving the child's general health, appearance, and disposition. Surgery to remove tonsils is advised in recurrent attacks of tonsillitis accompanied by swelling of the neck glands. The operation, tonsillectomy, is so common and has been so well perfected that complications are exceedingly rare.

In older persons or in the presence of heart disease and other cases in which anesthetic is not possible, tonsils are sometimes treated with radiation by X-ray. X-ray and radium are also occasionally used to treat fragments of tissue that may be left after tonsillectomy and when there is regrowth of secondary adenoidal tissue.

torticollis. Commonly called wry neck, a spasmodic movement of the neck muscles which causes the head to be pulled toward one side. In some instances, shortening of neck muscles is present at birth or may occur from an injury, but in the majority of cases the origin of this disorder is unknown.

Wry neck begins suddenly without warning. The neck muscles unexpectedly contract and the head is pulled to one side in irregular jerks. It may follow a nervous reaction due to tension, worry, or anxiety. At this stage the movements can be suppressed by the person, but as the condition grows worse the movements recur involuntarily and cannot be controlled.

Psychotherapy has been successfully tried in treatment of some cases. In more stubborn cases, this treatment is combined with a nerve block, a procedure in which the cervical nerves are blocked with procaine or novocaine. Light exercises also help to relax the muscles. Frequent periods of spontaneous relief occur, but the condition generally returns, even after long intervals of relief. Use of collars or casts is not recommended. Medication includes drugs of the belladonna group and sedatives. Surgery has brought only temporary relief at best, and is not widely employed.

toxemia of pregnancy. A somewhat unscientific term that covers a series of conditions affecting women in pregnancy. The symptoms are vomiting, elevated blood pressure, chronic nephritis, acute yellow atrophy of the liver, pre-eclampsia, and eclampsia.

toxoplasmosis. A recently discovered parasite that is thought to be one cause of mental retardation among newborn infants.

trachoma. A highly contagious chronic disease of the eyelids, caused by a filtrable virus. Trachoma was once an almost universal affliction and the most common cause of blindness. Trachoma has affected many American Indians and may still be found in the southern mountainous areas of this country. Sulfonamide drugs and antibiotics have made possible control of the spread of trachoma.

tranquilizing drugs. *See* BARBITURATES.

transverse lie. During labor, the baby presents itself by the shoulders, one arm appearing first.

trauma. An injury or wound.

trench mouth. *See* VINCENT'S ANGINA.

trichinosis. A disease caused by eating pork infected by *Trichinella spiralis,* a slender roundworm that is barely visible to the naked eye. If the worms have not been destroyed by proper cooking, they may develop in the intestines and later invade the muscle tissue, where they produce stiffness and painful swelling.

Tiny cysts, encasing immature worms, are present in contaminated pork. The human digestive process liberates them in the intestines, and they mature within a few days. The developed males fertilize the females, which then burrow into the intestinal wall and subsequently release larvae.

These larvae, carried through the blood circulation, lodge in the muscles, encysting themselves within a shell-like substance that they secrete. There they cause the pain and muscular irritation which are characteristic of the disease. Other symptoms are headache, fever, sore throat, general illness, and painfully swollen eyes. Specific treatment for the disease is not yet known. In time, the tissues of the body surround the organisms and wall them off.

Protection against trichinosis is possible in at least two ways. Since the trichinae cannot survive freezing or more than a certain degree of heat, they can be killed by freezing the meat at 0° F. for twenty-four hours or at 5° F. for twenty days, or by cooking at 140° F. or more for half an hour per pound of meat.

trichomonas vaginitis. A troublesome kind of vaginitis caused by a specific organism. There is often discharge and irritation. It can be treated with antibiotics, but it can recur with intercourse.

trigeminal neuralgia. *See* TIC DOU-LOUREUX.

tuberculosis. An infectious disease characterized by the production of tubercles, small rounded nodules which may appear on almost any part of the body. It is caused by the germ commonly called the tubercle bacillus, of which there are many varieties.

The past decade has seen tremendous advances in the control and treatment of tuberculosis. The death rate in the United States has dropped from 250 out of every 100,000 persons to rates as low as 5 in many states.

Tuberculosis remains a chronic disease and if healing is not complete, relapse may occur. Although in the acute phases of the disease, the new drugs act quickly to promote healing, treatment of the tuberculous patient may require a long time. The discovery and application of new drugs, like streptomycin, para-aminosalicylic acid, and isoniazid, has virtually revolutionized the management of tuberculosis, and patients can now be treated by a combination of hospital and home care rather than being placed in sanatoriums.

Although pulmonary tuberculosis is the most common form, the glands, covering of the brain (meningeal tuberculosis), the spinal fluid, the eye, and many other tissues may be affected. In acute miliary tuberculosis of the generalized type, the tubercle bacilli may be disseminated throughout the organs of the body. Acute active pulmonary tuberculosis, "galloping consumption," may be difficult to diagnose at the onset. It may attack suddenly, with coughing of blood-stained sputum, and in such cases a doctor should be promptly consulted. This form, which was once rapidly fatal, has now yielded to modern drugs. A person may have tuberculosis of the lung and some other form of the disease at the same time.

The cough is the best-known symptom of tuberculosis, and is an indication of infection of the lung by the tubercle bacillus or by some other germ. Any cough that persists for three or four weeks should always be brought to the attention of a physician. The cough is frequently accompanied by expectoration, and in some cases enough destruction of lung tissue has occurred for blood to be expectorated. Furthermore, fluid may pour out into the walls of the chest, an example of the way the body attempts to control infection. Another way the body tries to check the infection is to cover or wall off the infection with scar tissue, a process known as fibrosis.

The tuberculous person is generally sick, loses weight, and feels weak. A slight rise of temperature in the afternoon, or fever and an increase in the pulse rate, may also appear, and night sweats are common.

X-ray examination will reveal the extent of involvement of the lung, and a physical examination of the chest determines any changes that have taken place in its shape or contour and movement.

The success of the treatment depends largely on recognition of the disease at the earliest possible moment.

Anyone who has symptoms of tuberculosis—loss of weight and appetite, nausea, persistent fever, persistent cough and expectoration, a prolonged cold or spitting of blood —should immediately consult a doctor.

tularemia. An infectious disease transmitted to man by infected rabbits or other rodents, through their bite or through handling them.

By far the most common source of infection is contact of the hands with the diseased rabbit. Rabbit meat, thoroughly cooked, is harmless when eaten, since a temperature of 130° F. will kill the germ of tularemia.

When tularemia appears on the body, an ulcerlike sore is usually found at the point where the germs have entered through the skin. This sore ordinarily appears several days after exposure. Following rapidly are headache, aching muscles

and joints, weakness, chills, and fever.

For those who hunt rabbits, it is well to remember that a rabbit which runs slowly is probably a sick rabbit and best ignored. Any rabbit which a child or dog brings home is likely to have been too sick to run.

In treatment of tularemia, streptomycin is rapidly curative, and other antibiotics including Aureomycin, Chloromycetin, and Terramycin, have been used effectively. Complications, including pneumonia, may arise and require hospitalization, intravenous feeding, and, for serious cases, blood transfusions and oxygen.

tumor. Literally a lump or swelling, although the term is not used to describe the swelling of normal tissues such as occurs in inflammation or edema, or the enlargement of organs such as the spleen, liver, or kidneys. Specifically a tumor is a mass of cells, resembling ordinary tissue, which develops independently as new growth and serves no useful function. When such newly formed tissue occurs in blood vessels, it is called an angioma; in fatty tissue, a lipoma or fatty tumor; in cartilage, a chondroma. Tumors composed of tissue unlike the host organ may sometimes occur, such as cartilaginous or fatty tumors which develop in a gland—for example, the carotid gland. A malignant tumor, or sarcoma, is composed of fleshy mass derived from connective tissue.

A large class of tumors do not have harmful effects, except as they produce pressure by their growth, and are designated as simple, benign, or innocent. However, a malignant tumor not only exerts pressure on adjoining tissue but actually invades and destroys it, or may disintegrate and produce new tumors in other parts of the body, a condition known as metastasis.

Any lump or swelling should be brought to the attention of a doctor who will diagnose it and determine the necessary treatment. Some tumors may be left undisturbed, whereas others should be removed. *See also* CANCER; LIPOMA; METASTASIS; POLYP; SARCOMA; XANTHOMA.

Turner's syndrome. A congenital malformation with sexual infantilism including retardation of growth, webbed neck, clubbed feet and internal failures of development.

twilight sleep. Partial anesthesia during childbirth. The patient responds to pain but memory afterward is dulled or effaced.

typhoid fever. An acute infection caused by the typhoid bacillus.

The germ is found in the blood of a person seriously ill with typhoid fever, and in 80 per cent of the cases is also found in the material excreted by the bowels. The germ of typhoid fever is spread through excretions of the body, by contaminated food, clothing, water, and milk. In spite of improved sanitation, methods of treatment, and immunization by vaccination, a primary menace remains, the typhoid carrier, a person who has had the disease and recovered but who continues to propagate the germs and to spread them. Administration of penicillin and removal of the gall

bladder of the carrier have helped curb the problem, but many typhoid carriers still exist.

Typhoid vaccine is highly effective, but not absolutely preventive against typhoid fever. It is administered subcutaneously in three weekly doses by a physician or trained nurse. A booster injection at suitable intervals will maintain a high level of immunity and should be given to persons who because of occupation or travel may be exposed to typhoid-contaminated food or water.

Although areas still exist throughout the world where typhoid fever is a threat, persistent attention to water supplies, pasteurization of milk, disposal of sewage, control of typhoid fever carriers, and general education of the public in hygiene can eliminate the disease entirely. *See also* CARRIER OF DISEASE.

typhus fever. An infectious disease caused by a rickettsial organism. Other names for it are jail fever, ship fever, camp fever, and louse typhus. It is carried by the body louse or rat flea and an epidemic may arise wherever overcrowding, famine, and poverty prevail. It occurs principally in cold weather and may follow in the wake of war and famine, and spread in slums, concentration camps, asylums, and prisons.

Symptoms appear about ten days after a person has been bitten by an infected louse. Severe headache, high fever, and aches and pains of the entire body develop. On the third to seventh day, a rash appears, first on the armpits and flanks, then on the trunk and later on the arms and legs. Mental faculties are dulled and prostration is severe. Odor from the mouth is foul and bronchitis and pneumonia often develop. In mild cases recovery is usually rapid, and one attack establishes long immunity.

Treatment of the typhus fever group consists of good nursing care. Antibiotics have been effective in decreasing the severity of the disease and in controlling its spread. *See also* IMMUNIZATION; RICKETTSIAL DISEASES.

ulcer. Any open sore, other than a wound, with an inflamed base. Such a lesion usually occurs in the skin or mucous membrane of some internal organ. Ulcers may result from infection, injury to the blood supply, damage to nerves, or from a wide variety of other causes. Ulcers require the attention of a physician who will not only endeavor to learn the specific cause but will plan the treatment accordingly. *See* PEPTIC ULCER.

umbilical cord. The connection of the fetus with the placenta. It is severed at birth but should not be cut or tied until the umbilical vessels have stopped pulsating.

umbilicus. Or navel, the depressed scar in the median (middle) line of the abdomen, which results from the separation of the umbilical cord in childbirth.

undescended testes. The development of the testes, or testicles, takes place in the abdominal cavity. Normally they descend into the scrotum soon after birth. If this descent fails to occur, the abnormality is designated as undescended testes.

Undescended testes usually atrophy—that is, waste away. If this occurs in both testes, the person becomes sterile. Undescended testes through functional failure also hinder proper development of the secondary sex characteristics, such as the beard, the low voice, and the flat chest.

The parents or pediatrician should, therefore, examine the child at an early age to be sure that the testes have descended into the scrotum. Ordinarily the testes can be felt. Rarely it may be possible to press them down gently to the proper position. In cases of any difficulty the advice of a doctor is absolutely essential. If the child is old enough to realize the situation, care should be taken not to arouse his curiosity or create anxiety.

Sometimes surgery is necessary to transplant the testes to their proper position in the scrotum. This operation should, if possible, always be performed before puberty. *See also* REPRODUCTION SYSTEM.

undulant fever. Known medically as brucellosis. A remittent febrile disease, caused by infection with bacteria. The infection may last weeks or months and during this time the fever rises and falls over periods of several days, and may be severe enough to cause death. Unfamiliar in the United States before 1927, undulant fever has now been reported in every state.

Undulant fever is also found in cattle, sheep, and goats, and human beings may contract the disease from infected animals, although more frequently from infected milk or milk products. Twelve to thirty-six days after exposure, fever and other symptoms are noted. The temperature rises steadily over a period of days, receding temporarily each morning, until a fever of 102° or 103° is reached. It remains at this point for a few days, then steadily drops down, and this cycle may persist for months. Fever periods are accompanied by general malaise, pain, constipation, sweating, and weakness. Undulant fever has occasionally been mistaken for other illnesses with somewhat similar symptoms, such as malaria, typhoid fever, and even tuberculosis.

Until recently, little could be done for the infection, but vaccines now exist which can effectively prevent it, and sulfonamides and antibiotics are helpful in some cases, and other measures, such as heat treatments, have yielded a certain amount of success.

uremia. The poisoning which results when the filtering and excretion of wastes from the blood by the kidneys is blocked so that these substances accumulate in the blood. It occurs in acute and chronic forms. The most extreme type is when both kidneys are removed or their excretory channels are blocked. Death then follows in a few days.

An early symptom of uremia is headache, which may be present in annoying severity weeks before other indications of disturbance are perceptible. When the headache is accompanied by restlessness, difficulty in sleeping, nausea, and vomiting, the possibility of uremia definitely exists, and prompt medical attention is imperative.

In its acute form, uremia may attack without warning. A convulsive epileptiform fit followed by coma may be the first manifestation. Sometimes the coma occurs without a fit and in some instances mania seizes the patient. Inflammation of the kidney may occur in children during or after another acute infection, with similar sudden convulsions preceded perhaps by rapid swelling of the tissues and face. The attack may happen so quickly and violently that death ensues. Because of this, doctors watch carefully urine changes in children who have major infections such as pneumonia, acute tonsillitis, or scarlet fever.

In the more slowly developing uremia, the early symptoms are followed by shortness of breath, attendant on accumulation of toxic materials in the body. It is often difficult to distinguish between failing breath due to heart weakness and that accompanying the later stages of kidney disorder. The patient may grow apathetic, drift quietly into unconsciousness, and finally die. Occasionally fluid accumulates, presses upon the lungs, and affects breathing. Similarly fluid may intrude upon the brain and have to be withdrawn by spinal puncture.

In general, treatment of chronic uremia is the same as for chronic nephritis. Acute uremia is often relieved by inducing sweating and by frequent liquid bowel movements, both of which tend to help the body rid itself of excess fluid and liquid wastes. Many uremic patients, with obstructive lesions, are cured by proper treatment, which can include injections of glucose to correct dehydration. *See also* NEPHRITIS.

ureter. A thick-walled muscular tube that passes the urine from the kidney to the bladder. There is one on either side of the pelvis. The ureter acts by a process of contraction or peristalsis that forces urine down the tube in spurts. It is about twelve inches long and about one-fifth of an inch in diameter.

The close relation of the ureter to the cervix, uterus and vagina makes it liable to damage during hysterectomy.

Sometimes a stone may block the ureter and require surgery for its removal. The tube may become twisted or infected, and occasionally it has been ruptured.

Disorders of the ureter or any part of the urinary tract are generally treated by a specialist known as a urologist. When the ureter is affected, X-rays are generally taken, after injection of a substance which causes the ureter to become visible.

urethra. The passage from the bladder through which urine is voided.

The female urethra is broader than that of the male and is subject to greater dilatation. Urethral carbuncles are small swellings peculiar to women, and if they do not give any discomfort are best left untouched. If they become tender and painful during urination, they can be removed surgically.

In the male, the urethra is approximately eight inches long, and only an inch and a half in the female. The male urethra begins with a prostatic portion which is surrounded by the prostate gland. It receives ducts through which prostatic secretion and semen are discharged. After a short second part comes the cavernous section which passes through the main body of the penis. It too receives ducts, and recesses emerge from it. Infection of the urethra frequently lodges in these side passages and is difficult to dislodge.

Urethritis, inflammation of the urethra, most frequently the result of gonorrhea, causes a swelling which narrows and partly closes the urethra. The inflammation impedes the flow of urine and the emerging stream may fork or twist. Sometimes the urethra is clogged by a kidney stone or a foreign body which may have to be removed surgically.

Stricture of the urethra requires regular stretching with an instrument designed for the purpose, but sometimes surgical treatment may be needed to open the passage. A stricture of long duration can react on the kidneys and ureters and on the bladder too, causing it to dilate and enlarge abnormally.

The urethra may be ruptured by a severe blow or by an accident, causing urine to escape into nearby tissues.

urination. Technically termed micturition, the passing of urine from the body by the kidneys. A complicated muscular action is involved. The wall of the bladder and another related muscle are contracted. Then a circular muscle around the neck of the bladder which keeps it shut and holds back the urine at all other times is released. The nervous regulation of urination is through a center in the spinal cord. Thus, even an unconscious person can urinate. Complete interruption of urination will bring death in a few days. The spinal center, however, is controlled by the brain, whether during sleeping or waking. Three or four times a day is a normal interval for micturition and ordinarily it is not necessary at night.

Many factors may increase the frequency of urination—for instance, pregnancy, and cold weather. Since less moisture is lost from the skin during cold weather, a greater excretory load is thrown on the urinary system. Other factors may be excitement; inflammation or irritation of the kidney, bladder, or urinary passage; or a growth or presence of a stone within them. In addition, excessive urine may occur in diabetes and nephritis, and acid or other irritants be present in the urine itself.

Partially or wholly uncontrolled urination may also arise from several factors. The bladder may have reached its capacity and be unable to hold more, or nervous disorders may induce or permit involuntary urination. Apoplectic or epileptic fits as well as unconsciousness may affect micturition, and sometimes the brain loses its power to regulate the special spinal center.

Occasionally a sense of need to release urine develops when actually the bladder is empty. This condition, dysuria, may come from irritation of the urinary tract or from nervous sources in locomotor ataxia, a disease of the spinal cord. *See also* BED WETTING; BLADDER; DIURESIS.

urine. The watery fluid excreted from the blood by the kidneys, stored in the bladder, and discharged through the urethra. In health, urine is amber-colored and contains urea, inorganic salts, pigments, and other end-products of the metabolism of both protein and minerals in the system. Urine has a somewhat aromatic odor and when it stands for some time ammonia is produced, which is easily recognized by its odor.

Urine examination is routine in prenatal care. It is checked for albumin which may indicate heart failure, nephritis, urinary infection, or liver trouble. Sugar may also be found, a symptom of diabetes.

The daily quantity of urine may vary in health. In cold weather it may be increased and conversely decreased in hot weather when perspiration removes a large amount of waste products. The quantity is also affected by certain diseases. In diabetes, pints of urine may be excreted each day. In fevers and acute nephritis, urinary output may be greatly lessened. If urine has an ammoniacal odor when excreted, it has undergone decomposition, as occurs in chronic inflammation of the bladder. In diabetes the odor may resemble that of new-mown hay. In certain diseases and disorders, it is essential to determine the quantity of both normal and abnormal constituents of urine, particularly urea. A diminution of urea occurs in nephritis and other disorders. Albumin in urine may be indicative of nephritis or another disorder, but sometimes, as in albuminuria, the cause is physiological. In diabetes the urine is tested to determine the amount of sugar, and another test indicates whether or not blood is present.

The acidity of urine is increased by an ample amount of meat in the diet; large amounts of vegetables make it alkaline. In dyspepsia, when copious amounts of soda are taken, it may also be quite alkaline.

Specific gravity is also tested in diabetes and in diabetes mellitus it is considerably raised. In diabetes insipidus or cirrhosis of the kidney, however, it is quite low. *See also* ALBUMINURIA; HEMATURIA.

uterus. A hollow, pear-shaped organ in the female pelvis commonly known as the womb. Within the uterus, the unborn child develops and grows for nine months, nourished by the blood from the mother's body. In the non-pregnant woman, the uterus is about three inches long and only weighs two ounces, but during pregnancy its elastic wall stretches. It returns to normal size after delivery. The uterus is suspended in the pelvis by ligaments and opens into the vagina by means of the cervix, a small hollow fibrous tubelike structure situated at the bottom of the uterus. The cervix is a protective passage which shields the rest of the uterus, especially during pregnancy. At delivery it distends to permit expulsion of the fetus. The uterus is a muscular organ, but its lining is a soft glandular material known as endometrium. Bleeding at menstruation comes from this lining. The ovaries are near the uterus, on each side, but do not connect with it. Eggs from the ovary reach the

uterus by passing from the top through two armlike projections known as the Fallopian or uterine tubes.

The uterus is prone to infection, especially after childbirth or criminal abortion. Occasionally severe inflammation after abortion may result in permanent sterility, because of destruction of the uterine lining.

Cancer of the uterus occurs most frequently in older women. The symptoms include bleeding, usually between periods or after menopause. Bleeding may occur from less serious sources, such as fibroid growths in the uterine wall. The doctor can usually make the diagnosis by removing tissue from the uterus for examination. This is done by scraping the lining of the uterus. In this procedure sometimes referred to as "D and C," the cervix is dilated and the uterus scraped or curetted. *See also* CANCER; CERVIX; HYSTERECTOMY.

urticaria. *See* HIVES.

vaccination. Inoculation with a preparation containing disease germs or viruses for prevention of ailments caused by these organisms.

When the germs are grown from secretions or blood taken from a patient, so that it contains the strain of organisms responsible for the disease, the vaccine is called autogenous. Usually a vaccine contains killed germs, but sometimes living organisms are used, or a mixed vaccine of a variety of germs or viruses. A vaccine containing several strains of the influenza virus is used to prevent epidemic influenza. The Salk vaccine, which has been widely and effectively employed in immunization for poliomyelitis, is an example of a killed virus. *See also* IMMUNIZATION; VIRUSES.

vagina. The female genital passage or canal which extends from the outer sex organs, or vulva, to the uterus. It consists of muscular tissue which can dilate tremendously during childbirth. It serves for the insertion of the penis, the reception of semen, and delivery of the infant after pregnancy. It is three to four inches long. Inflammation of the vagina occurs in certain venereal infections, such as gonorrhea, or it may be a complication of some other infectious disease, such as scarlet fever or measles. Vaginal discharge is commonly known as leucorrhea or the whites. Vaginismus is a painful spasmodic contraction of the muscles at the entrance to the vagina. Bleeding of the vagina may occur after the eighth week of pregnancy due to venous congestion. *See also* DOUCHE; FISTULA; LEUCORRHEA.

vaginal discharge. In pregnancy a mucous discharge may occur from the fourth week onward.

vaginal smear. Also known as the "Pap" smear. A diagnostic test to discover precancerous or cancerous cells.

vaginismus. A painful spasm of the vagina from contraction of the vaginal walls, preventing coitus. It may indicate neurotic aversion to the act.

varicose veins. Veins which become dilated so that they project in lumpy fashion above the surface of the skin. They are caused by a breakdown of the valves which ordinarily serve to maintain a continuous flow of blood to the heart. These valves cease to function properly, and the blood tends to accumulate at intervals, causing the appearance described.

Varicose veins appear most frequently in the legs, for in this area the blood is required to climb almost straight up on its way to the heart. For the same reason, varicose veins, or hemorrhoids, often develop in the lower part of the bowels.

People who suffer most frequently from varicose veins are those whose blood, for some reason, is failing to circulate in a normal manner. Fat people are susceptible and also pregnant women. After the birth of a child, the interference with normal circulation may terminate. By that time, however, the valves have been broken, and once broken do not repair themselves.

Varicose veins are dangerous because dilation leads to clotting of the blood and therefore to secondary infection.

Occasionally varicosity of the veins can be prevented by proper attention to clothing. The habitual wearing of tight belts or tight garters, for example, should be avoided.

The treatment varies with the patient. Small varicose veins are sometimes emptied of blood and then filled with a fluid which causes the walls of the vein to grow together. In treating the legs, the physician may block off a large vessel in the upper part of the thigh, and so prevent the downward flow of blood into veins which might otherwise become dilated. In some cases this condition can be controlled by the wearing of elastic bandages or stockings.

The current treatment of varicose veins is surgical removal, by stripping and segmental excision. This has largely replaced injection in severe cases; mild cases are generally left untreated. *See also* HEMORRHOIDS.

veins. Vessels that return blood to the heart, as opposed to arteries which carry blood away from the heart.

The blood in veins is a dark purplish color, except the blood of the pulmonary veins which is red. It is purified blood carried from the lungs to the heart. All the venous blood from the rest of the body is poured into the heart through two large veins, the vena cava.

Veins generally follow the same course as arteries and many are named after the arteries they accompany.

A wound of the vein is ordinarily less dangerous than a wound of an artery, because the bleeding can be controlled more easily. However, a wound of one of the large veins in the neck or in the armpit is dangerous not only because bleeding may be profuse but also because air may enter the vein and form an embolus, or obstruction. Breathlessness and discomfort may ensue, followed by death within a few seconds if the embolism reaches the lung.

Varicose veins are dilated, hardened, and twisted. Inflammation of a vein that is septic (affected by general reaction of certain bacteria) or simple is phlebitis. *See also*

HEMORRHOIDS; PHLEBITIS; THROMBOSIS; VARICOSE VEINS; WOUNDS.

venereal disease. See separate entries for the five venereal diseases, CHANCROID; GONORRHEA; GRANULOMA INGUINALE; LYMPHOGRANULOMA VENEREUM; SYPHILIS.

vermiform appendix. Vermiform means worm-shaped, and vermiform appendix designates the worm-shaped tube or sac extending from the cecum. The vermiform appendix is commonly referred to simply as appendix. *See also* APPENDICITIS.

vertebra. One of a number of small movable bones which make up the spinal column or backbone.

Various disorders involve the vertebrae and vertebral discs. Mechanical imperfections may affect the sacrum and the fifth lumbar vertebra. At the joining site, the nerves may become the seat of low back pain. Spondylolisthesis, also known as swayback, affects the stability of the lower spine, and a slipped disc or injury may affect the intervertebral disc, also causing low back pain. Fractures or protrusions may also occur in connection with intervertebral discs. Tuberculosis of the spine or calcification can implicate or even destroy the discs. *See also* DISC; SLIPPED DISC; SPINAL CORD.

vertigo. When a person has the sensation that the outside world is revolving around her, or that she is moving in space, she has vertigo. There are various causes for vertigo. For example, a common type occurs when a person looks down from a height or up at a height. Other types are epileptic vertigo and intestinal vertigo. Vertigo is not the same as dizziness or giddiness, which designates a feeling of disturbed relation to the surroundings.

Vincent's angina. Variously known as trench mouth, Borrelia, and ulcerative stomatitis, an infection of the mouth and throat due to a peculiar spiral organism. Apparently the infection is found only in man. Infants or adults who have lost their teeth are seldom affected.

In Vincent's angina, sores or ulcers occur on the lining of the cheeks and gums, sometimes also on the tonsils and in the back of the throat. The ulcers may become so large as to incapacitate the infected person. A typical unpleasant mouth odor accompanies the ailment. While the disease often begins with local symptoms, headache and a general feeling of illness may also be present. Pain in swallowing, membrane in the mouth and in the throat are characteristic. Because of this membrane, the disease was once often mistaken for diphtheria.

Vincent's angina is easily spread to other persons through kissing and through contaminated articles such as towels and eating utensils. Cases have been reported in which it has been spread by improperly sterilized dental instruments. An infected child should not go to school until he is cured, although isolation in the home is not necessary.

Prevention of Vincent's angina demands constant watchfulness of the condition of the mouth, teeth, and gums. Persistent bleeding of the gums, the appearance of an unpleasant odor, or occurrence of ulcers in the mouth demands consultation with a dentist or physician.

Control of the infection is much easier in the early stages than later when the condition has become chronic.

Poor teeth and negligence of mouth hygiene are the prime causes of Vincent's angina. Conditions such as scurvy, diabetes, lead or bismuth poisoning, and syphilis may produce ulcers and damage to the mouth and gums, with Vincent's angina as a secondary condition.

The infection is treated according to the symptoms. Crystalline penicillin has proved beneficial, and solutions of hydrogen peroxide or perborate of soda are soothing as a mouthwash and of aid in destroying the Vincent's organism. In some instances, injections of arsenical preparations directly into the veins are beneficial. Care, however, is imperative, because of danger of chemical burns of the tender gums and lining of the cheeks.

virilization. Female hermaphrodites have defective adrenal glands. Feminization does not occur. They never menstruate and usually have excessive hair on face and body. Administration of cortisone early prevents the condition permitting feminization at puberty.

viruses. The smallest and most elusive of the infectious agents, have been established as causative of more than fifty different infectious diseases of man. All forms of life may be affected by virus infection —animals, plants, birds, and insects, and even bacteria, are subject to injury and disintegration by viruses, known as bacteriophages.

Viruses are so infinitesimally small that they can pass through porcelain filters which hold back ordinary bacteria, though the larger viruses pass through with difficulty. Most of them can be seen only through a powerful electron microscope. Viruses are composed of tiny particles and differ from each other in total size, structure, and stability, from the smallest organism, responsible for foot-and-mouth disease and poliomyelitis, to the largest, which causes parrot infection or psittacosis and which can be seen with an ordinary microscope to resemble the larger bacteria. The shapes vary from the spherical head and long tail of the bacteriophage to the sphere of the influenza virus and the cube of the smallpox virus.

Viruses thrive in the presence of living cells, becoming an intimate part of living body tissues which they damage, and are parasites, completely dependent for their existence upon this close intracellular association. They multiply only in young susceptible living cells and cannot be grown in artificial media unless living cells are present. This has made it difficult to study their growth habits, or to prepare vaccines for preventive treatment.

Each virus shows its specific type of action only upon certain tissues. For example, the virus of rabies does not become active in the body until it reaches the tissues of the nerves and brain. Different viruses which attack the human body are classified according to the part of the body for which they have an affinity. Dermatropic viruses affect the skin; pneumotropic viruses involve the lungs; neurotropic viruses attack nervous tissue; and viscero-tropic viruses harm the internal organs or viscera. Among the more familiar diseases caused by viruses are the common cold, measles, German measles, chickenpox, mumps, rabies, poliomyelitis, influenza, encephalitis, smallpox, and yellow fever. A number of other ailments, among them the so-called "virus pneumonia," glandular fever, and epidemic nausea and vomiting, have also been attributed to viral infections.

Virus diseases are conveyed in a variety of ways. The common cold, measles, smallpox, chickenpox, and influenza are probably transmitted by direct contact, as well as by airborne droplets of nasal and salivary secretions. Rabies is carried through the bite or wound produced by an infected animal. Mosquitoes, fleas, ticks, and other insects are carriers, as in yellow fever and in some of the encephalitic infections. Rarely have viral infections been spread by contaminated water or food, although transmission of infectious hepatitis has been traced to water, as well as milk, in some instances.

The fact that the virus becomes an intimate part of the cells of the body has made treatment of viral infections more difficult. Those substances which have thus far been found capable of destroying virus can, unfortunately, also damage body tissues and are too toxic for practical use. Some of the newer antibiotics, such as Aureomycin, Terramycin, and Chloromycetin, have proved effective in treatment of psittacosis and trachoma. The antibiotics may have some value in treatment of measles, chickenpox, and influenza, if not directly upon the virus, at least in combatting any secondary invasion by bacteria, which often occurs in viral infections and aggravates the condition.

Until now, the most encouraging efforts to combat virus infections have been directed toward the establishment of immunity to viral diseases. Immunity is the ability of living tissue to resist and overcome infection. One way of acquiring immunity to a viral disease is to have had that infection. Measles, chickenpox, smallpox, and a few other viral diseases confer a lasting immunity. Immunity for flu, cold, and herpes simplex or fever blisters has not yet been found.

Immunity may be produced artificially by two means. First is the introduction into the body of a vaccine. This substance is composed of weakened viruses which have been submitted to a chemical or other process and are called attenuated viruses. While the virus can still produce diseases in the body, this ability has been materially weakened. However, the vaccine stimulates development in the body of antibodies, a process known as vaccination or active immunization, and in general it induces a high degree of immunity and tends to be lasting.

The second means of producing an immunity is by injection of an immune serum, gamma globulin, or the blood serum of an immune animal or man. Production of immunity by this method is called passive immunization because the person involved does not take an active part in the development of resistance to the disease, but rather receives into his body a substance already containing the essential antibodies. Passive immunity is temporary.

The use of gamma globulin in measles, provided it is given early in the incubation period, has been successful in modifying the severity of that disease. It has also been helpful during the early stages of infectious hepatitis. In poliomyelitis, gamma globulin has been used in children in an attempt to prevent the disease or at least to avert the paralytic complications. The work of Dr. Jonas Salk of the University of Pittsburgh Medical School and his associates has led to the historic development of a polio vaccine that furnishes active immunization—that is, the vaccine causes the body to set up its own defenses against the disease. This is the type of immunization that has overcome smallpox, diphtheria, and whooping cough. *See also* INFECTIONS; IMMUNITY; IMMUNIZATION; POLIOMYELITIS; VACCINATION.

vitamins. Substances which are found in foods in minute quantities and which are indispensable to the normal functioning of the body. When they are deficient or lacking in the diet, or lost through cooking or processing, certain specific disorders, known as deficiency diseases, occur. About seventeen vitamins are known, and deficiencies of about half of them are definitely causative of disease in human beings. The seventeen vitamins are: vitamins A, C or ascorbic acid, D, E, K, P, and the members of the B complex group, including B_1 or thiamine, B_2 or vitamin G or ribo-flavin, nicotinic acid or niacin, B_6 or pyroxidine, pantothenic acid, biotin, folic acid, B_{12}, choline, ino-sitol and para-aminobenzoic acid.

Vitamin A is manufactured in the body from carotene, which is found in fish liver oil, green vegetables, egg yolk, butter, and many orange-or yellow-colored foods. One of the first signs of a vitamin A deficiency is night blindness, reduced capacity of the eye to adapt to the dark. A characteristic disease of the eye, usually called xerophthalmia, re-sults from this deficiency, and a thickening of the skin, hyperkerato-sis. Vitamin A deficiency usually occurs in persons who subsist largely on a starchy diet, but dis-turbances of the intestinal tract which prevent effective absorption of vitamin A can also cause it, as well as conditions of pregnancy, infancy, and lactation, when the need for vitamin A increases. If a generous serving of a yellow or green leafy vegetable cannot be in-cluded in the daily diet, a teaspoon of fish liver oil instead insures an adequate supply of vitamin A.

B vitamins are found naturally in vegetables and grains, meat and milk. Each vitamin in this group has a particular function to perform in the complicated metabolism of the body. Part of these vitamins are destroyed by cooking or proc-essing, but generous portions of vegetables and grains in the diet provide adequate amounts.

Thiamine is useful to correct and prevent the loss of appetite that accompanies many forms of diges-tive disorder. Frequently conditions are noted in which thiamine, al-though taken into the body, is not properly absorbed. For example, in case of vomiting, when the person must be fed by tubes, when a paralysis of the muscles associated with swallowing is present, or in the case of excessive alcoholism, it may be imperative to inject extra amounts of thiamine directly into the body. Other conditions in which extra thiamine is required are ex-cessive action of the thyroid gland, fever, or vigorous muscular activi-ties, which use more thiamine than is ordinarily available.

Most symptoms of thiamine defi-ciency disappear when the vitamin in pure form in combination with other vitamins is administered. Yeast, whole-grain cereals, liver and pork are good sources of thiamine.

Vitamin B_2, riboflavin, deficien-cies are found most frequently among persons who live on diets largely composed of starches, and the deficiency is common in the southeastern United States.

Symptoms of riboflavin deficiency may be weakness and disturbances of the vision, skin, tongue, mouth, lips, and face. To correct the defi-ciency, foods high in riboflavin, such as liver, egg, milk and whole-grain cereals, must be added to the diet. In treating acute cases, pure riboflavin alone is seldom effective, since, as in most deficiency condi-tions, more than a single vitamin is lacking.

An inadequate amount of nicotinic acid, or niacin, in the diet can cause pellagra.

Cobalt is a chief chemical in-gredient of vitamin B_{12}, which has a blood-stimulating activity, similar to that of the anti-anemic factor of liver. It is therefore especially valuable in treating pernicious anemia and sprue, as well as anemia resulting from its deficiency. Although inadequate diets are occasionally responsible for deficiencies of vitamin B_{12} and folic acid, more often the deficiency is caused by some impairment in absorption or utilization of the vitamin in the body.

Other vitamins of the B complex group are vitamin B_6, pantothenic acid, biotin, choline, inositol, and para-aminobenzoic acid. A deficiency of vitamin B_6 can cause neuritis, skin eruptions and sore tongue, nervousness and depression. It is widely employed in the treatment of nausea and vomiting in pregnant women.

Ascorbic acid, vitamin C, the antiscurvy vitamin, is found abundantly in citrus fruits and juices, tomatoes, potatoes, and leafy vegetables. This vitamin is responsible for the manufacture by the body of the material which cements teeth into position. An infant with a vitamin C deficiency is likely to suffer from fever, diarrhea, loss of weight, vomiting, and have a generally low resistance and probably intestinal bleeding. In children, the bones may be malformed. Most of the symptoms of the deficiency disappear rapidly when the vitamin is administered. All fresh fruits and vegetables contain some vitamin C and to prevent recurrence of the deficiency the diet must include these foods.

Vitamin D, or ergosterol, is manufactured in the body from a combination of chemically related substances, and is essential for the formation and growth of bones and teeth and for the utilization of calcium and phosphorus in the body. It is often called the sunshine vitamin because of the abundance supplied by the sun through its action on the skin, and the person who gets enough sunshine each day receives sufficient amounts of vitamin D.

Vitamin D deficiency causes rickets in children, and in adults it results in improper utilization of calcium in the bones and produces a condition known as osteomalacia. These disorders can be corrected by adequate amounts of calcium and vitamin D. Cod liver oil, vitamin D concentrates, and sunshine or ultraviolet irradiation are effective in promoting a rapid improvement in rickets. Other good sources of vitamin D are eggs, salmon and tuna fish, and milk.

Vitamin E is found abundantly in wheat germ oil, and in adequate amounts in liver, eggs, whole-grain cereals, and lettuce. Experiments with animals have indicated that a deficiency of vitamin E may be associated with sterility and miscarriages; however, it has not been determined whether or not vitamin E deficiencies occur in human beings.

Vitamin K has significant antihemorrhagic properties, and deficiencies of it usually involve the clotting of blood. It is useful in treating obstructive jaundice, hemorrhage which results in certain intestinal disorders, and in hemorrhagic conditions affecting newborn infants. In treating coronary thrombosis, vitamin K together with the drug dicumarol is also of value, since dicumarol affects the action of vitamin K and consequently the clotting of blood. Green vegetables are rich in this vitamin.

Also known as hesperedin, vitamin P is found in the rind of citrus fruits. Whether a deficiency of vitamin P can exist has not yet been determined. The vitamin has been used in connection with vitamin C in cases of abnormal bleeding.

The significance of vitamins cannot be overemphasized, and certain basic foods should appear in the diet each day, notably milk, meat, green leafy vegetables, citrus fruits, and whole-grain products. If the diet furnishes adequate quantities of vitamins, vitamin supplements are not necessary for the average person. A doctor should be consulted if any deficiency exists.

vitiligo. A pigmentary disorder in which the coloring matter disappears in spots from the skin. These spots then appear white, in contrast to the normal coloring of the rest of the skin. Sometimes this condition is an indirect result of another disease of the skin, but usually it occurs without apparent cause.

Vitiligo occurs commonly among Negroes. While not generally considered dangerous, it is often badly disfiguring. This disease sometimes disappears spontaneously.

In about 15 per cent of the cases of vitiligo, repigmentation can be induced by a drug derived from an Egyptian plant called *Ammi majus,* together with treatment by exposure to sunlight or artificial ultraviolet rays. This must be prescribed by a physician. Persons who have been so treated have relatively small areas of depigmentation when the spots have been present less than five years.

If 80 per cent of the skin surface is depigmented, it is often practical to extend the condition to the entire body by treating the skin with a special compound. The hair and eyes are not affected as in albinism.

vocal cords. *See* LARYNGITIS; LARYNX.

voice box. *See* LARYNX.

vomiting. The forceful ejection of the contents of the stomach through the mouth. The possible causes are innumerable. Vomiting by a person who is seasick is probably caused by a disturbance in the organs of balance. Vomiting may be set off by a severe pain, such as a sharp blow to the abdomen. Psychological factors related to the senses may also produce vomiting, such as an unpleasant smell, a displeasing sight, or even an unkind remark.

When vomiting is imminent, certain nerves are stimulated and a valve in the lower part of the stomach, customarily employed to pass food to the bowels, is then automatically closed. Following this, a chain of waves passes through the wall of the stomach, moving not downward as usual but upward. The person inhales deeply and the climax is a powerful contraction of both the diaphragm and stomach. Whatever happens to be in the stomach is then thrown through the esophagus and out of the mouth. Vomiting may happen so suddenly that some of the material emerges through the nose.

While vomiting is not a disease, it is often a symptom of illness. If vomiting is severe during pregnancy, it may be a sign that multiple births can be expected. If vomiting persists, or the matter ejected has traces of blood, a doctor should be consulted to locate and treat the cause.

vulva. The external sexual organs of the female.

Inflammation of the vulva, or vulvitis, may result from infection, but often is associated with various skin disorders. In children and in obese women, acute vulvitis results from uncleanliness and from constant irritation. It is characterized by redness, swelling, burning, irritation, and sometimes by itching which may spread to the surrounding areas. The treatment depends on the cause.

In leukoplakia, white thickened areas of the skin are found, usually in the region of the clitoris, labia, or perineum. This condition may also be accompanied by itching. Proper medication is needed promptly to cure these conditions.

In the rare cases of cancer of the vulva, leukoplakia is often the forerunner. Early diagnosis is essential for a successful treatment by X-ray, radium, surgery, or combinations of these methods.

Wassermann test. A test used to determine whether or not a person has syphilis. Only a modification of the original test is now used. Various modifications, such as the Kahn test, the Eagle test, and the Hinton test, are also used. It is required by law before marriage and is routine during the first prenatal examination.

In the test, the blood serum and sometimes the cerebrospinal fluid are examined. A positive reaction indicates the presence of syphilis. Tests are also made at frequent intervals during the course of the disease, to determine its progress and the effectiveness of treatment. *See also* KAHN TEST.

wen. A sac formed in the skin when the sebum, the fatty material excreted by the skin's sebaceous or oil glands, is obstructed and cannot escape to the skin surface normally. Physicians call such a sac a sebaceous cyst. If not removed, the material within the sac or cyst interacts with the blood and changes from a rather solid mass to one that is semifluid, and may develop an offensive odor.

Since a wen may continue to grow as long as the blockage continues and infection does not occur, it may reach the size of a golf ball or even larger. With a minimum of surgery a doctor can drain the material from the cyst and eliminate the blockage which caused it.

If, however, infection has occurred, merely cutting an opening for drainage is insufficient. Sebaceous matter will continue to be secreted by the inner wall of the sac which will harden, collect, and repeat the initial process. Removal of the entire internal wall of the cyst by surgery may be essential to prevent recurrence of an infected wen.

white blood cells. *See* BLOOD.

whooping cough. Or pertussis, a disease characterized by a convulsive cough, and affecting the mucous membrane of the respiratory system. The cough leaves the patient out of breath and the resultant deep inhalation produces the whooping sound.

The disease is not a trivial affliction of childhood. Coupled with a secondary infection, such as bronchopneumonia, whooping cough can be fatal, especially in young children or the aged. The most frequent victims, however, are children under five.

During the first ten days of this disease, the incubation period, the child exhibits the symptoms of an ordinary cold. The cough, however, does not improve. The second stage begins with the onset of the whooping sound. During a coughing spell the face may grow scarlet while the facial veins swell and tears appear in the eyes. The cough may be followed by vomiting.

The prevention of whooping cough primarily involves immunization which is now accomplished by a series of injections which combine immunity against diphtheria and tetanus as well. Only infants and children need to be injected.

If a child develops whooping cough, isolation of the child is necessary, chiefly to prevent secondary infection in the child and exposure of other children. In some cases of children under two or three years of age, antibiotics are used, but older children generally recover without the use of drugs. If convulsions occur, as sometimes happens,

the doctor may place the child in an oxygen tent and sedative drugs such as phenobarbital may be given. Treatment requires complete rest as well as constant protection of the patient's lungs from atmospheric irritants such as tobacco smoke or cold drafts of air. The inhalation of steam is sometimes advised, as well as certain drugs which relieve the severity of the coughing attacks. If coughing places a great strain on the stomach muscles, a rubber binder may be worn around that area. It is better to praise the child for coughing less than to pity him for coughing more. Commiseration is not the best medicine.

Finally, special attention should be given to the patient's diet, particularly to that of children, who are susceptible to vomiting and therefore to undernourishment. Generally speaking, the child requires nutritious food which is also easy to digest. The best time for meals is approximately a quarter of an hour after a coughing spell. The child should eat in small amounts, perhaps several times a day. To feed her a large amount of food at any one time is likely to stimulate coughing, whereupon the food which has been eaten will be regurgitated.

Starchy foods—bread, pastries, and potatoes—should be avoided, as well as any dry and crumbly foods which might tickle the throat and produce a cough. Vegetable soup is recommended, and also meat in small amounts, provided that it is carefully chopped or strained. Fresh fruit juices and plenty of plain drinking water are also to be given.

Wilm's tumor. A malignant growth that affects the kidneys of children, usually under six years of age. It may grow to great size and cause the child's abdomen to protrude. Sometimes the doctor can feel the tumor with his fingers before such symptoms as pain or blood in the urine appear. Other symptoms are weakness and vomiting.

Removal of the affected kidney followed by radiation is the best means of curing this condition. If the tumor is large, it may be necessary first to treat it with radiation, then follow with surgery and post-operative radiation.

womb. *See* UTERUS.

worms. Several types of worms live parasitically in the human body, usually in some part of the digestive tract. Although the United States has relatively high sanitation and hygienic standards, various kinds of worm infestation are common in some areas. A study of children in the District of Columbia, for example, revealed that 35 to 65 per cent of certain groups had pinworm infestation, and another study reported that 50 to 60 per cent of children in different parts of the southern United States had intestinal worms.

Some worms attain remarkable size, such as the beef tapeworm which may reach a length of fifteen feet; whereas others, such as the worm which causes trichinosis, are so thin and small that they are barely visible to the naked eye. Often worms are present in the bowels without causing any serious

symptoms. However, sometimes they may produce general and far-reaching disturbances.

The pinworm is easily the most widely distributed of worms which live as parasites in human hosts. Known also as the seat or thread-worm, it exists only in the form of a human parasite.

The drugs used against pinworm can be given only by a doctor's prescription and under his care. Enemas with a chemical called hexyl-resorcinol are given; a dyestuff, gentian violet, may be given internally; and antiseptic ointments for affected external areas may be prescribed by the doctor. The amount and manner of application of these remedies will vary with each case and must always be determined by the doctor.

After the pinworm, the parasite which most frequently infests the human body is the giant intestinal roundworm, scientifically known as *Ascaris lumbricoides.*

Several effective substances are available which can be used by the physician to rid the host of tapeworms. As in the other treatments, the person must abstain from food for a day or a few days while taking the drug. Recovery of the top end of the worm from the bowel waste usually is considered to constitute elimination of the worms. A person who has a tapeworm may have only a few mild symptoms or she may have more severe attacks. The condition often begins with diarrhea, which then alternates with constipation. False hunger pains are characteristic, although the appetite may sometimes diminish. The person loses weight and secondary anemia appears, and still later symptoms may disappear entirely. The victim of beef tapeworm is likely to experience discomfort when the proglottids pass through the rectum. In every case, the diagnosis can be made easily and with certainty by examination of the excrement.

wounds. Any injury that breaks the skin, mucous membrane, or inner surface of the tissues of the body is a wound. Minor wounds can be treated with various antiseptic preparations, such as tincture of iodine, Metaphen, Merthiolate, boric acid, and others, and then covered with a clean snug bandage or compress. If the wound is more serious, only the bandage should be applied and the cleansing and disinfection of the wound done by a doctor, since amateur efforts can cause serious damage.

xanthoma. A flat yellow tumor which may develop on the surface of the skin. Xanthomas are caused by the deposit of a fatty substance which the body has failed to dispose of in the normal manner. Most frequently they are seen in the vicinity of the eyes, especially on the inner part of the lower lid. A surgeon can remove these "yellow spots," as they are sometimes called, with relative ease, leaving only slightly visible scars. Xanthomas may tend to recur, but are seldom cancerous. *See also* TUMOR.

xeroderma. A disorder in which the skin becomes rough and dry, and sometimes discolored, with fine scaly shedding.

xerophthalmia. A disease in which a severe dryness of the eye occurs, resulting from a deficiency of vitamin A. The cornea becomes clouded and inflamed; ulcers of the cornea may develop. Permanent blindness may result in the advanced stages of this disease if it is not promptly and properly treated. The administration of vitamin A is effective for this condition.

xerosis. A disease in which abnormal dryness of the skin caused by vitamin A deficiency is a symptom. This condition may be corrected by taking liver oil extracts and making sure that the diet includes enough leafy green and yellow vegetables, as well as egg yolks, butter, or vitamin A-enriched margarine.

xerostoma. Decreased salivary flow; it is a symptom which arises from a number of causes rather than a disease. In many instances it is temporary, as in fever or in a state of fear or anxiety. Atropine, a drug often administered to patients before a surgical operation, may produce a dry feeling in the mouth.

In chronic cases, lack of saliva may cause the mouth to become rough and dry, and painful cracks and fissures which bleed easily may develop. A stone in the duct of the salivary glands may cause obstruction, swelling, and pain that will interfere with the intake of food and predispose the gland to infection. Surgery is the only means then of removing the stones.

X-rays. Radiation produced by the vacuum tube, similar to light but of much shorter wave length and possessing special penetrating and tissue-ionizing power.

One of the chief uses of the X-ray continues to be for the diagnosis of broken bones. Today pictures are made from different angles so that the exact relationship of the broken bones to the tissues may be determined.

An X-ray of the skull shows the presence of disease of the bone, sometimes the presence of a tumor or changes in the blood vessels in the brain.

By the use of accessory materials one may visualize various organs and tissues. These substances include various dyes which may be taken into the body and which localize in certain organs and tissues. Then by the use of the X-ray these tissues and organs are made visible.

By the use of the X-ray the exact size of the heart may be determined. The X-ray is also used in the treatment of disease, particularly in the treatment of tumors, conditions affecting the skin, inflammations of various kinds, and for a wide variety of purposes where radiation therapy is called for.

yaws. Also called frambesia, pian, bubos, and leishmaniasis, a disease caused by a spiral micro-organism, the *Treponema pertenue,* related to the *Treponema pallidum,* the agent of syphilis. Yaws is rarely found in the United States but is a disease of tropical regions, especially where sanitation is poor. Raspberry-colored growths on various parts of the body, especially the face, feet, legs, hands, and around the external genitals are characteristic signs. The growths may join to form large masses and may become ulcerated.

yellow fever. An acute infectious disease caused by a filtrable virus which is transmitted by the bite of an infected mosquito, *Aëdes aegypti,* in whose system the virus lives and breeds. The illness strikes suddenly, usually three to six days after the mosquito bite. The face becomes flushed and swollen, the eyes suffused, the lips and tongue a bright red, and a high fever appears, with pain in the head and back, and a feeling of extreme exhaustion. In two or three days, the temperature drops below normal, the pulse slows down, and the skin grows cold and assumes the yellow jaundiced hue, which gives the disease its name. A characteristic "black vomit" occurs, indicating internal bleeding. As the patient recovers, the temperature returns to normal, generally by the seventh or eighth day, and convalescence begins, leading to rapid, complete recovery. Complications are rare, and one attack gives lifelong immunity.

The greatest precautions are taken to prevent introduction of infected mosquitoes onto airplanes and ships. Crews are vaccinated against the disease and ships are fumigated. Persons who are infected are isolated in a screen-protected room for at least the first four days after development of symptoms of yellow fever. The United States Public Health Service, the World Health Organization, and quarantine agencies all over the world are constantly alert to the threat of mosquito disease carriers. Breeding places are sprayed with DDT or oil to kill the larvae, and such measures in recent years have kept the spread of yellow fever at a minimum.

yellow jaundice. *See* JAUNDICE.

INDEX
Page numbers in **bold face** indicate illustrations